Sociomedical Perspectives on Patient Care

Jeffrey Michael Clair
Richard M. Allman
Editors

THE UNIVERSITY PRESS OF KENTUCKY

Copyright © 1993 by The University Press of Kentucky

Scholarly publisher for the Commonwealth,
serving Bellarmine College, Berea College, Centre
College of Kentucky, Eastern Kentucky University,
The Filson Club, Georgetown College, Kentucky
Historical Society, Kentucky State University,
Morehead State University, Murray State University,
Northern Kentucky University, Transylvania University,
University of Kentucky, University of Louisville,
and Western Kentucky University.

Editorial and Sales Offices: Lexington, Kentucky 40508-4008

Library of Congress Cataloging-in-Publication Data

Sociomedical perspectives on patient care / Jeffrey
    Michael Clair and Richard M. Allman, editors.
        p.   cm.
    Includes bibliographical references and indexes.
    ISBN 0-8131-1815-8 (cl : alk. paper) : ISBN
0-8131-0819-5 (pa : alk. paper) :
    1. Physician and patient.   2. Medical care—Psychological aspects.
3. Interpersonal communication.   4. Communication in medicine.
I. Clair, Jeffrey M., 1958–   .   II. Allman, Richard M., 1955–   .
    [DNLM: 1. Comprehensive Health Care—trends.   2. Physician-
Patient Relations.   W 62 S6785 1993]
    R727.3.S63   1993
    610.69'6—dc20
    DNLM/DLC
    for Library of Congress   92-48516

Contents

Figures and Tables

Figures

Tables

Foreword

A Social Perspective

I spent two weekends steeping myself in the 13 chapter manuscripts that comprise this intriguing and rich book. In its implications for medical education and practice, for the social-behavioral sciences, and for public debate on health care, this book could not come at a better moment. It reminds us of how much more there is to medical care than the technical means to carry it out and the economic means to pay for it—important as those factors obviously are.

In current public debate, thoughts, anxieties, and strategies overwhelmingly fasten on economic issues. How can we provide medical services for the underserved segments of the population? If there is to be true public rationing—not simply market allocation—how can we frame priorities that reflect a public consensus? How can we contain aggregate costs and tame the rampant inflation? How should we conceptualize benefits, and how can we get more benefit per dollar expended?

Aside from the economic issues that capture the headlines, the public has many long-standing doubts and grievances about its medical care, centering on problems in communication and relationships. Patients want less hurried, more communicative, more caring doctors who will recognize them as individuals. Even when definitive medical intervention is not possible (e.g., for chronic or terminal illness), or necessary (e.g., for self-limiting illness), they still want such doctoring. Medical care with these superadded qualities of caring becomes patient care. The latter embraces and goes beyond the former. Patient care distinguishes human medicine from veterinary medicine. Relating to a sentient patient with communicative capacity and self-awareness directly establishes an accountability for the doctor that goes beyond the requirement of technical proficiency and conscientiousness.

This book deals forcefully with patient care issues and only glancingly with economic issues. It is thus a valuable counterpoise to the blinding focus on economics; at the same time, patient care has an essential connection with economic issues, as shown in the following considerations.

With 42% of the health care dollar coming from public funds, and another large chunk coming from employer funds, there is rising concern about value-for-money and a call for critical cost-benefit analyses. The first, almost "fun" part of such analysis is to identify the harmful, downright iatrogenic practices that have no redeeming virtues for the recipient. Next comes the category of "wasteful" practices—so-called needless surgery and medication, and needless or needlessly prolonged hospitalization. Finally, one moves into the more difficult terrain of deciding which of the many beneficial medical services—whether diagnostic, curative, palliative, supportive, or rehabilitative—justify, and which do not justify, the requisite expenditure of resources.

In the foregoing argument, the benefits to be assessed are tangible, measurable outcomes, such as postponement of death or incapacity, relief of pain and distress, and improved quality of life. Medicine can in varying degrees yield these vital benefits. From its perspective, this book deals, however, with those less tangible, measurable, and categorizable benefits that inhere in the processes of patient care. These benefits contribute to the satisfaction of the patient's need for information, guidance, care, and recognition.

In its many-sided concern with communication and relationships, this book deals with the patient care components of the overall benefit package. One would be rash to reckon too precisely in economic terms the value of good communication in the doctor-patient relationship, yet it is worth a great deal. If forced to choose, patients might prefer the technically superb surgeon who is brusque or inarticulate to a sensitive bumbler. In effect, the present system has—without consulting anyone—already made exactly that choice for us: it values and inculcates technical proficiency and disregards, almost systematically, communicative skill.

Why can't patients have a doctor who does his or her job well *and* who also cares and—better still—who talks and listens? These latter two qualities of patient care are not "free goods" in the sense of being part of the genetic endowment ("some docs have it and some don't") or early training of pre-doctors. Medical care organizations and medical training programs should emphasize, encourage, reward, and instill a sense of responsibility as well as skill in patient care. Further, the individual physician cannot be expected to function as a single-minded "patient care practitioner" against the tide of a depersonalizing environment; rather, the atmosphere, social structures, and policies of the organization must be reoriented toward the practice of good patient care.

This book carries a spirited patient care message to leaders in medical education and medical care. It diagnoses prevalent obstacles to good communication, tells some tales of patient woe and resentment in the face of the communicative dereliction of doctors, and describes efforts to improve the generally lamentable situation in both medical education and medical practice.

Social scientists working in medical environments have keen interest in the improvement of doctor-patient communication. They possess a growing array of techniques, skills, paradigms, and perspectives for bringing into clearer relief the elements of medical practice as it appears from the patient's standpoint. Social scientists also are prepared to function as the protector, advocate, and formulator of the patient's welfare in medical care situations. I do not mean that there is an inherent zero-sum clash between the doctor's interest and the patient's welfare. Short of actual conflict, it is bad enough that the inertial thrust of medical care leads to active, often imperious doctors and passive, often resentful patients. In the face of this typical imbalance, it is no wonder that some social scientists are at work on patient empowerment programs—teaching and training patients to be more questioning, probing, and discerning in their dealings with doctors. Social scientists also assist doctors in the development of more sensitive modes of communication and relationships with patients. Progress in this latter direction can obviate to some extent the need for patient assertiveness, but a certain minimum is probably desirable for the sake of the patient's autonomy in varied and complex medical settings.

Identifying and addressing patient needs—delineating the province of patient care (as distinct from medical care)—is a massive agenda that currently engages many sociomedical scientists. This much can be seen by examining the chapters of contributors to this book. Their work also unifies them across the otherwise disparate concepts and methodologies of sociology, anthropology, psychology, economics, law, and other social-behavioral disciplines.

In addition to their unifying focus on patient needs, a number of social scientists are at work on two subcategories of concern.

The first of these is the application of the distinction between the patient's *disease* and the patient's *illness*. Varying terms are used by social scientists to capture this familiar distinction, but the general meaning is clear enough. The patient's disease is what the doctor pronounces; it is the pathological entity, the CAT-scanned lesion, the biopsied tissue, or the blood-gas chromatograph that objectifies the patient's distress. Because diagnosis has become so precise and so externalized, sometimes it disconfirms the patient's own sense of what's the matter, as with the patient who thinks he or she has a bad migraine but is told that the problem is a brain lesion. More startling perhaps, the patient's disease is often not what doctors would have diagnosed on the basis of their own physical examination and clinical intuition. Doctoring also has become subservient to technology.

Standing in contrast to the patient's disease is the patient's illness—the pain and sense of unease, the symptoms and self-observations, the sense of self altered under the impact of illness. Although the disease is not the same as the illness, the latter can accommodate to encompass (or to reject) what the doctor avers as the truth—the biomedically characterized disease.

Working out the implications of the disease-illness contrast and understanding its implications are part of a broad new frontier in thinking about patient care.

The second subtheme is the microanalysis of doctor-patient verbal (and gestural) interaction, variously called conversational analysis or discourse analysis. Using refined tools and codes, the social scientist as discourse analyst is in a position to dissect and to illuminate what goes on in doctor-patient relationships—to take our understanding of it beyond our personal experiences of patienthood and our convenient or prejudicial stereotypes, and to move toward characterization of good and poor communication profiles at the level, virtually, of "speech molecules."

The reliable, quantifiable techniques of discourse analysis would probably impress even those biomedical investigators who are heartily disdainful of the striving of social science for rigor and reliability. More important, however, than this emblematic claim to objectivity is the potential of discourse analysis for opening up a new scientific interest on the part of medical educators and medical practitioners in communication with patients. Its procedures, methods, and findings can be adapted to medical undergraduate courses in interviewing, to postgraduate education, and to the self-education of doctors who consciously want to understand their communication with patients.

Jeffrey Clair and Richard Allman, and their contributors, have set out to personalize medical care—to convert it into patient care. This goal will not be achieved by accident or indirection. The prevailing winds may even point in the opposite direction, toward a greater gap between patient and doctor as a result of more impersonally efficient modes of medical care organization and relentlessly stronger reliance upon sophisticated technology. Yet it is also clear that, whatever the prevailing indications, both the public expectation and the hope of the individual patient for humane, communicative, compassionate doctoring will not die out. These expectations and hopes find powerful endorsement in this wise, humane, and singular book.

Eugene B. Gallagher

A Medical Perspective

There is little doubt that a young person choosing to become a physician today enters a profession under siege. The causes are all too easy to identify: the high cost of medical training and care, difficult access to medical care, poor communication, intimidating facilities, extraordinarily complex diagnostic and therapeutic regimens, and the increasing emergence of chronic illness and aging as the focus of "caregiving." Solutions are harder to define. However, one thing is clear: the introduction of science into medicine, which had its roots in the yearnings of Láennec, Pasteur, the Curies, Ehrlich, and Roentgen to know "why," has led inevitably and correctly to an increasing emphasis on a philosophy of medicine based solidly on quantification and, thus, to the need for specialization to solve complex problems. One can scarcely doubt the enormous contribution of this epistemology. Tuberculosis no longer devastates the previously healthy. Plague is a threat only from a megalomaniacal dictator who would use it as a weapon. Smallpox has been conquered. Typhoid fever is mostly of historic interest, as is poliomyelitis. Many cancers are cured. These accomplishments escaped humankind for centuries when our philosophical roots were mired in mysticism and ignorance.

Now that schizophrenia, coronary artery disease, and cancer have become incompletely conquered modern plagues, our society, impatient for solution, risks rejecting those philosophic roots that have resulted in the very progress that leads us to decry our unsolved contemporary problems. As a consequence of both the enormous contributions of quantifiable science and its limitations, we have entered an era of antiscience that masquerades as the very science it castigates. Our society blames special knowledge and skill instead of acknowledging and understanding their contribution. We confuse confounding influences with necessary causes. We demythologize medicine and its practitioners while yearning for a godlike physician. And we want all this at low cost!

It is little wonder, then, that those interested in a more rational (and therefore more quantifiably scientific) understanding of society have begun to add their views to the views of those who espouse "high touch" (sometimes, unfortunately, at the expense of high tech), and those who believe that some new legislation will cure the ills afflicting our system and its practitioners.

This volume of social science—oriented opinion must be viewed in such a context. Its authors do not want to throw out the baby with the bathwater, merely to add to our view of health the understanding that quality of life is not simply the absence of a disease with a pathophysiologic basis that, for the moment anyway, seems to explain its cause, natural history, therapy, and prognosis. Complex as this concept may be, they contend an even more intricate context is necessary to develop a fuller understanding of what promotes illness and what relieves misery. Although today's practitioner may have an increasingly accurate view of disease processes, these processes still occur in human beings whose experiences and beliefs critically affect the outcome. What kind of *patient* does the disease have? Now we must add a new level of understanding—that the patient with an illness is a member of an increasingly complicated society whose influences may be as profound as those of individual experience.

This book promotes cross-fertilization by bridging the gaps between the many disciplines interested in patient care issues. The emphasis is on using the techniques and analytic capacities of a "softer" and perhaps "kinder" science to elucidate problems, suggest solutions, and point in directions that might alleviate the current level of stress, distrust, and sequential faultfinding that afflicts our society as it faces its health care crisis. Thus there are chapters on the dynamics of patient-physician interactions and on the ways that technology, finance, and litigation affect these interactions. Improving communication in a variety of increasingly common circumstances, such as those encountered by handicapped children and aging adults, draws appropriate attention.

Finally, of course, when a suitable body of relevant knowledge has been defined, it must enter the curriculum of the future caregiver. And so it is hoped that we will come full circle. If the lessons, directions, and insights of those experts whose views are incorporated here are appropriately adopted by those aspiring to educate or become tomorrow's caregivers, we will be both less likely to discard the contributions of "hard" science and more likely to meet the needs of the sick whose illnesses are those of "real" people living in "real" societies. We are all, of course, imperfect but we can improve, if ever so slowly. Perhaps then the intensity of the siege will diminish, and as physicians become better advocates for their patients, their patients will no longer find the medical environment quite so adversarial. If so, this book will have made a signal contribution to our society and, most important, to medical practice.

John R. Durant

Acknowledgments

This project received support from the American Sociological Association Fund for the Advancement of the Discipline, with sponsorship from the National Science Foundation. Individual chapters herein were produced while the authors were receiving support from various sources. Jeffrey Clair acknowledges the support of the AARP Andrus Foundation. Richard Allman and Jeffrey Clair received support from the University of Alabama—Birmingham Hospital Continuous Innovations in Patient Care Program. H. Hughes Evans completed her chapter while under the support of a MacArthur Foundation Grant to Harvard Medical School for M.D./Ph.D. training in the social sciences relative to medicine. Howard Waitzkin's work is partially supported by grants from the National Center for Health Services Research (R01-HS02100), the National Institute on Aging (1-F32-AG05438), the Division of Medicine of the U.S. Public Health Service (PE-19154), the National Endowment for the Humanities (FA-22922), and the Academic Senate of the University of California, Irvine (Honorary Faculty Research Fellowship). Robert Pearlman acknowledges the support of the Geriatric Research, Education and Clinical Center and the Northwest Service Research and Development Field Program, Seattle VA Medical Center, and the Program in Ethics and the Professions, Harvard University. Jan Wallander was supported in part by research grant R01 HD25310 and Research Career Development Award K04 HD00867 from the National Institute of Child Health and Human Development at NIH. Data for Marie Haug's paper are derived from research supported in part by the National Institute on Aging (AM-20618), National Institute on Health (AG-05876 and GS41347), the National Science Foundation (HS01849 and HS0268), and the National Center for Health Services Research. Richard Frankel and Howard Beckman would like to thank Charles Whitten and R. Stewart Robertson for the support and encouragement to develop the year

2 communication skills teaching experience, and Robert Burack, Richard Butler, and Howard Schubiner for their participation as course faculty at Wayne State University.

Various readers have reviewed some or all of the chapters in this book. Thanks are offered to Patricia Baker, Stephany Borges, B.K.E. Hennen, Radha Holavanahalli, Thomas Huddle, Paul Lawrence, James Lewis, J. Hillis Miller, Michael Morrisey, Mark Poster, Leslie Rabine, John Carlos Rowe, Jerome Tobis, Kenneth Wilson, William Yoels, and four anonymous reviewers for helpful comments. We also would like to thank Krisenda Clair, Elaine Daunhauer, Susan Hancy, Barbara Harlow, Radha Holavanahalli, D.C. Peoples, Jackie Skeen, Michelle Stone, and Georgia Taylor for technical help. Finally, we are indebted to the doctors, patients, and family members enmeshed within this work.

Introduction

This book has its origins in an examination of patient care relationships and ethics undertaken by a group of multidisciplinary scholars who came together to discuss their ideas in December of 1990. The enterprise was funded by the American Sociological Association/ National Science Foundation Fund for the Advancement of the Discipline, and by the Department of Sociology and the Department of Medicine at the University of Alabama at Birmingham. The project provided the opportunity to explore the theoretical and empirical contributions of the social sciences to medicine, particularly as they relate to patient care. We were united by the common assumption that medical practice can be enhanced by an understanding of the basic social, economic, political, ethical, and legal processes affecting patient care relationships. Each chapter focuses on issues that have both social and medical significance.

Papers prepared for this book will challenge and stimulate anyone concerned with the human interactions that constitute medical practice. The authors come close to representing the almost bewildering number of disciplines currently offering suggestions on improving patient care. They include researchers and practicing physicians from the specialties of family, general, geriatric, pediatric, and oncological medicine; from disciplines within the social and behavioral sciences such as sociology, psychology, history, and social psychology; from the humanities as represented by English; and from the economic and ethical concerns of public health.

Many issues raised within the following pages are only now receiving proper attention from multiple perspectives. The social and medical sciences can agree that, in judging health and illness, humanistic patient care and quality of life are issues of overriding social concern. We feel that neglect of what is found in this book has had grave effects on American medicine.

The current lack of convergence among scientific perspectives on patient care issues results from the absence of interdisciplinary collaborative efforts. Such efforts are rare for many reasons, but conceptual language differences across disciplines remain the most formidable obstacle. This edited collection represents a beginning effort to bring together within one volume the seemingly disparate parts of patient care research. Each chapter is both detailed and broad in scope, yet specifically focused. We reveal a unified objective from multiple perspectives, with the importance of social issues in patient care as the common thread. Each writer attends to issues shaping the social content and quality of patient care.

Although the strength of disciplinary perspectives is noticeable, the concerns raised, when combined, cut across disciplinary boundaries. We codify much of the literature on the patient-doctor relationship and generate new questions in a language free of jargon. The issues should be accessible to scholars and students in many disciplines, even those outside the specialized backgrounds of the authors.

In the most specific sense, this volume focuses on the need for attention to social exigencies and influences in the doctor-patient relationship. The various authors all pay attention to the medical encounter and how this social interaction affects patient physical and mental health. We aim toward putting the reader in touch with the possibilities for a properly informed therapeutic practice of medicine, a modern-day practice building on the time-honored tradition of hand, head, and heart.

Our approach also attends to relationships beyond the doctor-patient relationship and includes variables describing caregiver roles (usually family members) in patient care. Inherent differences between each member of the doctor-patient-family triad can lead to marked differences in the conception of the problem for which help is being sought, the possible solutions, and the degree of reciprocity each is willing to offer. Here we introduce additional challenging issues from the medical encounter.

Social change has placed new demands on the practice of medicine, thereby altering almost every aspect of patient care relationships. Mandates toward changing biomedicine are transforming this social institution. Just as medicine was encouraged to embrace the biological sciences some 100 years ago, recent directives suggest the importance of the social sciences for understanding biomedical practice. Humanistic challenges necessitate changes in purely biomedical curative and technological imperatives. Social scientists contribute to such challenges by producing social evidence concerning the appropriate goals, objectives, and process of health care in the context of a changing environment.

Organization and Content

In varying degrees, each chapter: (1) addresses social behavior in patient care as a venue for thinking through theoretical issues of general interest to the social and medical sciences; (2) employs social variables and findings to gain new insights or make important observations about humanistic patient care; (3) asks new questions and opens up new areas of sociomedical inquiry; and (4) suggests new approaches to medical practice, education, and research.

The first section of this book, "Issues and Perspectives," is concerned with: (1) establishing the legitimate need for the application of social science to medical practice, education, and research; (2) reconciling the agendas of physicians and patients; and (3) predicting future patterns of the physician-patient relationship.

Chapter 1 focuses on establishing medical encounters as fundamentally social enterprises. Clair argues that communication processes between patients and their physicians require the appropriate attention to "social" as well as medical complaints, thus establishing the need for the application of social sciences to medical practice. He suggests that the social sciences can help reformulate medicine to emphasize, in an appropriate manner, the patient's experience and understanding of illness (disease). He specifies how such an interface can be accomplished through a sociomedical research agenda on patient care. The outcome of such an interface is what Clair calls a social science "with" medicine. A "social science with medicine" perspective promotes the institutionalization of the medical social sciences as special fields within, yet independent of, medicine. The objective is to advance initiatives that generate and test social theory and data, while expanding collaboration with medical clinicians, researchers, and educators to maximize the application of social evidence to patient care.

Chapter 2 examines the nature of the divergent definitions of the medical situation as constructed by doctors and patients. Allman, Yoels, and Clair argue that before the problems intrinsic in doctor-patient relationships can be resolved, physicians, patients, and social critics must develop a common language. They examine the fit between what patients want and what they get upon visiting doctors' offices. They also explore how the traditional clinical method, employing a biomedical model of disease diagnosis, often ignores social variables that critically affect physicians' abilities to identify the problems most important to patients. Attention is paid to some of the critical parameters of doctor-patient encounters: heavy patient loads, brief office visits, and the pervasive uncertainty of medical diagnoses. Allman, Yoels, and Clair conclude by examining a number of unresolved issues in patient care, such as the relationship between patient satisfaction and health outcomes and the need for triangulated, multimethod research designs employing both quantitative and qualitative approaches.

In chapter 3, Cockerham examines the changing pattern of physician-patient interaction in the United States and suggests that the traditional guidance-cooperation model is being replaced by the mutual participation model. Cockerham's position is that this change is part of a general worldwide trend associated with modernity. Growing consumerism on the part of patients, questioning of authority, the desire for greater personal control over one's life and health, and the high prevalence of chronic disease are all an outgrowth of modernity. He suggests that each trend points toward a modification of the traditional physician-patient relationship, in which status and power once favored the physician exclusively. Cockerham argues that change in the doctor-patient relationship is a logical and predictable outcome given the spread of formal rationality in society and the emergence of relatively large numbers of well-educated people who are competent and experienced in dealing with professionals and with modern technology. He sees physicians and patients as moving toward greater partnership.

The second section of this book is "The Social Context of Medical Practice." From a historical perspective, two chapters explore the development of laboratory sciences and technology, illustrating their effect on the modern doctor-patient relationship. The current economic context and legal realities of the doctor-patient relationship also are addressed.

Chapter 4 explores the history of the doctor-patient relationship and reveals its central role in defining medical practice and theory. Borst suggests that in the years before the development of laboratory "bench" medicine, each patient served as the physician's "laboratory." Up to the end of the nineteenth century, the doctor-patient relationship was based on the physician's understanding that disease entities were not common to multiple patients. Patients and patient symptoms were unique, and thus each patient had to be seen in a holistic way. Medical practice and medical theory relied on concepts developed by ancient Greek philosophers as early as 500 B.C. These concepts were based explicitly on the doctor's relationship with the patient, and they provided consistent theoretical and practical applications. Beginning in the Paris hospitals in the 1830s, and accelerating with the development of physiology and other laboratory sciences, Borst suggests, the doctor-patient relationship changed dramatically. Medical science had moved to the bench, and this new laboratory orientation gave consistent, quantifiable, reproducible results. For physicians, an understanding of disease and a decision about therapeutics no longer depended on the idiosyncrasies of each patient. With the move from the bedside to the bench, the physician's professional identity became linked with scientific knowledge rather than with the extent of experience with patients. Though this change is sometimes rued by those seeking a romantic ideal of the physician-patient relationship, Borst concludes by suggesting that medicine's link with bench laboratory science has the potential for freeing medical practice and medical theory from gender, racial, and class biases.

In chapter 5, Evans traces the roots of medical technology as a prominent feature in American patient care. She shows that instrumentation introduced in the nineteenth century fundamentally altered the process of medical professionalization, the understanding of disease, the ways medical knowledge is retrieved and interpreted, and the doctor-patient relationship. Evans reminds us that because of concerns about the effects of medical instruments on their status within society, doctors were wary of accepting medical technology. Proponents of new instruments emphasized their convenience, accuracy, and reliability. They advocated new ways of organizing medical information that reflected the use of instruments. Evans uses case studies of the stethoscope, thermometer, and sphygmomanometer to highlight these changes. Her conclusion is that the availability of instruments shifted interest in disease from what is felt and experienced to what is seen and measured.

In chapter 6, Ohsfeldt focuses on the financial aspects of physician-patient relationships. He points out that patients seek the advice of physicians and pay them to ameliorate the effects of illness. The nature of the financial incentives entailed in contractual arrangements between physicians and patients or their intermediaries may foster conflict between physicians and patients. Ohsfeldt provides an overview of agency theory as it applies to physician-patient relationships, which indicates that a truly incentive-neutral contract arrangement cannot be constructed. He reviews empirical studies concerning the impact of different types of physician financial incentives on the level of services provided to patients. These studies indicate some apparent physician responsiveness to changes in broad financial incentives, such as fee-for-service payment or a fixed salary, with a much stronger apparent response to more specific financial incentives, such as referrals to ancillary service providers in which physicians have an investment interest. The roles of peer monitoring and regulation also are discussed. Ohsfeldt concludes with some conjectures regarding prospects for the future.

In chapter 7, Ritchey discusses how the threat of medical malpractice lawsuits in the United States poses special problems for a profession whose status is derived from the uncertainty and esoterica of its craft. Through a review of existing studies, Ritchey focuses on how the "malpractice crisis" influences the physician-patient relationship generally, and especially the nontechnical aspects of the patient encounter. He examines the risk management industry to ascertain ways in which it helps shape the practitioner's frame of mind about potential malpractice liability.

Evidence suggests that physicians' fears of litigation have led them to alter patient care behavior drastically even though assessment of malpractice claims experience suggests that much of this is misplaced effort. Ritchey argues that in this atmosphere of uncertainty of law, compounded by medical uncertainty, "defensive medicine" has become an institutionalized part of medical practice. He describes how some patients are more likely to be stereotyped as suit-prone, leading physicians to alter patient management procedures and clerical practices in ways that raise serious ethical dilemmas. Ritchey questions the advice proposed by risk management counselors and concludes with proposals for future research.

The third section of this book, "Communicating with Patients and Caregivers," addresses fundamental issues during the medical encounter. These chapters focus on particularly understudied medical encounters. Old-age and pediatric encounters are addressed as well as triadic relationships. Special attention also is given to end-of-life decisions.

In chapter 8, Waitzkin, Britt, and Williams ask how older patients and their doctors deal with social problems in the discourse of routine medical encounters. Their conceptual work extends narrative analysis to focus on elements of ideology, underlying structure, and superficially marginal features of discourse. Based on a critical review of prior research on patient-doctor communication, they develop an interpretive method with systematic criteria to guide sampling, transcription, and interpretation. They applied this method to 50 encounters selected randomly from a larger data base of 336 randomly selected encounters of patients and primary-care internists. To illustrate the authors' interpretive approach, this chapter presents two encounters reflecting the variability observed in discourse involving older patients. The authors show that the structure of discourse tends to marginalize contextual problems, to leave them incompletely expressed, and to reinforce ideologies of stoicism and individualism. Contextual problems include social isolation, financial insecurity, loss of community and material possessions, death of family members, and retirement from work.

In chapter 9, Silliman argues that an aging population, and the increasing numbers of frail older persons, require physicians to develop a family-centered care approach to meet their complex and intertwining needs. She states that physicians must think of the context of care as the triadic doctor-patient-family caregiver relationship. Using two case studies, Silliman explores what is known about family caregivers of frail elders and the difficulties they experience; the expanded clinical database required for providing care in the context of the doctor-patient-family caregiver relationship; the dynamic and evolving nature of the relationship over time; and the pitfalls that should be anticipated when entering into this relationship.

In chapter 10, Wallander and Hardy raise issues about pediatric patient-parent-physician medical encounters. They suggest that parents of children who have a chronic physical illness or disabling condition often report dissatisfaction with their interactions with health care professionals. To illuminate this problem, Wallander and Hardy discuss the differing perspectives of parents of disabled children and those of health professionals. The authors examine the factors contributing to these differing perspectives. They suggest that part of the problem may be attributed to the health professional's typical adoption of the "clinical perspective," as well as to natural consequences of the interactional process. Special attention is paid to problems in information sharing by the professional. Wallander and Hardy provide suggestions for improving the parent-professional relationship, with the ultimate goal of providing better services for both the disabled child and the parents. In particular, they argue that adopting the "social system perspective" may better meet the needs of parents and lead to better care for children.

The focus of chapter 11 is on quality-of-life concerns and end-of-life decisions. Pearlman argues that enhancement and maintenance of quality-of-life are principal objectives of patient care. In providing patient care to older patients, quality-of-life considerations are pervasive. In part, this occurs because many treatments have both marginal benefits and appreciable burdens. Pearlman points out that a common task for surrogate decision makers (acting on behalf of mentally incapacitated patients) is to infer whether available treatments are in the patient's best interests. Advance care planning, as mandated by the Patient Self Determination Act and the Joint Commission on Accreditation of Health Care Organizations, encourages patients and health care providers to discuss the treatment preferences and values that should be considered in future patient care decisions. Pearlman argues that to promote optimal health care, health care providers must understand what is beneficial from the patient's perspective. They should avoid imposing judgments about patient quality of life that undermine respect for the patient's role in medical decision making and for the value of human life.

The final section of this book addresses the fundamentals of "Future Educational Considerations." We are used to mandates calling for physician education but still rare is work on patient education. Both important perspectives are addressed in our closing section.

In chapter 12, Haug presents informal as well as survey findings revealing that physicians' authority is being challenged in both developing and industrialized countries, including the United States, Japan, Great Britain, the former USSR, China, and Cuba. She argues that in each country those with more education are the most likely to exhibit attitudes and report behaviors that indicate a decline in unquestioned faith in doctors. She points out, however, that the pattern of education's effects may vary according to a country's stage of development and, within a country, by cultural characteristics. Haug concludes that such findings require the reconceptualization of sociological theories about professional power.

In chapter 13, Frankel and Beckman offer the reader insights on proper medical training. They acknowledge both a public and a professional crisis in American medicine today. They argue that traditional medical education has fundamentally failed to address the current crisis. They describe three dimensions of doctor-patient communication—historical, research, and educational—with the goal of providing an integrated view of the prospects and problems we face in preparing physicians to practice in the twenty-first century. They offer recommendations for teaching communication skills to medical students, residents, and practicing physicians. Their hypothesis assumes that students and residents who are respected, nurtured, and empowered in their educational process will become physicians who will bring these same skills, and the attendant positive outcomes, to the practice of medicine. Frankel and Beckman believe there is reason to be cautiously optimistic about the skills, attitudes, and values of future physicians regarding the doctor-patient relationship and its importance to health care process and outcomes

The "Concluding Commentary" was commissioned as a critique of this collection and to identify possible avenues for the development of a social medicine. Lewis and Bennett advance some provocative arguments, the most striking of them focusing on the experience of physicians, which the authors see increasingly as an ordeal of frustration. They do not see medicine in social science terms as a powerful institution, allied with hospitals and insurance companies, involved in regulation of occupational and institutional licensing, courted by multinational pharmaceutical companies, and forcefully affecting national health care policy through professional associations and interlinkages.

While some social scientists have an exaggerated view of a physician's power—as if the expansion of biomedical power has gone on ad infinitum—most are aware of the historical dynamics over the last 20 years (recent examples being PPS/DRGs and the RBRVS), in which physicians and medical establishments are facing increasing limitations imposed by the larger social system. Given these facts and the proclamations by an embattled medical establishment, most medical social scientists characterize medicine's influence as contracting, but this is only so relative to its past history of rising power.

Lewis and Bennett voice an appreciation for the social importance of the doctor-patient relationship as a therapeutic key to patients' physical, mental, and social well-being. They also see the practicality of communication skills for the sustained viability of medical practices. Interestingly, even as social and medical scientists offer perspectives on how much the overall environment of medicine has changed, training and research on the doctor-patient relationship remain enmeshed in traditional perspectives and methods.

Preparing physicians to practice requires a balance between the technical and human standards of care. This is in the best interest of patients as well as medical practitioners. If the trend continues toward physicians' loss of discretion, then their work will become more mechanical and inflexible. The more mechanical physicians' work is, the greater the likelihood that they will focus on technical standards of care. The more medical encounters are of a technical nature, the higher the probability that patients will lose their uniqueness as individuals. An informed patient care process manifests mutuality—a medical encounter based on a high degree of both physician control and patient empowerment.

The themes of biomedical power and physician control epitomize the need for, and provide the substantive basis of, a social medicine dialogue across disciplines. We should not be shocked to find that many in medicine view some of the social science perspectives presented here as providing illusory solutions. There is much to be done before a full-scale rapprochement can be realized. Disciplinary jargons do not help us solve evidence problems, but rather confound important issues. We need to deal with differences in our conceptual languages before we can identify mistaken ideas and move toward the development of a systemic interdisciplinary medicine.

The papers here call attention to the importance of sharing with one another among scholars in diverse fields. We hope they stimulate further efforts in this direction.

Jeffrey Michael Clair
Richard M. Allman

Issues and Perspectives

1

The Application of Social Science to Medical Practice

Jeffrey Michael Clair

The doctor-patient relationship is often portrayed as one of care, compassion, and trust. Many students of medicine are familiar with the nineteenth-century painting *The Doctor* by Sir Luke Fildes (1891). The scene is a dimly lighted cottage living area with the physician seated, like Rodin's *The Thinker,* at the makeshift bed of a child. The elderly doctor presents an image that at once combines concern, sensitivity, and intelligence. The illusion of this moment is that he is in control of the situation. In the background the father looks at the doctor with an expression of solicitude. The mother reflects despair, slumped at a table with her face buried in her folded arms. The doctor, with a solid working knowledge of pathology and a lifetime of professional experience, foresees how the disease will run its course. Having already arrived at a terminal diagnosis, he is observing the patient. He has delivered the bad news to the family in language they understand, and despite the gloomy outcome, at the moment of the painting he is engaged in the art of medicine—communicating that he is there to provide all possible support.

In contrast to the above characterization, a contemporary short story, "The Bag Lady," captures the spirit of Lady Cassandre, the patient who teaches anyone who will listen (LaCombe 1991). Cassandre, upon entering the hospital, has a compelling effect on the doctors. She moves with a calm grace, and to the medical observers who are accustomed to the brisk pace of hospital activity, her manner seems phlegmatic. Each doctor who sees Cassandre gets caught up in a strange empathy, each having the feeling of being scrutinized, dissected, and laid bare by the person before them. The doctors are compelled to learn from Cassandre and each other. No one who enters her room is left untouched. To what degree Cassandre's calming presence touches the spirit of each doctor depends in varying degrees on the doctor's own desires and defenses.

These depictions illustrate both sides of the doctor-patient relationship. From *The Doctor* we understand the importance of the doctor's influence on the patient and family. "The Bag Lady" reminds us of the strong influence patients can have on doctors and even on physician-physician relationships. And while patients are seen as having an increasingly stronger influence on health care providers in our current system, the public still yearns for the sensitive and supporting physician-icon portrayed by Sir Luke Fildes.

In this paper I examine the physician–patient care process. I begin from the position that the practice of biomedicine has special importance as a moral enterprise between an ill person receiving and a healer providing a precious service (Freidson 1989; Kleinman 1988; Zaner 1990). Such encounters reflect core assumptions and values derived from socially structured systems of meaning (Clair 1990a; Maynard 1991; Strauss et al. 1985). Persons' experiences of illness unfold within a matrix of interpersonal relationships in both informal and formal contexts. In other words, patients bring their informal experience to socially situated medical contexts in which physicians provide formal social support. By viewing medical practice as the organization of the ongoing, dynamic communicative exchanges among physicians, patients, and family, we can analyze the relationship between language, the illness process, and social behavior. My assumption is that until the *social psychological* contexts of medical encounters are given explicit attention in research and training, doctors, patients, and caregivers will be mystified about the ingredients of effective patient care (Eisenberg 1988; Shorter 1991). Franz Kafka (1971) in his short story "A Country Doctor" concisely summarizes the problem: "It is easier for a doctor to write a prescription than to come to an understanding with people."

My more specific objective is to represent medical encounters as fundamentally social interactions. I argue that communication processes between patients and their physicians require the appropriate attention of "social" as well as medical practitioners. The need for the application of social sciences to medical practice will necessitate newly conceived collaborative research. I will specify how such an interface can be accomplished through a sociomedical research agenda on patient care.

The Quarantine of Scientific Data Thought Applicable to Medical Practice

American medical education has increasingly become dominated by applied scientists and researchers (Starr 1982). Despite the incredible impact of the biological revolution on patient care, some critics conclude that, as a result of an overreliance on technical procedures, medical practice suffers from "too much science" and lacks the human touch. This argument often confuses science with technology and mistakes biomedicine as the only science relevant to medicine (Eisenberg 1988; Evans, chap. 5 of this book).

Investigations into patient care relationships must involve a panoply of disciplines far more extensive than those found in biomedicine (Engel 1977, 1980; Hellman 1991; Howell 1991). Too narrow a view of the sciences relevant to medicine has hampered the progress of patient care (Ludmerer 1985; Strahlman 1990). Recent mandates call for medical education and clinical research to involve the social and behavioral sciences (Lonergan 1991) in order to contribute to the proper development of humanistic qualities in physicians (American Board of Internal Medicine 1991; American Medical Association 1991a).[1]

The origins of these mandates can be traced back to the nineteenth-century German physician Rudlof Virchow, who maintained that medicine was a social science and should be used to help improve social conditions (Rosen 1979). Some 50 years ago medical historian Henry Sigerist (1946:130) advocated the incorporation of social science perspective into medical school curriculum, arguing that "Social medicine is not so much a technique as rather an attitude and approach to the problems of medicine, one which I have no doubt will some day permeate the entire curriculum. This, however, will require a new type of clinical teacher and new textbooks." Richmond (1992) points out that Sigerist would be disappointed if he could look in on us today, for "unfortunately we are still waiting."

Social science theory and methods must be integrated into the medical educational and research establishment if physicians are to be able to respond effectively to patient illness as a human experience. The social sciences can help medicine to be reconceived to provide an appropriate emphasis on the patient's experience and understanding of illness. Eisenberg (1988:483) writes: "Are those of us who celebrate the contribution of science to medicine merely deluding ourselves that the recent history of clinical medicine is one of progress? Why, in John Knowles' trenchant phrase, 'are we doing better and feeling worse'? " He goes on to argue that medical education suffers from too much emphasis on memorizing evanescent facts and too little on the social sciences as a way of framing questions and gathering evidence. The intellectual diversity of the social sciences is capable of inspiring efforts to knit together, empirically and conceptually, the seemingly disparate factors contributing to the patient care experience and its outcome.

Proponents of various patient care philosophies must recognize that many people enter clinics with illnesses that represent tragic personal experiences with the social world (Waitzkin 1991). Some estimate that more than 50% of all outpatient visits have social psychological roots (Howell, Lurie, and Woolliscroft 1987). A critical discourse asks what medicine might become if, beyond its biomedical goals and values, we begin to recognize how unmet needs, longings, and the social stresses of everyday life can manifest multiple illness symptoms within people (Scheper-Hughes 1990:194).

Many health care providers are indeed beginning to notice how much their success with patients is affected by social psychological factors. Although there is a growing awareness of the relevance of the social contexts of patients' interpersonal behavior, social networks, and economic circumstances, many physicians ordinarily see these factors as being outside their professional expertise (Freeman and Levine 1989; Mechanic and Aiken 1986; Maloney and Paul 1991; Stoeckle 1988; Waitzkin 1991). As Levine (1987:3) notes, accounting for the relevance of social factors to patient care acknowledges that medical decisions "do not emanate from a routine, scientific calculus, but are made by people playing social roles, guided by social values, and located in particular social settings or contexts." Few, if any, patient care decisions are purely medical (Zola 1991).

The social and behavioral sciences and the humanities should be involved along with the many subdisciplines of medicine and biology in patient care research and medical education (Fox 1990; Robert Wood Johnson Foundation Commission on Medical Education 1991). Social science perspectives can help physicians to recognize the distinction between disease and illness (*dis-ease*), between pathophysiological processes and the patient's experiences of being ill. Physicians are taught to conceptualize medicine as an applied biology (Zaner 1990) and disease as an abnormality in the structure and function of body organs and tissues (Eisenberg 1977, 1988; Hahn and Kleinman 1983). From a social science perspective, on the other hand, patients suffer from illnesses, during which they experience disvalued changes in states of well-being and social functionability. A patient's social class, social support, and interactional abilities illuminate illness and health-related behaviors as experienced social constructions that are unaccounted for by purely biological factors. In other words, social science perspectives demonstrate the particulars of how to treat a patient as a person, rather than the person as a patient (Clair 1990a). In this way, social scientists working "with" medical practitioners can replace the "promise" of the social sciences with hard evidence of their utility (Freeman and Levine 1989; Fritz 1991).

The Social Sciences Working "With" Medicine

The social sciences have produced a cogent body of data relevant to understanding health and medical services (Mechanic and Aiken 1986:1). Over the last few decades, we can trace the growth of basic, clinical, applied, and evaluation research in the social sciences in addressing concerns about medicine such as: (a) the broad determinants and correlates of health and illness, especially morbidity, disability, mortality, and distress; (b) social and behavioral processes affecting the etiology, course, and outcome of pathology; (c) the functions of, effects of, and interplay among the political-economic, ethical, professional, and organizational dimensions of medical services; (d) the processes of interaction among physicians, patients, and their families; and (e) the ways in which people care for their health, identify illness, seek help and information, and react to the health care system.

Despite these well-established data focusing on social science, medicine, and health, social scientists often feel overlooked because there is no one-to-one correspondence between the flow of new knowledge and its application (Mechanic and Aiken 1986:2). The theoretical and methodological contributions of the social sciences to patient care are not sought out or well understood by many medical administrators, researchers, educators, and practitioners (Niklas 1982). Much of our social knowledge is thought to be too abstract and uncertain to be helpful in a meaningful way (Lemert 1991; Light 1992; Seidman 1991). Social insights and data occasionally inform the clinician's view of the problem, but more often applicable findings remain on the periphery of medical practice. Expanding collaboration with medical clinicians, researchers, and educators is vital for the effective application of social scientific evidence to medicine in action, or patient care.

During the early development of the medical social sciences in the United States, it was common to differentiate between the applicability of social sciences "in" medicine and "of" medicine (Straus 1957).[2] The question of the appropriate relationship between the social sciences and medicine persists today. The relationship began with social scientists' provision of information solicited from the medical profession. Social scientists working "in" medicine is the phrase given to research structured more to serve medical interests. Mechanic (1990:87) has recently written that sociologists "in" medicine "work as applied investigators or technicians, seeking to answer questions of interest to the sponsors." This work usually stresses research design and data collection, with an emphasis on chronic diseases and their impact on mortality; on mental illness; on benefits derived from technological advances and therapy; and more recently on prevention (Susser,

Watson, and Hooper 1985). Within the disciplines of sociology and anthropology, social practitioners engaged "in medicine" often raise suspicions because their purely applied activity lacks theoretical substance and development (Freeman and Levine 1989). Recent arguments claim that such descriptive social science work is failing to fulfill its larger responsibility to understand medicine as a social enterprise, thus being "ripe for takeover by psychologists, epidemiologists, and/or clinicians" (Light 1992:910).

Critics of social scientists in medicine prefer to view medicine as a source of data for generating and answering social rather than medical questions. They have an "of medicine" perspective that is concerned with using the institution of medicine as an arena to study important social processes, such as stratification, organization, control, and professional socialization, within the broad context of social values and policy. In other words, the social scientist focuses on the medical arena as the dependent variable in an effort to contribute to the development of theory. There often is no particular concern about developing insights applicable to medical practice, with theory being produced and consumed almost exclusively by social science theorists. This is the one major distinction between "in" and "of" medicine: whether the social scientist works with a medical definition of problems or with social definitions (Larson 1990; Wardell 1982).

Within the last 10 years, it has become increasingly popular to view the whole issue of medicine more critically. Many social scientists are advocating a broad, "of health" perspective rather than what they see as a narrow, "of medicine" one (Conrad 1990; Twaddle 1982). Proponents of an "of health" perspective suggest that "of medicine" connotes a more bounded field, implying a focus on institutionalized structures, including occupations, organizations, power relationships, and structured interactions. Those operating from an "of health" perspective feel that they are not restricted to models viewing health as a function of the medical care system and practitioners. Rather, they see health as a multidimensional concept including physical, social psychological, emotional, and even spiritual aspects of subjective experience. Focus extends to all social structures that affect subjective experience, including family, industry, education, the environment, and biomedicine (Wallace 1990).

These seemingly disparate parts of the social-medicine-health relationship actually can be unified more easily than factional accounts sometimes portray, partly because many social scientists have become more practice-oriented. We have learned that "the interplay between theory and practice improves both" (Mechanic and Aiken 1986:3). Clinical studies of practical problems sharpen theoretical thinking and bring it closer to reality; good theory suggests dimensions of applied problems that enrich investigative comprehension (Clark, Fritz, and Rieker 1990; Larson 1990).

Working "with" medicine encompasses the various components of the social sciences described here. This approach emphasizes the independent pursuit of research on the medical system, its practitioners, and the personal experience of illness to generate and test social theory and evidence. Furthermore, the social scientist practicing "within" a medical context also is interested in problem solving and serves some broad medical interests by working toward developing specific insights applicable to medical practice for improved patient care. In this sense, the social practitioner continually reveals pertinent evidence that maintains the independent interests of social and medical practitioners, as well as those of patients.

My conception of the research relationship of social science "with" medicine, although not limited to it, will be specified in a practice terminology that follows. Suffice it to say here that such collaborative projects can generate fruitful social evidence. Social scientists can take into consideration interactional, organizational, professional, political-economic, and ethical processes while examining such concepts as distress, control, uncertainty, labeling, and psychosocial resources. Medical practitioners gain valuable information for medical education, clinical training, and clinical efficacy, as well as data on patient utilization and adherence patterns, and an appreciation for social context. Evidence on the patient care process, when properly implemented in practice, benefits the people receiving care through better health, improved well-being, satisfaction, and increased social support.

In developing a perspective of social sciences "with" medicine, the institutionalization of the medical social sciences must be promoted as special fields within, yet independent of, medicine. Our aim should be to promote initiatives that generate and test social theory and evidence, while expanding our collaboration with medical educators, clinicians, and researchers to maximize the application of social scientific data to patient care (see Bloom 1990; Light 1992). From this perspective, the medical sociologist combines through a research agenda the interests of social scientists, medical practitioners, and patient experience, with proper attention to disseminating results that have high applicability to practice settings.

The development of social sciences working "with" medicine is being sustained by a broad shift toward observing the linkages between social and patient care contexts. Representatives from the different perspectives within the medical social sciences have all come to agree that we are not concerned only with what medicine does "to" its patients but also about its actions "with" them (Zola 1991:11). An integrated social-medical-health emphasis is evident in a movement from a preoccupation with interventions thought to improve health status, to a recognition that the efficient and humane delivery of medical care must be sought. Because of concerns about costs and societal perceptions, medical practitioners, researchers, educators, and administrators are developing a broader view of humanistic patient care and quality of life. Freeman and Levine (1989:4) suggest that increasing collaboration between the social and medical sciences is evident now in the emergence of quality of life as an overriding social dimension of judging health, illness, and the patient care process. Sociomedical concerns about the quality of life are stimulating integrated measures to evaluate physicians' use of technological interventions and health care in general.

Social scientists and physicians now realize that living beyond the years of functional independence is equivalent to compromised health and social well-being (Brody 1989), or "dysquality" (Weiss 1985). Current multidisciplinary dialogue pays increasing attention to preserving the quality of care and of life (Fink et al. 1987) and to achieving an ideal mix of patient care and social support (Clair 1990b). There are calls for medical science and technology efforts that emphasize "healthy aging," or years lived independently without limitation on social function. We need measures that combine data on health, morbidity, disability, and mortality data as a way to indicate "active life expectancy" (Katz et al. 1983; Manton and Stallard 1990) or "life expectancy free of disability" (McKinlay et al. 1989:39). The implication that patient care decisions are prolonging life of less than optimal quality is certainly worthy of all the current attention it is receiving, and more. ·

Functions of the Clinically Applied Social Scientist

While the role of social scientists in clinical settings should be fundamentally research-oriented, in actuality most social scientists in these settings can simultaneously serve the three roles of *researcher, diagnostic-consultant,* and *educator* (Lee 1979; Straus 1979; Wirth 1931). Balancing these three roles is a dynamic process.

For instance, the social practitioner can bring quantitative and qualitative research skills to bear on data gathered through participation in clinical settings, thereby generating diagnostic and educationally useful information (Mechanic 1989). Our own clinical work includes utilization of triangulated research skills to conduct field observations, interviews, discourse analysis, and quantitative assessments of satisfaction and mental and physical health outcomes (Clair

1991). Besides collecting basic sociodemographic data on patients and primary caregivers, our strategy includes collection of data on variables such as depression, locus of control, social activity, informal support, and strain; information on daily-life activities; baseline morbidity data on hospital admissions and stays and emergency room visits; number of days confined to bed because of illness; and physical, social, and psychological well-being indicators.

We also function as participant-observers and make audio recordings of medical encounters. To assess the larger social context of illness, postencounter assessments of the physician-patient interaction are conducted by interviewing the patient, and when present, the caregiver, while the doctor answers the same Likert scale items through a self-administered questionnaire. Patients are then followed to obtain information on adherence to medication and referrals, as well as physical and social psychological health, through both telephone interviews and medical record review at one- and six-month intervals. Such detailed data are not collected by clinical social workers and psychologists as part of their patient contact.

Our data contribute to the diagnostic-consulting aspect of our role, which includes assisting other health care and service providers in parts of their work about which the social scientist has special knowledge. The consultative responsibilities are intermittently requested as the social scientist participates with practitioners in the study of cases and their treatment. Thus, the social scientist is included in making the rounds of patients and in discussing their cases with the health care team members.

The educator component is equivalent to systematic instruction. The social scientist can provide practical clinical information for assessment team members and also theoretical instruction for residents. For instance, just as a clinical psychologist can train health care providers to recognize and treat mental disorders, the social scientist can train these providers to recognize and help patients cope with social problems. The social scientist also can help physicians interact more effectively with patients and with one another. Utilizing transcripts, residents can be taught to develop greater awareness and more humanistic qualities. In general, instruction focuses on continually sensitizing physicians and other health professionals to the ways in which the implicit, unstated values of biomedicine affect the patient's experience.

Generating Applicable Sociomedical Data

I have already argued that the social scientist's research perspective generates social evidence that contributes to medicine in several important ways: (1) in the diagnostic workup, which benefits patients and their family members; (2) in the overall clinical efficacy of patient care; and (3) in the continued training of physicians.

Successful generation and application of social evidence to medical practice requires a distinctive methodological approach. First, a pragmatist epistemology explicitly recognizes that knowing is the act not of an outside observer but of a participant inside the social scene (Dewey [1929] 1960:196; James [1909] 1970:80; Shalin 1986:18). The goal in practice, therefore, becomes that of approximating the accounts of meaning that social reality represents to those participating in its production (McHugh 1968), by studying the patient care process *in situ*, in its natural milieu.[3]

Second, I suggest a multiple data collection strategy because no single methodological technique is uniformly superior. I acknowledge that each technique has inherent strengths that are unmatched by other techniques, but suggest that every technique suffers from inherent weaknesses that can only be rectified by cross-checking with other sources of data. The generation of social theory and evidence from multiple data sources improves our probabilistic opinion (Lieberson 1992).

Third, a grounded theory approach, in which theory is generated from the data should serve as the foundation for research. This approach allows for the discovery of concepts and hypotheses that are relevant to the issues at hand (Glaser 1978; Glaser and Strauss 1967; Turner 1981). The grounded theory approach endorses fundamental strategies: (1) discovering and analyzing social and social psychological processes structures one's inquiry; (2) data collection and analysis phases of research proceed simultaneously; (3) analytic processes prompt discovery and theory development; (4) theoretical sampling refines, elaborates, and expands conceptual categories; and (5) systematic application of analytic techniques leads to more abstract analytic levels of evidence (Charmaz 1983:125).[4]

This perspective does not compromise quantitative verification. In fact, even structural-equation, traditional model testing can be incorporated into social practice. The distinction is that closeup, first-hand knowledge of issues related to doctor-patient communication, by means of observational and in-depth interviewing formats applied to varied subcultural groupings, forms the basis for generating questionnaire-based instruments in which the questions posed have both relevance and saliency for the populations being studied. Insofar as current knowledge of doctor-patient communication derives heavily from reliance on single research technique—either purely qualitative treatment of transcripts or closed-ended questionnaires—we have trouble ascertaining the degree to which findings are generalizable, a difficulty that may simply be an artifact of the methodology employed. To the extent to which different methodological techniques point toward similar evidence, we can have more confidence in the validity of results.

I recently began studies with a field-developed instrument that isolates the contribution of the physician to patient mental and physical health. This research started in response to the question of whether doctor-patient communication really matters (Hughes 1991). This seemingly simple question shakes the foundation of the current work in this area, because it lacks theoretical grounding.

My perspective treats physician communication as an instance of formal social support. The effect of social support in alleviating life stress is conceived almost entirely in terms of informal support from family and friends. There is a virtual absence of any assessment of the physician's role as a social support resource. These facts point to the need for study of the extent to which physician support mitigates life stress and enhances patient mental and physical health.

My major premise is that psychosocial resources, such as formal physician support, informal family and friend support, and personal coping abilities play a direct and significant role in mediating or reducing the detrimental effects of social stressors on distress. Stress is the relationship between external conditions and the present state of an individual; and distress is the biopsychosocial response to this relationship.[5] The general formulation is that external stressors such as undesirable life events, role strains, and situational stressors, if not mediated, disrupt an individual's psychosocial equilibrium and induce distress responses. An absence of psychosocial resources contributes to negative psychological states such as depression. In turn, these psychological states may ultimately influence physical health, either through their direct effect on physiological processes—influencing the susceptibility to disease—or through behavioral patterns that increase the risk for disease (Cohen and Wills 1985).

An individual's psychosocial resources affect this process by modifying conditions leading to problems or altering the meaning of external stimulus, thus moving toward neutralizing any incongruent life events. In other words, psychosocial resources are conceptualized as change elements in the stress process that are mobilized in order to directly deter distress, or to mediate or buffer the potential adverse consequences of stressful conditions and situations, thereby enhancing well-being (Ensel and Lin 1991).

Undesirable life events (ill health, loss of a job, death of a loved one, family conflict, and the like) and situational stressors (the daily hassles of one's life circumstances) disrupt the individual's life and challenge his or her psychosocial resources. For example, the death of

Figure 1.1. Psychosocial Resource Model

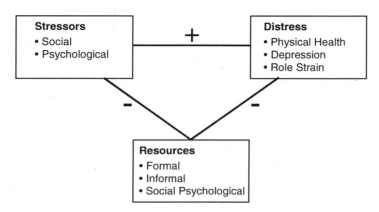

a spouse disrupts an individual's ongoing aspects of life, since the confidant the person depends on for shared response exchanges is lost (Burke 1991). The result of such a loss is distress.

This distress and psychosocial resource model can be expressed by the following propositions: (1) the frequency of undesirable life events and daily hassles (stressors) experienced by individuals is related positively and directly to the extent of mental and physical symptomatology (distress); (2) the frequency of undesirable life events and daily hassles is inversely related to informal and formal social support and an individual's coping skills (psychosocial resources); and (3) the extent of an individual's informal and formal social supports and coping skills is related inversely and directly to the extent of mental and physical symptomatology.

The contribution of formal support by a physician in the distress process still needs to be specifically identified. What doctor-patient care relationship evidence indicates for patients in general is that desired outcomes are associated with a communication style that provides a high level of information and opportunities for participation in decision making. Additionally, patients want doctors to respond favorably to their questioning, and show sensitivity to their well-being. In this sense, isolating physician communication strategies as a special form of formal social support should focus on factors such as physician information giving, reciprocity, affect, and personalization (Clair 1991).[6] Physicians who manifest these humanistic communication qualities can expect to contribute to an individual's psychosocial resource stock, thus providing the person with more opportunity to mediate the potential harmful consequences of stressors. This formal support should enhance an individual's overall physical, psychological, and social well-being. The benefits are direct and additive when considering informal social support and coping skills. Deciphering the unique contribution of psychosocial resource factors remains an empirical question.

There are enormous potential benefits in generating research evidence that will allow successful medical interviewing skills to be integrated into teaching curricula (see Frankel and Beckman, chap. 13 of this book). Patient and caregiver satisfaction depends in part on the quality of the medical encounter (Cleary and McNeil 1988; Comstock et al. 1982; Haley, Clair, and Saulsberry 1992; Lipkin, Quill, and Napodano 1984; Starfield et al. 1981; Weinberger, Greene, and Mamlin 1981). The accuracy of the information elicited is a function of medical interview techniques (Carter et al. 1982). With effective communication techniques, the physician's spectrum of concerns expands (Engel 1980). When the physician learns to focus on listening to the patient rather than directing the patient, much new information becomes available. For instance, major complaints beyond the initial ones can be clarified and addressed (Barsky 1981). Psychosocial complaints and maladjustments can be put into proper context in the care process (Bellet and Maloney 1991; DeVries, Berg, and Lipkin 1982).

Medical practitioners also can be taught to become more aware of sociolinguistic differences among social classes and age groups. With this sensitivity, treatment strategies can be used with enhanced comprehensiveness and compliance (Kimball 1982). From a practical standpoint, the best diagnosis is worth nothing if patients fail to follow through with treatment. All the resources of the medical establishment are rendered impotent by a simple act of noncompliance, such as not taking medication (Blascovich 1982; Kessler 1991).

Unraveling the dynamics of labeling and the operation of stereotypes is another important aspect of research and application. Like other human beings, physicians are likely to treat patients in stereotypical ways, depending on the patient's sex, age, race, and occupation. We know that persons of lower socioeconomic status are reluctant to ask questions during the medical encounter, suggesting that more information should be volunteered for them (Waitzkin 1984). There also is documentation that communication difficulties exist between doctors and their geriatric patients (Beland and Maheux 1990). And recent research shows that physicians are less willing to interact with AIDS patients (Kelley, Lawrence, Smith et al. 1987; Rizzo, Marder, and Willke 1990).

The contents of the medical record and the attitude of caregivers also can contribute to the labeling of patients (Clair 1990a). Does information in the medical record bias even new patient-physician interactions? Do caregivers unintentionally establish patients as unreliable historians, thus undermining the patient-physician relationship (see Silliman, chap. 9; Wallander and Hardy, chap. 10, this book)? Physicians can benefit from knowing statistical generalizations about categories of patients. But this knowledge should stimulate questions, rather than lead the physician to draw unfounded conclusions. Research findings on at-risk populations must be used astutely to benefit an individual patient. Physicians, through techniques that must usually be taught, must learn to establish whether a specific patient fits the statistical pattern.

An awareness of subtle labeling processes is one way to make the achievement of reciprocal communication more probable. It remains to be seen whether an expansive mode of communication, one requiring attention to the social psychological as well as physical aspects of illness, can be developed within medicine (Cook, Coe, and Hanson 1990). These are sociomedical questions that can be appropriately addressed to by integrating social research practitioners into medical settings through a triangulated, grounded-theory research approach.

Conclusion

Sociomedical attention to quality patient care should focus on a host of empathetic and egalitarian *social psychological* variables beyond traditional medical models based on the symptomatology and etiology of the patient's illness. A sociomedical perspective acknowledges that when patients approach a physician for help, they represent (*represent*) a social context along with their physical problem(s). Because of a lack of training in the social sciences, when social issues arise in the intimacy of the patient-doctor relationship, they often get dealt with in "unwitting" and "unintended" ways (Waitzkin 1991 and chap. 8, this book). Although patient care rarely involves straightforward technical solutions, physicians typically focus on physical complaints, often failing to address patients' underlying concerns.

The possibility of physicians' working to improve social contextual sources of distress is overlooked in professional training. The style of instruction in the traditional clinical history is that of "high control" (Waitzkin 1991). While the traditional format of the medical interview conveys a fairly accurate sense of the technical structure, it discourages sharing by the patient and masks or marginalizes the underlying sociocontextual structure. Medical education requires a rethinking and a critical evaluation of what traditional history taking accomplishes. If we fail to modify the educational process, adverse patterns of medical discourse will remain entrenched (see Haug, chap. 12; Frankel and Beckman, chap.13, this book).

As social scientists, we are continually challenged to generate distinctive contributions to our respective disciplines and, more recently, to medical practice as well (Colombotos 1988). Our contribution is dynamic, best accomplished by generating research questions that are field-validated, uncovering valuable evidence through innovative triangulated approaches to data collection. The ideal situation proposed here is one where social scientists work "with" medical providers in applying empirical knowledge to patient care activities. Clearly, there is a growing need for social scientists to work in this capacity.

We must remember, however, that clinical involvement is often the response to an invitation. Social scientists may have difficulty in obtaining an invitation, since such an offer implies that others in the medical context clearly understand our distinct offerings (Bloom 1989; Hunt and Sobal 1990). Some raise doubts about whether a social science interest can develop within the prevailing paradigm of medical practice (Niklas 1982). While some social scientists will "request inclusion" and thus gain access in clinical practice settings, "invitations" from innovative medical leaders help ease entry into such settings, while legitimating the body of social knowledge.

The legitimation of social scientists in clinical settings relieves the pressures of dual loyalties (Kleinman 1980; Scheper-Hughes 1990). Social scientists in clinical contexts must take a stance that is intrinsically divided. We face demands that we be collegial by expressing concern about the practical resolution of clinical problems, yet at the same time we must remain autonomous by generating social theories and evidence of illness and care that can stand on their own. Although invitations run the risk of making us indebted to medical interests, the clinically applied social scientist is justified in shifting between patient care concerns and medical practitioner objectives, being a sympathizer of both. This holistic, pragmatist research approach allows the social scientist to generate data on patient care processes even though the interests and goals of doctors and their patients do not always coincide (see Allman, Yoels, and Clair, chap. 2).

The sociological imagination and language represent an additional frame of reference that allows help-seekers and help-givers to construct a useful reciprocal language. Delineating how these social actors conceive and conceptualize their experience is a significant contribution of a "social science with medicine."

I am not suggesting, as some have strongly argued, that the social scientist become a counseling clinician. In fact, I stress the research orientation of social scientists. We must admit that most persons in our society expect to go to a doctor to heal the body, a dentist to fix the teeth, and a clinical psychologist or psychiatrist to ease mental distress. Nobody wakes up in the morning and says, "I need to go see that medical sociologist today." It is not desirable that the social scientist should displace other health care practitioners (Wirth 1931). Rather, it is suggested that we need to bring to the clinical setting the unique theoretical insights and methodological skills furnished by social science perspectives.[7]

Placing social scientific ideas in the crucible of clinical practice and education can help to clarify, refine, and broaden the patient care process. The broader significance lies in encouraging open social debate by deepening the notion of critical discourse that moves toward a humanely representational sociomedical practice (Richardson 1991). This process will enhance the disciplines of the social and medical sciences while ensuring that members of society receive more informed, comprehensive, and humane patient care.

Notes

1. The definition of humanistic here is consistent with that of the Committee on Humanization of Health Care of the Medical Sociology Section of the American Sociological Association, which set out eight conditions as "necessary and sufficient" for humanized patient care: viewing patients as autonomous, unique, and irreplaceable persons, who should be treated with empathy and warmth, and should share in decisions with health care providers in a reciprocal and egalitarian relationship (see Howard, Davis, Pope, and Ruzek 1977).

2. Parts of my discussion in this section on the development of the medical social sciences also appears in J. Clair, "The Contribution of the Medical Sociologist to the Geriatric Assessment Unit: A Sociology 'With' Medicine," Sociological Practice, in press.

3. In contrast to rationalist epistemology, a pragmatist epistemology does not see adjudication, or the systematic reduction of things to logical categories, as a technical problem, but rather as a substantive problem that requires direct and continuous examination. In this sense, "all social particulars . . . are marginal and situationally emergent" (Shalin, 1986:20). Thus, classifactory categories are treated as probabilities to be ascertained by direct observation in the present situation.

4. To develop grounded theory, close attention needs to be paid to the processing of qualitative data as originally presented by Glaser and Strauss (1967) and elaborated on by Charmaz (1983), and Turner (1981). The schematic list of nine stages is as follows: (1) developing categories; (2) saturating these categories; (3) abstracting definitions of the categories; (4) utilizing these definitions; (5) exploiting these categories fully by being aware of additional categories; (6) noting, developing, and following up links between categories; (7) considering the conditions under which the links hold; (8) making corrections, where relevant, to existing theory; and finally (9) using extreme comparisons to the maximum to test emerging relationships.

5. Stressors are both social and socioenvironmental (see Burke 1991). The distinction is that social stressors challenge coping abilities and an individual's sense of mastery over life circumstances, while socioenvironmental stressors not only challenge an individual's psychosocial resources but also threaten the person's biological system (e.g., criminal victimization).

6. Quantitative factor scale items developed from discourse analysis and field observations may be obtained from the author.

7. I am not suggesting that counseling clinical sociologists are illegitimate practitioners. In fact, many sociologists also are marriage and family therapists and have a legitimate claim to research and insurance-billable service privileges. My position is that we make our most unique, autonomous, and beneficial contribution through the research-oriented role. I acknowledge that both styles of social practice can develop legitimacy and coexist within academic affairs social and behavioral science departments. Medical practitioners should eventually clearly see the contributions that both kinds of clinical social scientists can make to their work.

2

Reconciling the Agendas of Physicians and Patients

Richard M. Allman, William C. Yoels, and
Jeffrey Michael Clair

Relationships between physicians and patients constitute the most intimate core of medical practice. Many researchers stress the clinical and theoretical importance of these interactions, as witnessed by an explosion in studies investigating doctor-patient relationships. James Hughes (1991) estimates that this topic has generated about 600 articles per year during the last decade.

There is increasing evidence that all is not well between physicians and their patients, and discrepant agendas may be one of the major problems in their encounters (Levenstein et al. 1989:119). Those outside the medical system argue that many physicians do not realize that patients have their own agendas when they go to see a doctor. Many of these outsiders, however, fail to understand the goals of the medical encounter from the doctor's perspective. Before the problems intrinsic to doctor-patient relationships can be resolved, physicians, patients, and critics must develop a common language.

An underlying assumption of this chapter is that the life worlds of health care providers and patients differ so widely as to render the formation of satisfying relationships problematic. To be sure, physicians and patients are united in the common pursuit of restoring patients to healthy life. But health is more than absence of disease, so achieving this objective remains an ambiguous goal in many cases (Clair 1990a).

We will discuss how the goals of physicians and patients in the clinical encounter may differ. We also will examine several issues that illustrate the interplay between the personal-cultural interpretations of the illness experience and the larger, structural features of contemporary medical care in the United States. We conclude by offering suggestions for future research and practice geared toward resolving some of the problems in doctor-patient relationships.

What Needs to Be Done When Doctor Meets Patient?

From the physician's perspective, the primary objective of the clinical encounter is to make a diagnosis or to define diagnostic possibilities. Other objectives include developing an evaluation and management plan, communicating those plans to the patient, and finally, developing a relationship with the patient.

Since the early 1900s physicians have used a specific approach to accomplishing the primary objective of the clinical encounter—making a diagnosis (McWhinney 1989; Stoeckle and Billings 1987). This includes eliciting a *chief complaint* from the patient. Although Beckman and Frankel (1984) have shown that the most important problem may not be mentioned until later in the clinical encounter, physicians generally use the first thing mentioned by the patient in identifying the chief complaint.

The physician then proceeds to obtain a *history of the present illness*. By exploring all the patient's symptoms relating to the chief complaint, the physician gains an understanding of the severity of the symptoms, the palliating and ameliorating factors for the complaints, and the timing of the symptoms, as well as their bodily location and associated symptoms. The physician then moves on to review the patient's *past medical history* including surgeries, hospitalizations, medication usage, allergies, immunizations, and health habits.

In the traditional approach the physician also obtains a *social history* related to marital status, education, work history, and living arrangements. A *family history* permits identification of any hereditary or contagious conditions. The *review of systems* involves asking a series of questions about the major organ systems to determine whether any symptoms that could assist in the diagnosis of the primary problem have been missed or whether there are other problems needing attention. Finally, a *complete physical examination* is performed; here the physician correlates the findings with all the other information available, constructs a list of potential diagnoses, and decides on the most likely problem. Thus, the physician can then decide on the most appropriate evaluation and/or management plan with the diagnostic possibilities in mind. These activities are all part of the traditional clinical method.

For medical students in the United States, the physical diagnosis course is usually the earliest and most comprehensive introduction to how to conduct the stages of the clinical encounter. This course is generally scheduled during the second year of medical school, while the students are being challenged with difficult courses in pathology and pharmacology. The diagnostic courses contain variable amounts of information on how to conduct an interview; unfortunately, the time to practice these skills is quite limited. Moreover, there is generally a shortage of faculty having the time, interest, or knowledge of interviewing skills to provide a high-quality experience in medical interviewing even if time were provided in the curriculum. Complicating matters even more, medical students also are expected during the physical diagnosis course to learn the technical aspects of the physical examination: using an otoscope, an ophthalmoscope, and a sphygmomanometer for blood pressures, as well as feeling for the spleen, listening to the lungs, probing for heart sounds, checking for reflexes, and other tasks. Much emphasis is usually placed on the student's ability to communicate, in a written and an oral presentation, the findings obtained in the clinical encounter.

After completion of the physical diagnosis course, the student begins clinical clerkships equipped with the methods of the traditional clinical approach: taking a history, performing a physical examination, choosing appropriate laboratory studies, and making a diagnosis. As Huddle (1991) notes in a critique of the literature on educating humane physicians, students are thrust into the commotion of inpatient and outpatient services, where they are taught by house staff who face competing demands for their time in caring for patients and conducting research. Often, because of the fast pace of clinical work, only essentials are attended to, those bearing on pathophysiology rather than social psychological aspects of the patient's illness experience. After graduation the student becomes a resident and is often exhausted to the point of minimizing attention to matters not directly related to physical diagnosis and treatment. In such an environment, the wonder may be not that many physicians fail to manifest appropriate compassion and empathy, but that at least some do so (Huddle 1991). Frequently, the development of interpersonal skills is left to chance as the students begin clinical rotations and go on to postgraduate residency training. The traditional medical approach, frequently called a "disease-centered" approach (Levenstein et al. 1989), usually allows the physician to accomplish the primary objective of the encounter: to make a diagnosis and thereby determine appropriate therapy; patients, however, consult the doctor for more than this.

What Does the Patient Want from the Clinical Encounter?

Most episodes of illness occur and resolve without the involvement of a physician; such episodes constitute what is referred to as the "illness iceberg" (Scambler and Scambler 1984; Last 1963). Zola (1983a:87) writes:

Consider the following computation of Hinkle et al. (1960). They noted that the average lower-middle-class male between the ages of 20 and 45 experiences over a 20-year period approximately one life-endangering illness, 20 disabling illnesses, 200 non-disabling illnesses, and 1000 symptomatic episodes. These total 1,221 episodes over 7305 days or one new episode every six days. And this figure takes no account of the duration of a particular condition, nor does it consider any disorder of which the respondent may be unaware. In short, even among a supposedly "healthy" population scarcely a day goes by wherein they would not be able to report a symptomatic experience.

In effect, then, doctors' offices would be overwhelmed if people immediately acted on the symptoms causing them discomfort. What happens here, as Kleinman et al. (1978:251) note, is that "an estimated 70-90% of all self-recognized episodes of sickness are managed exclusively outside the perimeter of the formal health care system. . . . (If, for example, 90% of all illness episodes are managed without resort to professionals, a shift of 10% of these cases could double the demand on medical institutions.)" More recent data presented in Scambler and Scambler (1984:34) indicate that as few as 5% of the symptoms expressed by persons over a six-week period eventuate in a medical consultation. Those who are not using medical professionals for help are most likely relying on alternative healers, self-help groups, self-treatments, and other elements of "folk" explanatory models for solutions to their medical problems.

We also might expect that reliance on folk medicine frameworks is a function of socioeconomic status, with those lowest on the social ladder relying on cultural values that make them more reluctant to visit doctors. Also critical here is the financial burden that our medical system entails for those who lack access to health insurance and/or proximity to medical facilities. According to Blendon (1989:2), 37 million Americans are currently uninsured, and this segment of the population has increased by 25% since 1980. Furthermore, the insurance held by sizable numbers of working-class and middle-class persons is inadequate for handling major medical problems. We can see, then, that the decision to consult a doctor about an illness is the result of an interpretive process that takes place in the context of the distribution of available medical services.

In presenting an illness experience to a doctor, what does a typical patient desire from the doctor? Given the significance of such a question for understanding patient experiences, it is surprising how little attention has been devoted to this issue. Often patients have reasons for coming to the doctor that remain hidden (Barsky 1981). Most patients who consult a doctor want an explanation for the cause of their illness, along with treatment and cure (Korsch et al. 1968).

In a recent study, Ende et al. (1989) examined patients' desire for autonomy, participation in decision making, and information. They found that while patients are not interested in being "principal decision makers," they do want to be kept informed by the doctor. In addition, the more serious the illness, the less likely the desire to make decisions, although even here it is important to realize that patient desires "should be regarded as dynamic, not static. Whatever decision-making powers they may forgo in acute illness they *may reclaim as health is restored*" (1989:28, emphasis added). Such a situation calls our attention to the importance of the ongoing interpretive process that all human beings engage in as they continually assess and reassess their life experiences.

Ende et al. (1989:28) present a very illuminating concept to describe their findings. They describe patients as "granting permission to the physicians to take charge of certain decisions. This is 'paternalism with permission' [a term borrowed from Cross and Churchill 1982] and may be typical of most medical encounters."

A question quickly emerges here about what patients are typically told in a medical encounter. Are patients' wishes to be informed actually fulfilled in visits with doctors? The news here is unfortunately not very heartening. Data provided by Boreham and Gordon (1978) cited in Matthews (1983:1373) indicate that fewer than 50% of patients get even a minimal level of explanation from doctors. In addition, physicians "seldom remark on the causes or expected course of the illness. In only half the cases is the patient told the name and effect of prescribed drugs. The authors find the majority of patients view information about their illness as an important facet of the medical consultation, yet few ask for a diagnosis or the name of a prescribed drug. They observe that a doctor's response to a patient's question frequently conveys to the patient he has implied lack of confidence in the doctor's judgment."

It also has been found that physicians overestimate the time they spend with patients, and underestimate the amount of information that patients want (Waitzkin 1984). Another study suggests that physicians and patients agree less than 50% of the time about the most important problem addressed during a clinic visit (Freidin et al. 1980).

Some patients may consult a doctor to obtain education about how to remain healthy (see Haug, chap. 12, this book). Many others come in need of help in understanding or dealing with life stresses, depression, and social isolation (see Waitzkin, Britt, and Williams, chap. 8). In many of these situations, a specific disease or pathologic condition does not explain the patient's problem. The problem may not be definable by a biopsy or an abnormality in the function of an organ, tissue, or cell of the patient. It may be better defined as an illness, the individual's social or psychological response to disease, grief, or just the pain of living (Novack 1987). The traditional clinical method does not ensure that the physician will pay attention to these issues.

Implications of Discrepant Doctor-Patient Agendas

The discrepancies in the agendas of patients and doctors during the clinical encounter may seriously impair the patient-doctor relationship. The failure of the traditional clinical method to ensure that physicians identify the problems most important to patients—whether emotional and social issues, patient educational needs, or illness behavior—is a serious problem when one considers the realities of primary care. About 30% of patients seen in primary care come to the doctor with significant psychosocial problems deserving of physician attention and as many as 85% have some degree of psychological distress (Bertakis et al. 1991). Patients report better outcomes when the physician and patient agree on the principal problem (Starfield et al., 1981).

An important aspect of primary care is preventing disease, not merely diagnosing it during the clinical encounter. A significant part of the physician's responsibility, therefore, is to encourage healthy behavioral lifestyle changes. Unfortunately, physicians often have not been taught to fulfill this responsibility in medical school or during postgraduate training. In addition, physicians often lack the knowledge and skills required to make the clinical encounter a therapeutic intervention for the many patients with depression, anxiety, somatiform and conversion disorders, and stress-related illness (Novack 1987). Time pressures on physicians as well as a belief, perhaps, that they possess little expertise in the realm of psychosocial matters, also may be at play here. As a result, physicians may fail to utilize family and social supports, community agencies, and other health care providers to relieve patients' distress precipitated by social problems (Novack 1987). The lack of such knowledge and skills may decrease physicians' satisfaction with their work.

Physicians in primary-care practice quickly learn that management has to be tailored to individual patients, whatever the diagnosis. Evaluation and management must accommodate the patient's ideas, expectations, and feelings to be of maximum benefit for the resolution of illness. If the evaluation and management plan is not understood by the patient and does not match the patient's desires, the plan is not likely to be followed (Levenstein et al. 1989). For example, if a patient believes an antihypertensive will lower the quality of life, adherence to the treatment regimen is likely to be poor. The patient may be reluctant to share such feelings with the physician, thereby making it difficult to know why blood pressure control is inadequate. Physicians have little experience or training in eliciting such information from their patients. The resulting difficulties in managing adherence problems in patients can be very frustrating for physicians.

Many physicians have been criticized for being uncaring because they fail to compensate for the problems of the traditional clinical method. They have not recognized the importance of attentive listening, eliciting a patient's responses when attempting to cure a disease, or providing education and recommendations for life-style change (Levenstein et al. 1989). When physicians fail to provide explanations for illness, many patients become dissatisfied (Korsch et al. 1968). Dissatisfaction may manifest itself in nonadherence (Francis et al. 1969; Roter 1977), withdrawal from health plans (Davies et al. 1986), doctor shopping (Kasteler et al. 1976), or malpractice litigation (Ritchey, chap. 7; Ware et al. 1978). On the other hand, some physicians have been able to adapt the traditional clinical method in a way that minimizes patient dissatisfaction.

Pressures on Physicians

To explain the gap between what patients want and what they are most likely to get, we have to focus on the pressures facing physicians in a system of medical care that is profit-driven (see Ohsfeldt, chap. 6). A gain-loss formula heavily influences what kinds of medical technologies providers purchase in an effort to remain competitive with other providers who are purchasing similar items. Such purchases, of course, lead to pressures to use the technology in order to provide better care as well as "justify" the original need for the item. As a result, patients may undergo needless testing, thereby increasing insurance fees in a dog-chasing-its-own-tail kind of medical cost escalation.

Perhaps the most significant structural constraint facing physicians in the current system of health care concerns the dimension of time. To maintain adequate income levels and pay the costs of doing "medical business," such as malpractice insurance, doctors must maintain certain levels of patient care loads. Such care loads lead to considerable time spent by patients waiting in offices or reception areas before actually seeing doctors and little time actually spent in face-to-face contacts with doctors. Earlier research indicates the average length of a doctor-patient office encounter to be about five minutes, with initial visits averaging about 30 minutes (Helman 1978:126; Zola 1983a:222). According to more recent work by Waitzkin (1991:286), typical medical encounters last about 17 minutes, of which doctors spend only about one minute, on the average, in actually giving information to their patients. Current Health Care Financing Administration billable-services standards recognize an average of 10 minutes for medical encounters.

Time limitations are particularly problematic for patients with complicated cases who may have a number of social psychological problems. Older patients are at particular risk for the negative consequences of such time constraints. Despite the greater number of problems for older patients, physicians tend to spend less, rather than more, time with them. This problem may be exacerbated unless policy is changed so that time spent in talking with patients is adequately reimbursed. Such "cognitive" services are generally undervalued, while procedure-related services tend to be overvalued under the current reimbursement policy. The Resource Base Relative Value System introduced in 1992 may reduce the disparity in reimbursement for cognitive services in the future, but current policies make it difficult for physicians to spend additional time with patients if they are to conduct an economically viable practice.

Given the brief time available for doctor-patient contacts, it is particularly important to recognize the uncertainty of the general conditions in which medical diagnoses occur. Based on work by Pickering (1979), Brody (1980:720) argues "that in about 90% of medical conditions there is either no specific remedy or effectiveness of the treatment is unknown." Physicians face the fundamental dilemma, then, of making judgments based on a biomedical explanatory model that operates within the structural constraints of the uncertainty of medical knowledge itself, coupled with the constraints on time available for a diagnosis. It is not surprising, then, that the more amorphous, social dimensions of patients' lives are paid minimal attention (Waitzkin 1991). The biomedical explanatory model orients the physician to the physical, organic, disease state of the person's *body*, thereby minimizing the *selfhood* realm of the patient's experience (Young 1989). In fact, recent data presented by Gerrity et al. (1992:1043) suggest that conditions of uncertainty prompt physicians to worry about their *own selves*, experiencing "the fear of personal inadequacy and failure."

We also might expect that in conditions of limited time, stereotypical thinking will most likely occur as a way to short-circuit the time-consuming interpretive process entailed by critical thinking and attention to individual uniqueness. In this regard, experimental studies reviewed by Jamieson and Zann (1989:387) suggest that "stereotype-based categories organized perceptions and biased judgments when subjects were situationally motivated to come to rapid decisions." During a typical office visit, then, when doctors are often rushed to make judgments and are faced with numerous illnesses having no single "cure," we would expect that the greater the disparity between doctors' socioeconomic status and that of their patients, the greater the likelihood of engaging in stereotypical thinking and of making a diagnosis focused on organic as opposed to social and psychological issues (Eisenberg 1979). No one to date, however, has empirically tested such a hypothesis; we offer it here simply as a way of making sense of some currently unrelated findings in the medical literature.

Time, and its usage and meanings for doctors and patients, serves as an ideal vehicle for thinking about the linkages between the social psychological process of interpretation and the larger structural setting in which such interpretations occur. From the doctor's point of view, time is a scarce and most valuable resource that is parceled out to patients in ways dictated by the doctor's position of power and status within the formal health care system. Waiting, as Barry Schwartz (1975) has so eloquently demonstrated, is something "lower-downs" are required to do in return for the services or expertise provided by "higher-ups." Given that doctors are the gatekeepers of medical knowledge, patients have little choice but to do what is required to get medical care, such as waiting, both for appointments to take place and, upon actually visiting the office, for the availability of the doctors. We might add here, however, that large numbers of people who are not availing themselves of traditional medical care may be demonstrating not only financial concerns but also a kind of "resistance" to the costs of such care in terms of time.

Patient Satisfaction and Health Outcomes

Studies that have examined associations between communication patterns during clinical encounters and patient satisfaction provide supporting evidence that the discrepancies between the physician's and the patient's agendas for the clinical encounter lead to problems in the doctor-patient relationship. Bertakis et al. (1991) have shown that communication patterns between physicians and their long-term patients correlate with a number of dimensions of patients' satisfaction. They found that physicians' counseling, physicians' questioning, and the experience of patients in talking about psychosocial issues were all positively correlated with patient satisfaction. Physicians' use of both open- and close-ended questions and patients' talk regarding biomedical topics were negatively associated with patient satisfaction. Patients also were less satisfied when physicians dominated the interview. Older, white patients tended to be more satisfied than other patients.

These findings are consistent with those of other investigators (Buller and Buller 1987; Stewart 1984). Hall, Roter, and Katz (1988) presented a metaanalysis of 41 studies and found that patient satisfaction was associated with the amount of information given by providers, greater technical and interpersonal competence, more social conversation, more positive and less negative talk, and more communication overall.

Perhaps one of the most intriguing questions to pose, given the current literature, is how to explain high levels of patient satisfaction with doctors in view of some of the medical care features we have analyzed in this chapter—such as brief office visits or little information giving. In a three-nation survey (United States, Canada, Great Britain) conducted by Louis Harris for *Health Management Quarterly* (Blendon 1989), for example, American respondents indicated considerable satisfaction in response to a question about their last doctor visit. Fifty-four percent of the American sample answered "very satisfied" and 32% answered "somewhat satisfied" to this question. Eighty-five percent of the American sample also were very or somewhat satisfied with their last hospital stay (Blendon 1989:4). It is important to keep in mind that these answers were given by respondents who had visited a doctor's office in the last 12 months or who had been overnight hospital patients during the past year.

In thinking about results such as those here, we also might consider the findings of Kleinman et al. (1978:25) presented earlier in this chapter: "70-90% of all self-recognized episodes of sickness are managed exclusively outside the perimeters of the formal health care system." Given that figure, it may very well be the case that most patient satisfaction studies, insofar as they deal with patients who have seen or are seeing doctors, may be tapping into a self-selecting sample that biases the responses toward the favorable end of the spectrum. Those who manage their illnesses independent of traditional medicine may have arrived at the decision to do so for a variety of reasons, possibly including negative experiences with, and negative reactions to, traditional medical care. Generalizing, then, to the population at large from current patient satisfaction bases may run the same risk as generalizing from clinically based samples to the non-help-seeking population.

Another significant finding from the Blendon (1989) three-nation survey of health care satisfaction is that sizable numbers of American respondents, in contrast to Canadians and Britons, would prefer to switch to a nationalized health care system in which "the government pays most of the cost of health care for everyone out of taxes and the government sets all fees charged by hospitals and doctors" (1989:5). So, despite high levels of satisfaction with doctors and hospitals, even those seeking traditional medical care are quite critical of the overall health care system in the United States. Given the growing rate of both uninsured and underinsured persons in this country, it is not hard to envision access to health care services becoming one of the major political issues of the coming decade.

Patient satisfaction, while important, has limitations as an outcome of patient-doctor communication. Patients may be satisfied with less than optimal health care or health outcomes. In assessing the quality and effectiveness of patient-doctor communication, health status outcomes should be assessed as well (Kaplan et al, 1989). The studies available that look at health outcome also suggest that aspects of communication that may be deemphasized by physicians may be those most closely related to patient compliance and other desirable health outcomes.

Roter (1989) conducted a metaanalysis of 80 journal articles published during the 1962-86 period to assess associations between doctor-patient interaction data and compliance as a health outcome. Only 10 of the 80 studies in Roter's sample actually reported data on correlates of doctor communication with patient compliance. The data available suggest that a personalizing dimension plays a role in compliance results. Roter finds that positive talk on the physician's part is significant, as is information giving. She indicates, however, that in general, "compliance showed a comparatively weak relation to physician behavior" (1989:92). This finding may reflect a number of other factors associated with compliance, such as financial problems, transportation, or problems with access to care (Kaplan et al. 1989).

In view of the fact, as noted earlier, that about 6,000 articles on doctor-patient relationships have been published during the last decade (Hughes 1991), it is quite remarkable that Roter's metaanalysis located only 10 studies empirically that investigated the effects of doctor communications on patient compliance. More surprisingly, the 80 articles in Roter's analysis were selected from studies published between 1962 and 1986, a time period for which the general universe of published doctor-patient studies may well number above 10,000. In short, one must proceed with great caution in making generalizations about how relationships with doctors affect health outcomes such as compliance, morbidity, and general physical and mental well-being.

Stiles (1989) has pointed out that the absence of correlations between specific interview characteristics and compliance or other health outcomes may not be surprising. He suggests that those patients who are perceived by physicians as requiring more information are likely to be given more by the physician. Those patients who require the most information may be the most likely either to be nonadherent or to have the most serious illness and the worst health outcome. Thus, correlation analysis may show a null, or even a negative, association between information giving and compliance or other health outcome. This suggests that in studies of patient-doctor communication, greater attention must be paid to assessing patients' needs for information and physicians' responsiveness to these needs.

Despite the difficulties in demonstrating associations between patient-doctor communication patterns and health outcomes, one such study by Kaplan et al. (1989) summarized results from clinical trials in which patients were coached in behavioral strategies for increasing their participation in care during clinic visits. These studies were performed in diverse practice settings and included subjects with hypertension, diabetes, or peptic ulcer disease. Greater patient control of the interaction, more negative emotional content (tension, anxiety, strain, self-consciousness, frustration, and impatience) by doctors, and more information giving by physicians during the office visits were associated with better health status reported at follow-up. Health status measures included self-reported overall health ratings, days lost from work, number of health problems, and functional limitations. Moreover, physiologic parameters of health status such as lower hemoglobin A1C levels in diabetics and lower blood pressures in hypertensives were similarly correlated with a greater degree of conversation control by patients and greater emotional exchange during the clinical encounter.

In summary, the data available on patient-doctor communication suggest that when patients' desires for health information and psychosocial issues are addressed during the clinical encounter, satisfaction, compliance, and health outcomes are improved. These associations have been found despite many other factors that may impact these outcomes, including physician and patient responsiveness to one another during the clinical encounter (Stiles 1989). This latter phenomenon would lessen investigators' ability to find associations between communication patterns and patient satisfaction, compliance, and other health status outcomes. The data suggest that improving patient-doctor communication during clinical encounters should be a priority for physicians, patients, and the health care system if we are serious about improving patient satisfaction, compliance, and health outcomes.

Future Research and Practice

In spite of the plethora of articles on doctor-patient relationships, much of the work is atheoretical, focusing on selected aspects of the relationship without regard to any overall, integrated picture of how doctor-patient relationships reflect dimensions of the larger sociocultural setting in which medicine is practiced. The works of Howard Waitzkin (1991, 1989, 1985) and Arthur Kleinman (1986, 1980, 1978) are notable exceptions.

Waitzkin, a physician and a sociologist, sees medicine as functioning largely as an agency of social control geared to promoting and sustaining a work ethic in the population. As such, medicine operates as a gatekeeper, certifying workers as "legitimately" sick and thereby excusable from work requirements, or patching up those needing "repair" so as to return them to the workforce in a "recharged" condition, so to speak. In his latest book (1991), *The Politics of Medical Encounters: How Patients and Doctors Deal with Social Problems,* Waitzkin argues that the personal troubles of patients—such as psychological stress and substance abuse—are "medicalized" by doctors and reduced to problems of *individual functioning* amenable to biomedical intervention. Waitzkin's position is that such personal troubles are really symptomatic of *public, political issues* stemming from the distribution of power and resources in the larger society.

Kleinman's work (1986, 1980, 1978) centers on cultural and social psychological dimensions missing from Waitzkin's more structurally oriented focus. For Kleinman, the patient exists in a world of social, humanly constructed meanings that are creatively organized by persons through shared communications with others into "explanatory models." This is the fundamental framework that patients use to make sense of their lives, especially the encounters they have with medical professionals, who are operating also within the framework of their own explanatory model, which is based on a biomedical interpretation of disease. The patient presents an *illness* to the doctor, a lived experience of discomfort, *dis-ease,* or a response to pain, for example. That lived, subjective experience is transformed by the doctor using a biomedically based explanatory model into a less ambiguous, more controllable entity called a *disease,* which is amenable to medical monitoring.

Waitzkin's work emphasizes social structure, while Kleinman's writing focuses on the role of individual patients in the clinical encounter. There is an urgent need for future research to examine both the role of individual patients and the social institutions of medicine.

As our discussion of Roter's (1989) metaanalysis indicated, it found only 10 studies correlating a health outcome variable, such as compliance, with third-party observations of doctor-patient interactions. Most studies of doctor-patient interactions rely on questionnaire-based, fixed-choice formats in which doctors and/or patients are asked to provide self-reports or reconstructions of what transpired during the encounter. Such questionnaire responses are then correlated with other self-reported health outcome variables. Researchers' observations, then, of patient-doctor encounters are lacking in the great bulk of studies on this topic.

Quantitatively oriented studies of doctor-patient interactions, employing some form of interaction process analysis, provide observational data, but generally fail to link such data to actual health outcomes. Qualitative approaches that both observe actual encounters in the office or clinic and then follow patients by means of in-depth, open-ended interviews are especially needed here. Such approaches would allow for the probing of the "meanings" that patients confer on their medical experiences. Given that persons act toward objects and events in terms of the meanings invested in them, it is essential to capture this dimension of patients' lives. Qualitative studies also may uncover dimensions of interaction overlooked in more narrowly focused analyses of interaction processes. Whatever the format, however, the most promising avenue for advancing our knowledge of this area is a linking of observational phenomena with some form of verifiable health outcomes. Ideally, of course, as Waitzkin (1991) has recently argued, studies should employ *both* qualitative and quantitative methodologies.

Another pressing issue in doctor-patient research is the problem of a possibly self-selecting sample of patients, as noted earlier. Recent work by Renee Fox (1989) in her wide-ranging overview of medical sociology is relevant here. She writes: "Social and cultural factors also affect decisions about to whom an illness is confided; what kinds of help, if any, are sought for dealing with it and from what sorts of persons in which statuses and roles" (Fox 1989:7). Fox provides no references to published studies on these issues although she does cite examples from the works of cultural anthropologists dealing with the instance of a Latin American "folk illness" called *Susto*. The critical issue remains, however, that we simply have no current representative data on characteristics of those seeking alternative health care as compared with those seeking traditional care. Numerous anthropological studies of folk medicine are available (see, for example, Simons and Hughes 1985; and Rubel et al. 1984), but no one has yet painted a comprehensive, integrated picture of the phenomenon.

In reference to those who seek medical help, Barsky's review (1981:492) of earlier work states: "Even more striking is the finding that those who do go to doctors are not necessarily sicker than those who do not. In fact these two groups are indistinguishable when one compares the number and type of their symptoms." Barsky refers here to previous work by Zola (1972), Wadsworth et al. (1971), and Ludwig and Gibson (1969). In the 20 years since the study by Wadsworth et al. (1971), few additional empirical analyses of this topic have been published. The fact that the works cited here indicate no significant differences in levels of physical sickness would seem to support our earlier argument that those seeking traditional medical care may be different from those not seeking such care in terms of the cultural meanings of medical care and their attitudes toward it. At this point, however, we can only offer that argument as a tentative hypothesis in need of much further study.

The phenomenon of the "personalization" of medical care also requires more attention. Empirical studies point toward empathy, information giving, and positive talk on the physician's part as being related to patient satisfaction. We would like to suggest here that the issue of "personalization" of medical care be broadened to encompass the patient's total experience of the medical setting. In a provocative analysis of doctor-patient relationships in an inner-city hospital, Ellen Lazarus (1988) argues for the importance of studying the institutional context in which medical care occurs:

Observations and interviews in clinical settings should include learning who works in the institution and what they do, as well as understanding clinical procedures. Interviews should not be limited to doctors and patients but should extend to other clinic personnel—for example, nurses, receptionists, and medical assistants. Staff meetings should be attended. The researcher must come to understand the difference between what is said and what is done and what the goals of the various participants are.... Multiple interviews and observations.... [make it possible] to distinguish between what was accidental or exceptional about each patient-clinician encounter and what was ordinarily to be expected. [1988:50]

Lazarus's work calls attention to the need for first-hand observation of both the doctor-patient encounter and the events and processes occurring outside that encounter but within the context of the broader medical setting.

In an observational fieldwork study now being conducted by the authors in a general outpatient clinic of an urban university medical center, we have begun to notice numerous instances in which admitting receptionists stationed in the first waiting area that patients enter may be playing an important role in putting patients at ease. They establish a personal connection to the clinic through first-name greetings and questions about what is happening in the patients' lives.

These receptionists seem to have detailed knowledge of patients' family situations, where patients go for vacation, whom they live with, how their children are doing, and the like. The nursing staff too play a significant role in patient experiences, and nurses' behaviors must be observed to help attain a deeper understanding of what patients are experiencing in clinics and doctors' offices.

Work by Katherine Young (1989) on the patient's experience of the doctor-patient examination as a shifting realm of self and body is relevant here. We might speculate in this regard that it is not only during the exam itself that patients experience this transformation; rather, the entire clinic or office experience involves variations and modulations on this dialectic. Patients enter the clinic and are greeted in varying degrees of "personal-ism" or impersonality by receptionists, thereby affirming their status as persons with social identities. They are then checked in by nurses who weigh them and take blood pressure readings, starting the patient on the route toward being treated as a body, although the nurses do engage in light, jovial, personal banter as well with the patients. The typically brief doctor-patient encounter itself then fully launches the patient toward the experience of self as simply a body. This is quite likely a typical patient experience, given the work by Waitzkin (1991) documenting the inability and reluctance of physicians to deal with patients' social and psychological problems. In the final passage out of the clinic, when the patient checks out at the reception desk, some personal conversation may occur, reestablishing the patient as a person with an identity as opposed to simply a physical body.

We need much more research on what patients are experiencing and the meanings they are constructing in response to the various encounters taking place in the broader medical setting. The ultimate question, of course, is how such experiences play out in terms of patient health outcomes and the quality of medical care. This is not to overlook the point, however, that good doctor-patient relationships are an end value in and of themselves, independent of any "measurable" health outcomes.

Changes in Education and Practice

The possibility of efforts by physicians to reduce distress resulting from the social context of the patient is often overlooked in professional training. Instruction in the traditional clinical history takes place in a "high control style" (Waitzkin 1991) or "physician-centered" manner (Smith and Hoppe 1991). While the traditional format of the medical interview conveys a fairly accurate sense of the technical structure, it discourages patient sharing and masks or marginalizes the underlying sociocontextual structure. Medical education requires a drastic rethinking and critical evaluation of what traditional history taking accomplishes. Waitzkin feels that if we fail to modify the educational process, adverse patterns of medical discourse will remain entrenched.

Richard Frankel and Howard Beckman (1989) suggest reformulating the traditional approach so that it becomes less disease-centered and more patient-centered. Such an approach can help physicians use time more efficiently to make a diagnosis and decide on appropriate management without missing important psychosocial problems or patient educational needs. Borrowing from Kleinman et al. (1978), Frankel and Beckman (1989) suggest asking questions during the clinical encounter that will help determine the social and emotional impact of the patient's problems. These include: What do you think caused your problem? Why do you think it started when it did? How severe is your sickness? What are the most important results you hope to achieve by coming today? What concerns you most about your sickness? These questions allow patients to express their fears, feelings, and ideas about their problems as well as expectations for the visit. Smith and Hoppe (1991) offer suggestions for physicians about integrating such patient-centered interviewing into the medical encounter. Attention to these issues will allow physicians to address their patients' concerns, obtain a more complete idea of their patients' problems, and identify the psychosocial concerns so common in the clinical encounter.

Despite the barriers to implementing change in patient-doctor communication, the potential is there for teaching future doctors how to make the clinical encounter patient-centered rather than disease-centered (Putman et al. 1988; Smith and Hoppe 1991). This goal will require recognition by all medical schools that there is a need for a formal medical interviewing curriculum. A policy statement on this subject was drawn up by the Task Force on the Doctor and Patient, Ad Hoc Working Group on the Ideal Medical Interviewing Curriculum, 1991; this statement, if endorsed by the leadership of appropriate professional organizations, will be a source of legitimacy particularly useful to medical interviewing faculty at institutions that may not recognize a need for such a curriculum. In the policy statement, we identify five key elements needed at a medical school if a medical interviewing curriculum is to be developed: (1) administrative support, (2) faculty development, (3) academic recognition and reward, (4) time, and (5) continuity of curriculum.

Without administrative support, the establishment and maintenance of a meaningful interviewing curriculum is not possible, financially or logistically. Administrative support should lead to a faculty development process that includes the selection, recruitment, and education of an interdisciplinary faculty. Maintaining an interested and involved faculty requires the proper academic recognition and reward. Medical interviewing faculty also must be guaranteed protected time for participation in the curriculum. Adequate time also must be set aside in the curriculum for learners at every level. Most important, from the learner's point of view, teaching institutions must be committed to the learner's continuous development. This process should occur throughout the medical undergraduate and postgraduate years.

Such a curriculum will do much to prepare doctors for the challenges facing health care in the twenty-first century. The need for attention to such matters was recognized many years ago by Francis Peabody (1927:877): "The most common criticism made at present by older practitioners is that young graduates have been taught a great deal about the mechanism of disease, but very little about the practice of medicine—or, to put it more bluntly, they are too scientific and do not know how to take care of patients. . . . One of the essential qualities of the clinician is interest in humanity, for the secret of the care of the patient is in caring for the patient." A patient-centered approach for clinical encounters may help physicians demonstrate such care and compassion to their patients.

3

The Changing Pattern of Physician-Patient Interaction

William C. Cockerham

The physician-patient relationship in American society is undergoing fundamental change. The physician's role in the health care encounter is evolving from that of an all-powerful, dominant figure to one emphasizing greater partnership with the patient. For most of the twentieth century, this has not been the case. Parsons (1951) perhaps explains it best in his concept of the sick role where he describes the traditional physician-patient role relationship as asymmetrical, with an imbalance of power and technical expertise extremely favorable to the doctor. The power of physicians rests in medical expertise that the patient lacks but needs to alleviate a health problem; thus, the patient has typically occupied a dependent and subordinate status.

Furthermore, as Freidson (1970b) explains, physicians create the social possibilities for the state of being sick because they are society's authority on what constitutes illness. They decide who is sick and what should be done about it. In essence, physicians are "gatekeepers" to most professional health resources (such as prescription drugs, laboratory tests, and hospitals) which cannot be utilized without their permission. Given their preeminent role in health care, how is it possible that physicians' domination of the physician-patient relationship is changing in favor of greater control by the patient? The purpose of this chapter is to examine this question. First, the models of physician-patient interaction developed by Szasz and Hollender (1956) will be reviewed to identify the current direction of change. Next, the spread of consumerism in health matters among patients will be discussed, along with its implications for the professional status and autonomy of physicians.

It will be argued that trends leading to lessened status and autonomy for physicians are a more or less inevitable outgrowth of modernity. As Giddens (1991) explains, modernity—the institutions and modes of behavior resulting from industrialization—is essentially a post-traditional order. Modernity promotes social relations that span the globe, moves social life away from traditional practices, and features the progressive use of knowledge to organize and transform society. In this context, medical science becomes less of a mystery as the knowledge it produces becomes increasingly accessible to laypersons (Cassell 1986). This situation, along with the desire of modern individuals to be in control of their lives, points toward a modification in the physician-patient relationship in the direction of greater equality between the two parties.

Models of Physician-Patient Interaction

The manner in which doctor-patient interaction is changing can be illustrated by referring to the three models developed by Szasz and Hollender (1956). The first is the activity-passivity model, which applies when the patient is seriously ill or is being treated on an emergency basis, in a state of relative helplessness. The state of helplessness results from the severity of the patient's illness or injury, or from lack of consciousness. Typically, the situation is desperate as the doctor works to stabilize the patient's condition. Decision making and power in the relationship are all on the side of the doctor, as the patient is passive and contributes little or nothing to the interaction. The quality of the doctor-patient relationship is not an issue, nor particularly relevant, as the physician works quickly to save the patient and restore the ability to regain health. This model is important because it accounts for emergency care, but it is not the typical form of doctor-patient interaction.

Second is the guidance-cooperation model, traditional in situations of acute illness. Freidson (1970b) explains that this is the model most people have in mind when they speak of the doctor-patient relationship. The patient knows what is happening, has chosen to visit the doctor, and cooperates by following the doctor's guidance. In this model, the physician makes the decisions and the patient acts as instructed. Although this has been the most common model of doctor-patient interaction, it is now being increasingly rejected by those patients who want to be more involved in decisions that affect their health (see Haug, chap. 12).

The third model, which this chapter suggests is becoming more characteristic of doctor-patient interaction in America, is the mutual participation model. In this model, the patient works with the doctor as a full participant in treating a health problem. It applies particularly to the management of chronic disease in which the patient modifies his or her lifestyle, as well as to acute illness. In the mutual participation model, the patient asks questions, seeks full explanations, and makes rational choices as an informed consumer about the medical services offered by the doctor.

According to Freidson (1970b), the interaction specified by the mutual participation model requires characteristics on the part of the patient that facilitate communication. It is not an appropriate model for patients who are immature, poorly educated, or mentally deficient. The most important social variable in physician-patient communication appears to be social class background, with the lower class identified as having the most communication problems with physicians (Boulton et al. 1986; Waitzkin 1985).

It has been found, for example, that poorly educated persons are the most likely to have their questions ignored and to be treated impersonally as simply someone with a disease, instead of an individual to be respected (Ross and Duff 1982). Upper-class and upper-middle-class persons, on the other hand, however, tend to receive more personalized service from physicians (Link 1983). They also are more active in presenting their ideas to doctors, seeking explanations in return, and receiving them (Boulton et al. 1986).

Waitzkin (1985), who studied information giving in medical care, agrees that social class differences are the most important factors in physician-patient communication. Waitzkin found that physicians did not usually withhold information from their patients as a means of controlling them; rather, some doctors were simply better at communicating with patients than others. Doctors from upper-middle-class backgrounds usually tended to communicate more information to their patients than doctors from lower-middle-class or working-class backgrounds. In turn, patients with high socioeconomic status and high educational levels usually received more information from doctors. In other words, the social backgrounds of both doctor and patient appear important in the giving and receiving of information.

Boulton et al. (1986) explain that the influence of social class on the doctor-patient relationship is best understood in terms of social distance. Those patients who are similar to physicians in social class are more likely to share their communication style and communicate effectively with physicians; those with dissimilar class backgrounds are likely to find communication more difficult because their communication style differs from that of the doctor and they lack the social skills to negotiate the medial encounter effectively. Ethnic minority groups, especially low-income and poorly educated Hispanics, can have serious communication problems because they speak little or no English.

Thus, the mutual participation model appears to be strongly affected by social class differences. Besides problems in communication, lower-class patients tend to be more passive in dealing with doctors as authority figures and to show a lesser sense of personal control over health matters (Cockerham et al. 1986; Cockerham 1992; Seeman and Seeman 1983). They tend to accept unquestioningly whatever the doctor suggests. Patients with upper and middle socioeconomic status tend to be more consumer-oriented, active, and assertive in the physician-patient relationship. That is, they view themselves as consumers and doctors as health care providers. They want to make choices about the services doctors provide in a manner similar to making choices about a major purchase, such as an automobile or a house.

Freidson (1970b) adds, however, that when the mutual participation model works well, it does so not only because of educational and experiential similarity but also because a collaborative status is present. Both doctor and patient must accept each other as relative equals in the search for a solution to the patient's problem. The influence of the doctor on the patient rests primarily on the doctor's ability to persuade the patient to take a recommended course of action.

This approach places the patient on a more equal basis with the physician, since the patient consults with the doctor about the options available and ultimately makes the decision on which type of treatment to accept. Or, if not satisfied, the patient can choose another physician for care. This form of interaction has the doctor and patient working together as a team, rather than the patient simply following the doctor's orders in a more or less automatic fashion. It gives the patient more control over his or her health situation. This empowerment is consistent with the finding that having control over one's life, including one's health, appears to be a major component of the larger societal trend known as modernity (Cockerham 1992; Gallagher 1988; Glassner 1988; Turner 1987).

The research supporting this change in the doctor-patient relationship, the parameters of modernity in this matter, and the implications of this development for the status and professional autonomy of physicians generally are discussed in the next three sections.

Patients as Consumers

Reeder (1972) was among the first to note the changing relationship between doctors and their patients. He identified three factors as important in this regard. The first is the shift in medicine away from the treatment of acute illness toward preventive health services intended to offset the effects of chronic diseases. A medical system that provides either "cures" or emergency care, Reeder explained, is a "seller's market," and physicians are more likely to totally dominate interaction with patients. But in a system focused on the treatment of chronic diseases, which cannot be cured but only controlled by medication and/or modification of lifestyles, the patient must be persuaded of the need for medical services. Under these circumstances, there is a greater tendency for a "buyer's market" to develop, as the patient exercises choice and shares responsibility for outcomes.

The second trend observed by Reeder is the growing sophistication of the general public about the manner in which modern medical bureaucracies operate, which has made people aware of how to negotiate care. The third factor is the development of consumerism, in which the social roles of physicians and patients can hardly escape modification. Reeder suggested that doctor and patient will interact on a more equal basis.

Cockerham et al. (1986) found, for example, that in nonemergency situations, the tendency among middle- and upper-class patients is greater involvement and control in dealing with doctors about their health. The poor reported that they visited doctors more or less routinely when ill, even for minor ailments, while the more affluent were more likely to engage in self-treatment or to recognize minor ailments as self-limiting—that is, likely to disappear in a day or two without a physician's services. Among the poor, a lesser sense of personal control over health has been reported in other studies (Seeman and Seeman 1983). Thus, lower-class persons seemed relatively passive recipients of professional health services, while the more affluent tended to have a significantly greater sense of control over their health and what was needed to maintain it.

Haug and Lavin (1981, 1983) found that better-educated and younger adults were more skeptical of physicians' motives in providing treatment than less-educated and older persons. Those in the first group were especially likely to question whether doctors' primary purpose in ordering tests and providing services was to help the patient and reduce clinical uncertainty or to make money. These persons strongly believed that decision making in the doctor-patient relationship should not be left entirely to the doctor. Rather, they felt they should share in decisions regarding their health.

According to Freidson (1989), patients are unlikely to be troublesome for doctors if they have a lower social status than the doctor, lack a higher education, are not exposed to a broad range of media information, and are not forced to make calculated choices. On the other hand, if a patient is of equal or higher social status than the doctor, considers himself or herself well-informed about personal health, and is experienced in dealing with professionals, that patient has the potential to raise serious management problems because of unwillingness to relinquish total control to the doctor.

As Cassell (1986) explains, the adage that the "doctor knows best" is no longer accepted among virtually all laypersons. Americans have become more knowledgeable about medicine, and while they do not believe they are doctors, they believe that they can understand their own health situation and perhaps apply certain knowledge that is equivalent to a doctor's. Yet Cassell observes that patients' acquisition of some degree of knowledge about medicine was not enough to displace doctors from their previous preeminent status. Rather, he cites as a factor the social turbulence associated with the civil rights movement and the Vietnam War during the 1960s, when the relationships of individuals to authority began to change in the United States. Americans became more questioning about the motives of those in authority, including physicians. Cassell concludes that social as well as personal forces have changed the doctor-patient relationship. Significant numbers of patients have gone from being relatively passive in interacting with doctors toward a state of believing themselves to be active partners in their own care. Cassell points out that they want to take part in decisions formerly reserved for the doctor and to exercise choice in therapy.

Consequently, when it comes to health care, the evolving pattern among many Americans is one of consumerism, with the consumer wanting to make choices about the services available and refusing to be treated as a subordinate (see Ohsfeldt, chap. 6). As American medicine moves into the twenty-first century, the most common type of patient-physician relationship is likely to be the mutual participation model, in which doctors and patients share responsibility for decision making and for the results of medical treatment. Such a development would reflect the following: (1) growing demands on the part of educated patients for doctors to treat them as informed consumers, (2) an increased tendency in society generally to question authority, (3) the desire for greater personal control over one's life and health, and (4) the increased prevalence of chronic disease, which requires a greater partnership between patients and their physicians.

Modernity

The developments just listed—growing consumerism, questioning of authority, desire for greater personal control, and high prevalence of chronic disease—are all associated with modernity. Modernity is the way of life that began to develop in postfeudal Europe with the onset of the industrial revolution and subsequently became worldwide in its influence (Giddens 1990, 1991). Traditional forms of social life based on an agrarian economy were shattered with the spread of urbanization and industrialization; social relations, as noted, became less local and more global in scope, preestablished concepts and practices were discarded in favor of practicality and efficiency, and societies were transformed on the basis of regularized new knowledge and technological development. Giddens (1990) points out that modern social life is reflexive; that is, social practices are continually examined and changed in response to new information about those practices.

Furthermore, states Giddens (1990), modern social life is a complex affair in which technical knowledge is absorbed in varying degrees by laypersons who apply the knowledge in their day-to-day activities. For example, aspects of medical practice are demystified when they become part of an individual's routine experience, or when they are the subject of self-study and education by health practitioners, the mass media, and schools. Cassell (1986) tells us that during the last generation the scientific knowledge of medicine has indeed become increasingly accessible to laypersons. Again, that does not mean they think their knowledge can approximate that of physicians; rather, it means that they can use their knowledge to be more informed consumers of health care and more active in the physician-patient relationship.

Another aspect of modernity is the questioning of authority. One characteristic of the late stages of modernity, which Giddens calls "high modernity," is the recognition that science and technology "are double-edged," in Giddens's (1991:28) view. They create new parameters of risk and danger as well as benefits. What emerges is widespread skepticism about claims that advanced technology invariably represents a positive outcome, and hesitance about following the advice of experts if there is danger to health and the environment. High modernity has ushered in an age of greater questioning of the capabilities and/or motives of business corporations, governments, and the professions, including medicine. The volume of malpractice litigation, for example, is clear evidence of the tendency to question medical decision making.

Modernity also brings with it the desire for greater control over one's body and one's life. Grounded in Weber's (1946) masterful analysis of the transition to modernity in Western society is the notion that the dominance of formal rationality (the purposeful calculation of the most efficient means to an end) produces a culture that devalues "mysterious, incalculable forces." That is, Weber maintains that modernity rejects magic and mysticism in favor of the principle that people can master all things by calculation. Modernity "disenchants" the world and substitutes formal rationality in its place.

Mastering one's life situation includes being in control of one's health (Glassner 1988; Turner 1987). This trend is expressed in society in two major types of behavior: (1) health lifestyles and (2) interactions as partners with doctors. Health lifestyles are ways of living that promote good health and longer life expectancy. Health lifestyles include contact with physicians at intervals to obtain checkups and to seek advice, but the majority of activities take place outside of clinics and doctors' offices. These activities typically consist of choices and practices concerning good eating habits, exercise, weight control, rest and relaxation, and the avoidance of stress, smoking, drug abuse, and the excessive consumption of alcohol.

Participation in health lifestyles has spread across class boundaries in American society and other Western countries, although the quality of participation remains greatest in the upper and middle classes (Cockerham, Kunz, and Lueschen 1988). Modern Americans pursue health lifestyles for a variety of reasons: to avoid disease, live longer, feel good, look good, and have greater control over their quality of life (Conrad 1988; Crawford 1984; Glassner 1988; Kotarba and Bentley 1988). As Crawford (1984) points out, there has been a growing awareness that the major diseases—such as heart disease, cancer, and diabetes—are not curable by medicine; that lifestyles themselves can cause disease; and that medicine is not the automatic answer to all threats to one's health. When such threats persist in the environment and medicine cannot provide a cure, Crawford suggests that self-control over the range of personal behaviors that affect health is one of the only remaining options.

To sum up, the coming of the twenty-first century shows a trend toward increased self-control over health, expressed by a partnership role with doctors in receiving medical care and by a healthy lifestyle. The emphasis upon a healthy lifestyle, as seen in the popularity of jogging and other forms of exercise and in greater attention to diet and the like, is not a new development in American society. What is new is the reawakened interest in health lifestyles that occurred in the mid-twentieth century because of the profound decline in infectious diseases and the increase in chronic diseases associated with certain behavioral practices like smoking, overeating, and lack of exercise.

Thus, an important feature of modern society appears to be the tendency for many people to adopt a healthy lifestyle within the limits of their circumstances and capabilities. Being in control of one's health outside the doctor's office likely extends to the interaction that takes place within that office since the basic concern (a healthy body) remains the same. Therefore, as previously noted, greater self-control over the medium of one's body has emerged as a major expression of modernity (Glassner 1988), and the modern person is one who exerts control in dealing with doctors and in being physically fit.

Finally, it must be noted that simply the changing nature of disease in advanced societies—from a preponderance of acute and communicable illnesses to a prevalence of chronic problems that cannot be cured—pushes physicians and patients toward teamwork. In the case of chronic problems like heart disease, cancer, and diabetes, lifelong measures must be taken by the patient in cooperation with the physician to control symptoms and maintain the patient's quality of life. To be successful, doctors and patients have to work together in partnerships that give the patients increased responsibility for their health status. The mutual participation model is undoubtedly the most effective approach in treating chronic disorders.

The increased prevalence of chronic disease in modern societies is clearly associated with modernity, since a regular sequence of health problems, corresponding to each stage of a nation's change in social organization from a rural to an urban society and from an agricultural to an industrial producer, can be traced (Cockerham 1992). As a society modernizes, the pattern of diseases changes as a result of improvements in lifestyles, diet, housing, public sanitation, and health care delivery. People generally live to the older ages, when chronic health problems are more prevalent. In 1900, for example, influenza, tuberculosis, and gastroenteritis were the leading causes of death in the United States; today, heart disease, cancer, and cerebrovascular diseases are the major killers.

It therefore appears that changes in physician-patient interaction are a logical outcome of the conditions of modernity. Why should it be expected that the physician-patient relationship would be spared from the forces of social change generated on a global level by modernity? To the contrary, health care and the practice of medicine are an integral feature of everyday social life and thus subject to the broad influences of modernization that reach into daily living.

Implications for Physician Status and Professional Autonomy

Greater control over their health by patients implies a gradual overall decline and readjustment in the social status and professional power and autonomy of physicians. As patients strive for greater equality in the doctor-patient relationship, doctors find their actions subject to increased questioning and negotiation by their clients. Physicians also find themselves subject to greater government regulation of health care and to the spread of corporate medicine. Tighter regulation of medical practice by the federal government has taken place largely because of public demands to reduce the cost of health care. The amount of money paid to hospitals for procedures used in treating patients with Medicare public health insurance is based upon the schedule of fees (Diagnostic Related Groups) set by the government. Other measures include the 1992 Resource Based Relative Value Scale (RBRVS), which pays higher fees to family practitioners and lower fees to some specialists, such as surgeons, to encourage greater use of less expensive care by Medicare and Blue Cross–Blue Shield patients. Professional Standards Review Organizations also have been established to evaluate medical treatment on a post hoc basis. The clear trend is toward increased government regulation of the work of physicians, including efforts to encourage more doctors to enter primary care.

Corporate medicine in the United States is the delivery of health services by profit-making business corporations (Starr 1982). Nearly 15% of all U.S. hospitals are owned by such businesses. Since 1970, these hospitals increasingly have been organized into multihospital systems and most operate in relatively affluent urban areas. According to Starr (1982), doctors who practice corporate medicine have less control over their practice because business corporations, not doctors, manage the hospitals and hire doctors as employees; yet doctors are willing to work in corporate medical settings because of high salaries, good facilities, and regular working hours. Nevertheless, there is a loss of professional autonomy for those physicians who do corporate work. On one side are the patients who insist on greater equality in the doctor-patient relationship, and on the other side are health organizations seeking to control costs, maximize profits, and provide efficient services in response to market demand; physicians are caught in the middle.

Ritzer and Walczak (1988) argue that medical doctors are experiencing a process of deprofessionalization—not in the sense of becoming less professional, but in the sense that the profession's autonomy and control over its clients are declining. Physicians retain the greatest authority in medical affairs, but that authority is no longer absolute, as medical work is subject to greater scrutiny by patients, health care organizations, insurance companies, and government agencies. As Light (1989) points out, buyers of health care wanted to know what they were getting for their money, and it did not take long for them to demand detailed accounts of the costs of services.

Utilizing a framework of analysis based upon the classical sociological theory of Weber (1978), Ritzer and Walczak (1988) argue that government policies emphasizing greater control over health care and the general public's perception of the rise of the profit orientation in medicine are part of a trend in medicine away from substantive rationality (stressing ideals, like serving the patient) toward greater formal rationality (stressing rules, regulation, and efficiency). Medicine existed for many years as a relatively unregulated sector of the economy, but the amount of money recently spent on health in the United States ($939 billion in 1992) attracted external forces and regulation into the medical marketplace. The result is greater control over physicians by the government and investor-owned corporations in the health field, lessening the professional power and authority of doctors through bureaucratic measures and various forms of fiscal control.

Conclusion

Increased consumerism on the part of patients and greater government and corporate control over medical practice combine to suggest that the professional autonomy of physicians is declining. That is, doctors are moving from being the absolute authority in medical matters toward a position of somewhat lessened authority. Pressure from both below (consumers) and above (government and business corporations in the health field) signals a decline in the professional dominance of physicians who are caught between. Doctors will remain powerful in health matters and will retain the final authority over medical treatment, but they have lost some autonomy as a professional group.

As seen from the patient's perspective, the doctor-patient relationship seems clearly headed toward the mutual participation model. While the extent to which patients and doctors will approach equality in dealing with each other remains subject to speculation, the process is nevertheless under way. The doctor-patient relationship in the next century is likely to be substantially different from that described by Parsons (1951) in his famous concept of the sick role.

Ultimately, however, it is the position of this paper that the changing pattern of physician-patient interaction in the United States is part of a general worldwide trend toward modernity. Growing consumerism on the part of patients, questioning of authority, the desire for greater personal control over one's life and health, and the high prevalence of chronic disease are all an outgrowth of modernity. And each development points to a modification of the traditional physician-patient relationship, in which status and power favor the physician exclusively. Change in this relationship is a logical and predictable outcome, given the spread of formal rationality in society and the emergence of relatively large numbers of well-educated people who are competent and experienced in dealing with professionals and modern technology, and who are oriented toward controlling their own lives to the greatest extent possible.

The Social Context of
Medical Practice

4

From Bedside to Bench:
The Historical Development of
the Doctor-Patient Relationship

Charlotte G. Borst

From the dim photos of Louis Pasteur in his laboratory to modern television videos interviewing AIDS researchers in France and the United
States, some of the most potent images of physicians focus on their role
in the research laboratory. Soberly clad in the uniform of science—the
white laboratory coat—doctors tell us news of the latest research
findings for curing disease. At the same time, however, television
programs, newspaper articles, books, and even professional medical
journals wistfully detail the life and times of the old-time general
practitioner. Almost always portrayed as a selfless caretaker of the
community, this historical physician is lauded for dedication to his
patients, a hero who made house calls even in the most extreme
circumstances.

It is an ancient commonplace among physicians that medicine is
both an art and a science, and the images of the researcher and the
family doctor reflect this longstanding dichotomy of the doctor as scientist versus the doctor as healer. From the ancient Greeks through
the end of the nineteenth century, doctors struggled with these conflicting images, particularly as they related to interactions with their
patients. This essay explores the changing relationship between the
two parts of medicine and the impact these changes have had on the
doctor-patient relationship.

The Physician's Dichotomy: Artist or Scientist ?

The potential causal relationship between the art and the science of
medicine has posed a problem for historians of medicine as well.
Traditional histories of medicine usually held that scientific discoveries led the way in changing the art of medicine. In this model, the
doctor first solved a medical-scientific question, and then took his

findings back to the bedside. More recent scholarship has begun to suggest that the relationship between the art and science of medicine is much more a two-way street—that, in fact, the doctor-patient relationship has a role to play in shaping medical science. In these histories, the patients become more than inert, inarticulate lumps, and their needs can instead be seen as molding physician practices. Indeed, as one medical historian has warned us, without the sufferers there would be no need for doctors (Porter 1985). We must recognize, however, that this debate has centered mostly on theories about medical practice; with only a few exceptions, we know very little about the actual interaction between doctors and patients in the past.

The one-on-one relationship between the doctor and the patient was particularly important in the prebacteriological era, and understanding why and how medicine was practiced in this era facilitates an understanding of how greatly medical practice was transformed in the late nineteenth century. Beginning in the Paris hospitals in the 1830s, and accelerating with the development of physiology and other laboratory sciences, the doctor-patient relationship changed dramatically. This essay suggests that in the years before the development of laboratory "bench" medicine, each patient served as the physician's "laboratory." But the move to the bench gave consistent, quantifiable, and reproducible results, and it demonstrated that an understanding of disease and a decision about therapeutics did not depend on the idiosyncrasies of each patient. The move of medical science away from the bedside to the bench also changed the physician's professional identity, which became linked with scientific knowledge instead of long experience with patients. Though this change is sometimes rued by those seeking a romantic ideal of the physician-patient relationship, this essay will conclude by suggesting that medicine's link with bench laboratory science had the potential for freeing medical practice and medical theory of gender, racial, and class biases.

The historical relationship between physicians and their patients raises several questions, namely: What was the nature of this relationship? (In other words, how did the doctor diagnose and treat patients?) How was this relationship shaped by the gender, race, and class of either the doctor or the patient? And, finally, how was this relationship affected by developments in hospital medicine and in experimental physiology in the middle and the end of the nineteenth century?

Up to the end of the nineteenth century, the doctor-patient relationship was based on the physician's understanding that disease entities were not abstract. Patients and patient symptoms were unique, and thus each patient had to be seen in a holistic way. This medical practice and medical theory relied on concepts that had been laid down by ancient Greek philosophers as early as 500 B.C. The concepts were based explicitly on the doctor's relationship with the patient, and they provided consistent theoretical and practical applications.

The beginnings of this worldview can be found with Pythagoras (who died about 500 B.C.) and several other contemporary Greek philosophers, who determined in their investigations of the natural world that equilibrium, or perfect balance, was the key to perfect health (Sigerist 1961:96-97).[1] Applying these philosophic concepts to medicine, the physician treated the ill patient by the application of "hygiene," a process that restored balance by moderating the patient's diet and stabilizing the level of stress. Since each person, male or female, young or old, had a unique body with singular needs, the doctor had to carefully balance each individual's hygienic regimen. This therapeutic ideology extended beyond the immediate physical state of a patient; exertion, nourishment, and even external circumstances such as the climate were part of a hygienic regimen that was monitored carefully (Edelstein 1967).

On the whole, Pythagorean philosophy was mystical and class-bound, appealing to upper-class Greeks, who could afford the luxury of a hygienic lifestyle. However, Pythagorean ideas were very influential in establishing a more concrete physiological system for medicine. Employing the Pythagorean mathematical idea of pairs of opposites, the philosopher-scientist Alcmaeon (first half of fifth century B.C.) contended that health was a harmonious balance of the qualities of wet and dry, hot and cold, bitter and sweet, and so on. Illness resulted when this balance was upset and one pair of qualities predominated (Sigerist 1961:101-3). The writings of the philosopher-physician Empedocles (middle fifth century B.C.) also reflected Pythagorean ideas. Frequently pictured as the founder of chemistry, Empedocles brought earlier ideas about the essential elements together with Pythagorean numerical ideals. He declared that the world was constituted of the four elements earth, air, fire, and water, and that differing quantities of these elements determined the quality of an object (Sigerist 1961:107-8).

Humoral Physiology: Emphasis on the Individual Patient

The literature attributed to Hippocrates (fourth and fifth centuries B.C.) expanded on the Pythagorean ideals of health, and established a humoral physiology that persisted under various guises until the late nineteenth century. The Hippocratic literature built on Empedocles' theory of the four elements, with the heart as the center of the blood vessels and the seat of the soul (Sigerist 1961:109). In addition, Hippocrates linked the four elements with the four primary fluids or humors, namely yellow bile, black bile, phlegm, and blood. Reflecting the influence of Pythagorean mathematical and philosophical ideals, Hippocratic physiology paired each of these humors with the dualistic qualities of hot or cold and dry or moist (Sigerist 1961:318-22).

The Hippocratic physiological and pathological systems were attempts at explaining the world in rationalistic terms. Explicitly rejecting magical or religious causes, classical Greek physicians understood disease etiology and treatment in rational, empirical ways derived directly from clinical practice (Edelstein 1937). But this physiological system did not lead to abstractions about disease or therapy, and physicians instead continued to emphasize the uniqueness of each patient. Furthermore, Hippocratic physiology and pathology were explicitly holistic—health depended upon the equilibrium and normal blending of the humors. Illness resulted from a disturbance or imbalance of the patient's humors, or from an improper mixing of the humors, or from an accumulation of a given fluid in one part of the body.

Therapeutics reflected the holistic consequences of humoral physiology and its emphasis on the individual patient. The physician treated the patient by restoring the body's humoral balance. However, the humors also were linked with the four qualities, hot and cold, wet and dry, which in turn were part of the larger world of nature, discernible in the passing of each season. Thus, the patient's humoral balance was influenced by the surroundings, and a holistic therapeutic regimen dictated that the physician study both the patient and the patient's environment. Hippocrates instructed the physician "to consider the seasons of the year, and what effects of each them produces. . . . Then the winds, the hot and the cold . . . the qualities of the waters . . . in taste and weight. . . . The rising of the sun . . . the waters which the inhabitants use . . . and the ground, whether it be naked and deficient in water, or wooded and well watered" (Hippocrates 1886:156).

It is important to emphasize how much this physiological system relied on the physician's relationship to and knowledge of the patient. Indeed, the patient's individual symptoms and surroundings precluded generalizations. Because each person's bodily sensations, the sole measure of medicine, were different, there could be no fixed dogma on which to base Hippocratic medicine. The individuality of each case made it very difficult to determine exactly the right thing to do. Thus, it was considered a matter of art to interpret bodily phenomena and to give general advice on how to treat the sick patient (Edelstein 1967:108-9).

This emphasis on the uniqueness of the doctor-patient relationship has led medical historians to question the "scientific" content of

Greek medicine. Indeed, this matter seemed even more problematic by the second and third centuries B.C. (Hellenistic Greece), when philosophical arguments about skepticism and the role of experience had divided medicine into at least two sects (Edelstein 1967:195-203, 349-66). Each sect grappled with the philosophical question of how to approach nature and gain knowledge, an argument that had substantial implications for the doctor's relationship with the patient. For the first time, physicians deliberated about the role of bedside practice in shaping medical thought. Would experience with patients or the use of logic, a process that could take place away from the bedside, shape scientific ideas?

Hippocratic medicine had emphasized the individual signs, symptoms, and environment of each patient, a uniqueness that denied the usefulness of the physician's experience. By the Hellenistic period, this idea of individuality, with its rejection of generalized knowledge, directly confronted the philosophical debates about skepticism and the role of experience. The Dogmatists argued that logic was the constitutive element, and they accorded only limited significance to experience, maintaining that nothing could be observed repeatedly in exactly the same way. Though they took individual conditions into account, they tried to comprehend them in general terms. The Empiricists, on the other hand, were not willing to move medical science or theory away from the bedside. They rejected the use of inference, arguing that disease and treatment could not be discovered by searching for hidden causes. Nature, they maintained, could not be understood. Thus, empirical physicians argued that experience alone taught the physician the correct way of approaching the patient, and that the repetition of similar experiences could direct an approach for the future (Edelstein 1967:173-91, 195-203).

Discovery of Hidden Causes Shifts Bedside Focus

The study of anatomy at the Greek medical school at Alexandria in the third century B.C. reflected this debate over the role of the individual patient versus the discovery of hidden causes. In a move away from the bedside focus on the individual patient, Alexandrian physicians began to investigate human anatomy by doing dissection and even vivisection. Explicitly Dogmatist in their philosophical beliefs, Alexandrian physicians saw knowledge of hidden causes as necessary for any treatment. Followers of Aristotelian ideas, they argued that nature was knowable, that form and function were related (Temkin 1953; Edelstein 1967:247-302). Knowledge of the internal organs of the body, they argued, was the prerequisite for correct treatment of internal diseases.

The Alexandrian school, due to the confluence of a number of intellectual and social currents, became the site of the first direct and comprehensive study of the human body (Edelstein 1967:247-302; Longrigg 1981).[2]

Though one historian has described the Alexandrian school as having "reached a level never achieved before, or indeed again until the seventeenth century A.D.." (Longrigg 1981), the anatomical discoveries of the school did not change the physician's practice, therapeutics, or most important, humoral physiology. Instead, the work of the Graeco-Roman physician Galen (who died in 199 A.D.) had the most long-term impact on medical theory and practice. Galen shaped classical medicine through reinterpretations of Hippocrates, and as historian Owsei Temkin explains, "by the fourth century A.D., he was considered the greatest medical authority next only to Hippocrates, and his true heir" (Temkin 1953). Indeed, Galen's death marked the end of the sectarian schism of medicine, and his synthesis of medical science and philosophy became the only medical science after the end of the classical period.

Galen was trained as an Empiricist, and this early preparation convinced him that physicians must rely extensively on their own senses. However, Galen went beyond the Empiricists in his high praise for logic, agreeing with the rationalists on the need for speculation about the nature of hidden causes (Temkin 1973:15-18). Reason, he maintained, enabled the doctor to go beyond the limits set by the contact with the patient. However, Galen cautioned practitioners that reason alone was not a sufficient basis for medical practice. For example, he pointed out that young doctors who were guided only by reason were severely handicapped by the lack of long experience with patients. The practicing physician, Galen argued, used reason that was not a pure mental construct, but reason that was related to knowledge based in clinical experience (Ballester 1981).

In advocating the use of reason to arrive at a diagnosis, Galen wanted to move medicine beyond the individual patient's signs and symptoms. In his tract on pulses, Galen elaborated (Ballester 1981:19): "Which of us has learnt the art of healing from the pleuritic John Smith? No one. Not even of curing a pleuritic patient. No, the arts consist in concepts of genera and species." Though he sometimes went to hyperbolic extremes, Galen's intent was to elevate medicine to what he understood constituted a science. Aristotelian logic, he felt, provided the physician-scientist with the idea of typification. Individual symptoms could better be understood and diagnosed by means of general principles.

For the doctor-patient relationship, however, there was a real danger to this approach, as the historian Luis Garcia Ballester has pointed out: Galen's tendency to typify laid the foundations for a withdrawal from the "reality" of the patient. The patient's role became secondary, reduced to that of "example." The physician who wanted to become a scientist reduced the complexities of reality with logical rules, building a knowledge base of genera and species. Ballester maintains that medical practice for this physician-scientist came to be an irritating necessity (Ballester 1981:23). In the end, Galen did move medicine away from the bedside, creating a place for logical inference. It must be remembered, however, that until the end of the nineteenth century, this logic was based on experience with patients, not on experience derived in some other way.

Though Galen attempted to build a scientific diagnosis using analogy and typification, as a practicing physician he understood the problems of variation, remarking that "in the last analysis the individuality of the patient cannot be expressed in any formula; it is ineffable" (Ballester 1981:24).[3] Further undercutting the attempts to move to an objective diagnostic system was the perpetuation of the idea of disease as somatic phenomena, related only to the body. Taken together, these clinical demands kept diagnosis and treatment inevitably tied to the individual needs of the patient.

This approach to the patient was evident in Galen's descriptions of arriving at a diagnosis. Galen focused diagnosis on what he termed "sensing" the patient. He argued that the physician must examine all the signs and symptoms that manifest themselves in the patient's body. In this respect, Galen's description of the clinical examination acknowledged its debt to many of the old Hippocratic ideals. In the best situation, the physician started out by having known the patient in a state of health. Lacking this knowledge, the physician, according to Galen, must carefully study the patient by use of the senses, in particular sight and touch. Though Galen devoted much of his attention to these two, other senses should also be employed, such as listening to the patient's signs and symptoms and even tasting them. In addition, as in Hippocratic medicine, the Galenic physician was instructed to use his senses to assess the patient's surroundings (Ballester 1981:24-30). Like the old Hippocratic physicians, Galen also insisted that treatment should vary according to the circumstances of the patient, the condition of the disease, and even the power of the treatment (Temkin 1973:10-50).

Galen's reinterpretations of Hippocrates and his extensive clinical and scientific writing established his system as the only medical science to survive the ancient period. He had also succeeded in elevating the social position of the ancient physician. Greek medicine had been considered part of a craft tradition, and for many Greek physicians, medicine was a practical art, learned by apprenticeship. As craftsmen, many physicians traveled from town to town seeking upper-class patients who could afford to pay for medical services. After Hippocrates, however, some physicians turned to philosophy for help in building some kind of system. By the end of the ancient period, Galen's medical system, based on an understanding of logic, astrology, and anatomy, elevated medicine to a learned discipline. This elevation had implications for the doctor-patient relationship; the physician had become a literate, educated practitioner, the equal of his upper-class patients (Temkin 1953).

Christianity and Medical Theory

The intellectual evolution of medical theory occurred within the social and political revolution of the acceptance of Christianity in western Europe by the early Middle Ages. In examining the historical aspects of the doctor-patient relationship, what is most interesting about the spread of Christianity is the degree to which Christianity accepted, modified, and then elevated Galenic ideas. Indeed, by the sixteenth century, Galen was portrayed in a painting in a monastery as one of the more important pagan sages who had foretold Christian doctrine (Nutton 1985a). Yet the pagan and materialistic Galenic doctrines that explained illness had to be reconciled with the spiritual doctrines of Christianity. These doctrines had a substantial impact on the doctor-patient relationship, particularly in terms of the understanding of disease and the physician's obligation to the dying patient.

Christianity introduced some very new ideas that related disease to sinfulness. In strict Christian doctrine, disease was punishment for transgressions, to be accepted by the patient as a penance to prepare for the next life. No such doctrine had been part of the pagan world, as historians point out. Greek temple medicine did not require penitence of patients, and disease could be understood on physical, not moral, grounds (Nutton 1985b). The New Testament, on the other hand, emphasized the healing power of Christ and his apostles, an ability passed on to church elders, who could help to heal through prayer and the laying on of hands. Christianity was not opposed to secular healing, but true Christians were expected to rely principally upon a more spiritual medical system. Divine providence, according to one monk, had placed remedies in nature, but the hope of healing should be placed not in doctors, but in the true Savior, Jesus Christ (Nutton 1985a:5).[4] Indeed, as historian Darrell Amundsen (1982) points out, Christian doctrine emphasized wholly new attitudes toward sickness and suffering. Pains in the body were a test of one's faith, something to be welcomed, not merely endured.

Despite this asceticism, which echoed older Greek Stoic doctrines, Christian spiritualism did not supplant secular medicine. Indeed, in at least three ways, medieval Christians in fact promoted worldly medicine, molding it to fit a new Christian doctrine. The increasingly close relationship between ecclesiastical orders and physicians is one example of early Christianity's influence on medicine. By the early medieval period, as historian Vivian Nutton states, medicine had actually achieved a higher public profile than it had previously enjoyed, in part because doctors had become bishops, church leaders, and even saints (Nutton 1985a:12). The priest-physicians probably helped to develop hospitals, another means by which Christianity helped to promote medical care. The growth in the number and importance of Christian hospitals, which offered medical care and other services to the poor and the old, bespoke a commitment to make secular as well as spiritual care available (Nutton 1985a).[5] Beyond hospitals and priest-physicians, Christianity also helped to promote medical care by extending the obligation of the physician to help the dying patient.

As several historians have pointed out, classical physicians were under no obligation to treat the dying patient. Indeed, the physician who treated hopeless cases was considered unethical. The physician-patient relationship in this ethical framework was considered to be a contract under which the patient and the physician collaborated in a common effort to make the patient well. When the patient could no longer fulfill his or her part of the contract, the physician was dutifully to withdraw (Amundsen 1977, 1978; Gourevitch 1969).[6] Christian doctrine, however, changed this professional obligation. Only God, it was argued, understood whether a patient would live or die. Because the physician did not know whether a miracle would intercede to postpone death, the physician, under Christian interpretations, was to stay with the patient until the end, and could licitly accept a stipend for the services (Amundsen 1981).

Medicine as Part of University Curriculum

The translation and dissemination of Galen's work in the Middle Ages owed a significant debt to the flourishing Arabic culture of Byzantium. Historians have found that it was Syro-Arabic commentators who added the three spirits to Galenic medicine—the natural spirit in the liver, the vital spirit in the heart, and the psychic spirit in the brain (Temkin 1977). In addition, Arabic commentators added the four temperaments to Galenic humoral physiology (Temkin 1973,1985). Beginning in Byzantium, where Galen's Greek manuscripts were translated into Syriac and then into Arabic, the transformation of Galen's work was completed in the translations made by Avicenna (980-1037) in his famous medical encyclopedia *al Qanun,* or *Canon.* A verbose but comprehensive collection, Avicenna's *Canon* codified all areas of the health field as then known by compiling earlier Greek and Arabic works, leaving out original contributions (Hamarneh 1971). This Galenic medical system reemerged as the *ars medica* or *tegni* in the Latin West by the eleventh century with the establishment of medieval universities (Baader 1985; Temkin 1973). The result was the integration of medicine into the university curriculum.

The incorporation of medicine as a university discipline in the Middle Ages had several significant effects for medicine and for the doctor-patient relationship. Because medical study took place within the university, practitioners learned both the theoretical and the practical aspects of healing, natural philosophy as well as therapeutic applications (Demaitre 1976).[7] One effect was to create a profession of medicine that established Galenic medical theory within the scholastic tradition (Bullough 1966). A second effect, very significant to the doctor-patient relationship, was the separation of medicine from surgery.

Ancient physicians undoubtedly practiced both medicine and surgery, as demonstrated by the several surgical treatises that are part of the Hippocratic corpus. By the twelfth century, the emergence of didactic literature had placed medicine within the mechanical arts. But the medical professors found that this mechanical tradition kept them from full incorporation within the university. In their fight for acceptance, some medical professors argued that medicine could best attain its desired status by eliminating its operative branch—namely surgery. By jettisoning surgery, physicians could maintain that they were not dirtying their hands, and that even their practical aspects could be cerebral. In some places, such as the University of Paris, this attempt at disassociating physicians from manual labor even led to physicians' distancing themselves from their patients. Parisian university physicians, it was later told, did not visit their patients, but sent a runner to collect information and urine specimens, which the physician analyzed. The runner then returned to the patient with the prescribed treatment (Amundsen 1979; Bullough 1959).[8]

Though the anatomical and other scientific discoveries of the Renaissance directly challenged Galenic science, they did not replace the ancient medical practice that had insisted on a holistic understanding of the unique aspects of each patient. Indeed, much of the "new" science of medicine was accepted because it could be fit within the ancient humoral tradition. For example, William Harvey's discovery of the circulation of the blood, which constituted a significant break with past understanding about the movement of the blood, also addressed important questions within the humoral medical tradition, namely, circularity and the primacy of the heart. Moreover, though Harvey's discovery employed the new philosophy of mechanical and quantitative reasoning, in the end it did not substantially affect traditional medical practice. Though after Harvey a practitioner might now know more about what happened when he opened a vein for bloodletting, the reason for performing bloodletting was a faith in ancient therapeutic ideals (Bylebel 1978; Temkin 1973).

The chemical philosophy of Paracelsus (1493-1541) also challenged ancient scientific authorities and what Paracelsus saw as an excessive faith in reason over experience. But even as Paracelsus questioned the moral and scientific validity of medieval Galenism, he did not overthrow all ancient authorities. Instead of Galenism, he was willing to base his practice on what he saw as the Hippocratic ideal of experience. Challenging Galenic humoral pathology, Paracelsus maintained that disease was ontological—that is, that disease was determined by a specific agent foreign to the body. His new ideas about disease led to new therapies. Employing measures specifically aimed at the disease agents rather than using general antihumoral procedures, Paracelsus argued for the use of essential parts of drugs. His therapeutic agents became famous for including both chemical and herbal remedies (Pagel 1974; Temkin 1973).[9]

Though Paracelsus has sometimes been lauded as a forerunner of "scientific" medicine, his natural philosophy was spiritual, magical, and Neo-Platonic. Indeed, he turned away from abstraction and rejected book learning, arguing that knowledge was to be gained from a spiritual union of the observer with the object (King 1963). Paracelsus's long-term effect was the challenge to Galenic physicians to find more effective remedies, and his legacy was to be found in the increased use of chemically derived drugs (Pagel 1974; Brockliss 1978). Indeed, one historian argues that the popular acceptance of these chemical remedies and their widespread use by surgeons forced physicians to employ them. Ultimately, the acceptance of chemical therapeutics, while not displacing Galen, moved physicians towards greater acceptance of innovation (Webster 1979a; 1979b).[10]

Though the discoveries in the physical sciences of the seventeenth and eighteenth centuries challenged and then replaced ancient science, the biological discoveries of this period had very little impact on the continuing acceptance of humoral medicine and its bedside focus. While some university medical schools such as the University of Leyden and even the University of Paris began to move away from a total reliance on Galen, their curricula still reflected Galenic beliefs (Temkin 1973; Brockliss 1978).[11]

The continuation of this ancient system, based on direct observations of the patient, demonstrated both its compelling philosophical power as well as the inherent problems of doing "laboratory bench" medical research. The lingering doubts about the low status of the mechanical arts kept some tradition-minded physicians away from the bench (Shryock 1979).[12] In addition, medical research posed many more problems than those faced by the scientist doing physics research. For seventeenth- and eighteenth-century physicians, the multiplicity of phenomena to observe, together with the difficulty of measurement, led to questions about the usefulness of pure medical science. Physicians asked themselves, for example, What good was it knowing that the pancreas had a duct if this could not help medical practice? The famous British physician Thomas Sydenham (1624–89) held that doctors should spend their time in sickrooms rather than in laboratories (Shryock 1979).

This intellectual skepticism was reinforced by the intense experience of bedside practice during outbreaks of epidemic diseases. Under the rampages of epidemic fevers, physicians were forced to decide quickly how to cope with the problems of many patients. Historians have argued that this experience shaped physicians' theoretical and clinical answers (Shryock 1979). Patients' needs dictated that something must be done, some remedy must be found, and quickly. As Richard Shryock explains, it would have seemed frivolous at best for Benjamin Rush to suspend scientific judgment on any possible cure for the rampages of yellow fever in Philadelphia in 1793. Instead, the good doctor grasped at any hint of a remedy in such circumstances, and tried desperately to believe that any cures that followed were the result of its employment (Shryock 1979; Ackerknecht 1948; Rosenberg 1962).[13]

Though medicine in the eighteenth century was marked by debates about the usefulness of mechanistic philosophy, mechanism did not replace Galenism. As Oswei Temkin, a leading Galen scholar, concludes, Galenism offered a unifying medical philosophy that went beyond the power of merely explaining phenomena. Galenic philosophy, suffused with Aristotelian holistic teleology, offered the best explanation for the strength of the relationship between the individual and health or disease (Temkin 1973).

The development of the French clinical "school" in Paris in the first half of the nineteenth century posed the first real challenge to the sterile hypotheses of medieval Galenic medicine. The French doctors argued instead for a radical empiricism. These ideologues emphasized the careful observation of phenomena and the avoidance of speculative hypotheses. The practical manifestations of this philosophy developed into pathological anatomy, in which bedside observations were correlated with subsequent pathological findings. The development of tools such as the stethoscope enabled physicians to examine, even measure, their patients, instead of merely observing them. Such measurements and the assessments of autopsies eventually led Xavier Bichat and subsequent Parisian physicians to postulate an ontological disease etiology—that is, they argued that disease in fact existed separately from the body, invading it from outside. The radical empiricism also engendered a skepticism about traditional therapeutics. Pierre Louis's statistical studies seemed to show that the absence of therapy was better than most of the treatments then in use (Shryock 1979).

Though French clinical medicine offered a very potent critique of traditional, Galenic-style medicine, it also challenged many physicians' ideas about what the practice of medicine really involved. For American physicians who flocked to France to walk the wards and crowd the autopsy rooms, French medicine seemed to threaten the foundations of what it meant to be a physician. As historian John Harley Warner (1986) states, "At the core of their anxiety was a distinction between knowledge and practice in defining the physician's role." American physicians were a practical lot—they acknowledged that a physician could be both a scientist and a practitioner, yet they maintained that science had to be subordinate. They feared that the scientific emphasis of French medicine, which they saw as understanding and observing disease rather than intervening in it, subverted practical medicine. Indeed, as one American physician remarked, "The triumph with these physicians is in the dead room" (Battey 1860).

Despite the implications of the Paris school for medical science, for most of the nineteenth century physicians continued to practice medicine in the ancient tradition of close, continuous monitoring of the patient within a specific context. The laboratory bench might demonstrate certain chemical or physical laws, and the autopsy might reveal subtle tissue changes, but medical practice, including diagnosis, treatment, and prognosis, relied on the physician's knowledge of the specific patient within a particular context. As American physician D.W. Cheever asserted in 1860 in an article in the *Boston Medical and Surgical Journal*, "Idiosyncrasy, or the peculiarities of the individual, are as anomalous and impossible to reduce to rule and measure, as the passage of the clouds. . . . What is true of one place may not be true of another" (Warner 1986:59).

In terms of the doctor's relationship with the diseased patient during treatment, the world of nineteenth-century medicine had changed very little from the ancient Greek period. Although nineteenth-century physicians understood the discrete anatomical parts of the body, though they had learned the universal laws of chemistry, and despite the claims of the French clinical school, most physicians still understood the disease and the therapeutic process in the holistic constructs first defined in the fifth century B.C. Their attitude would change only after the discovery of the bacterial connection to disease, which confirmed an ontological understanding of illness. Until then, a good doctor was one who had a wealth of experience and was known to have good judgment. Most important, at least to physicians, the physician derived status and authority from the relationship with sick patients. Knowledge about scientific matters was desirable, but knowledge about practice, about how to deal with the idiosyncrasies of individual patients, was essential to a physician's sense of professional identity and his or her assumption of public confidence (Warner 1986: 11-36; Rosenkrantz 1985).[14]

A South Carolina physician, Thomas Cooper, who translated Broussais's physiological findings from French into English in 1831, expressed his concerns and those of many of his colleagues about the importance of relationships with patients. While he acknowledged Broussais's contributions to the study of pathological anatomy, he argued for a fundamental distinction between the universality of findings in the basic medical sciences and the need for specific, patient-directed therapy. In a quote concerning climate that ancient Greek physicians would have understood, the South Carolina doctor contended: "The Southern climate of the United States seems to require more bold and decisive practice, than the Northern climate of Paris and London: hence, to us, the therapeutics of Broussais . . . appear feeble; but the *principles,* founded on the physiology and pathology of the tissues, are undeniable and universally applicable" (Warner 1986:59).

American physicians in this period, particularly those practicing in the southern United States, were adamant supporters of the idea of patient-specific diagnosis and therapy. They still believed that a single disease could take on a variety of forms that depended upon the "constitution" of the individual patient. Disease entities were not fixed but fluid, and thus two patients with identical diseases could require different, even opposite treatments. As in ancient Greece, the good nineteenth-century physician followed the accepted medical science of treating his or her patient's unique circumstances. Indeed, well into the nineteenth century, disease-specific treatments were ethically suspect, unscientific, even professionally illegitimate. As Warner (1986), put it, "No scientific physician willingly admits the existence of specifics. . . . Such an admission is a germ of quackery" (Booth 1849-50).[15]

As the quote from the South Carolina doctor demonstrates, the old Hippocratic idea of differing climates, particularly the quality of hot versus cold, was of major importance in distinguishing the course of disease and the kinds of treatment. David Hosack, a professor at the College of Physicians and Surgeons in New York City at the turn of the nineteenth century, explained to his students: "Inhabitants of Hot climates will not bear the same mode of treatment as those of Cold." He explained that "in warm countries or tropical climates the inhabitants are more subject to debility....Their diseases are of low grade" (Warner 1986:71).[16] Such patients were to be treated with stimulants, the direct opposite of the treatment for patients of cold climes, whose very robust constitutions demanded depletive therapies. As Warner (1986) stresses, this emphasis on climate and patient topologies demonstrates the deep roots of the notion of patient uniqueness in medical institutions, thought, and practice.

American medical schools, more than any other medical institutions, helped to inculcate the idea of local diseases and individualized therapies. However, this intellectual discourse was shaped by the swirling political and social debates of antebellum America. Thus, it is not surprising that southern and western American doctors were among the most ardent supporters of the idea of local knowledge. As one southern physician argued in 1844 (Warner 1986:76): "It is precisely because diseases are *not all entities,* and do not preserve the same features, wherever met with; and that remedies are *not all specifics,* or uniform and invariable in their effects, that it becomes necessary to *study* them where they prevail."

The medical graduate who ignored this advice risked great peril, both to patients and in terms of establishing a practice. One story describes the graduate of a Philadelphia or New York medical school who, after returning home to the South "in high spirits and with bright anticipations, 'sticks out his shingle' ready and very willing to go to work." But despite his knowledge of medical science, he is destined to fail in practice because he treats his first patients in accordance with northern teachings. By practicing general bloodletting and dispensing sedative medicines, he produces dire results: "Now his bright anticipations are clouded; disappointments discourage him; and a sad experience teaches him that the instructive lessons of a northern institution will not answer, in the treatment of southern diseases. He cannot now under the circumstances establish an extensive practice. . . . The confidence of the people in him is shaken, he is neglected, despised, and soon forgotten" (Warner 1986:77).[17]

Regional differences were compounded by the ancient ideas of constitution and temperament. The Massachusetts physician D.W. Cheever, writing in 1861, explained the nineteenth-century idea of constitution, a definition that had not changed much since Hippocrates: "The 'constitution' of the patient. . . is the sum of all of the influences of locality, station, hygiene, occupation, habit, diet, or accident, which have acted upon the individual from the time of his birth, until the period of the disease we are treating" (Warner 1986:64). Because heredity and life experiences helped shape a constitution, each person's was unique. As if the vagaries of constitution were not enough, a patient could also be classified and treated according to his or her temperament, of which there were four: sanguineous, choleric, melancholic, and phlegmatic. Each temperament was associated with a characteristic physique, behavior, type of disease, and therapeutic needs (Temkin 1973).[18] A person's temperament interacted with the characteristic temperament of the climate, the region, and the country where he or she resided. Beyond the treatment of disease, the entire concept of constitution and temperament provided a rationale for believing in the essentialism of class, gender, race, and national origin.

Gender-Based Theories of Doctor-Patient Relationship

Though most women in ancient Greece probably consulted other women for their medical and obstetrical care, some of the works of the Hippocratic corpus devoted attention to "women's complaints," namely gynecological or obstetrical problems. Other parts of the corpus, particularly *On Airs, Waters, and Places,* discussed sexual differences in response to climate and the incidence of disease (Lloyd 1983).[19] Galen's biological system of explaining differences between males and females built on the Hippocratic model and promoted hierarchical Aristotelian biological ideas. For example, women were less perfect than men, women were colder and wetter than men, and women produced a seed that was colder, wetter, and scantier than the seed of men; thus a female was herself the product of a colder, wetter seed (Lloyd 1983; Laqueur 1987). Galenic distinctions between the sexes persisted even after the anatomical discoveries of the sixteenth and seventeenth centuries. By the eighteenth century, the concepts were used to create separate places in society for men and women, based on their biological capacities. As Jean Jacques Rousseau explained: "The male is male only at certain moments. The female is female her whole life. . . . Everything constantly recalls her sex to her" (Laqueur 1987). To Rousseau and eighteenth-century physicians, it followed from this theoretical construction that men were active and strong, while women were passive and weak, possessing a natural modesty, with less passion than men. Even the late-eighteenth-century feminist Mary Wollstonecraft subscribed to this principle, arguing that passionlessness made women more moral than men (Laqueur 1987).

By the early nineteenth century, these traditional theoretical ideas were supplemented by the discovery of spontaneous ovulation in dogs and in other mammals. Though no evidence of spontaneous ovulation in humans was shown until the early twentieth century, physicians focused their treatment of women patients on the ovaries and on ovulation. Ovaries were defined as the driving force of the whole female economy, with menstruation the outward sign of its power. The female body operated in a kind of closed loop, with a finite amount of energy available. Energy dissipated by the brain, for example, deprived the reproductive organs. A therapeutic regimen for women followed from this model. Nineteenth-century physicians viewed the reproductive part of women's lives (puberty to menopause) to be fraught with danger. Thus, for women of childbearing age in particular, the diagnosis and treatment of disease differed from that for men. Women's reproductive organs were seen as the seat of any problem, so physicians responded to most illnesses of women with local treatment of the uterus or vagina, or they ordered special rest cures to allow the reproductive organs to replenish their fixed store of energy (Laqueur 1987; Smith-Rosenberg 1973).

The construction of a gender-based theory of the doctor-patient relationship also extended to the gender of the practitioner. Though childbearing women turned increasingly to physicians by the early nineteenth century, many worried about the breach of female modesty represented by the attendance of a male physician, which, it was believed, could counteract the good of any therapy (Leavitt 1986).[20] In reaction, some men and women called for the training of women physicians, and a few women responded. Dr. Harriot Hunt, a Boston physician who began her practice in the late 1830s, was typical. She and other female physicians based their practice on working with women to protect them from the possible compromise of female delicacy represented by male treatment (Morantz-Sanchez 1985).[21] Though women doctors later embraced medical science for its own sake as much as for what it could do for women, historians agree that the dominant point of view in the nineteenth and early twentieth centuries was that women belonged in medicine because of their special talents. Dr. Ella Flagg Young, for example, observed that "every woman is born a doctor. Men have to study to become one" (Morantz-Sanchez 1985:5). Medicine seemed especially suited for women because it combined the assumed authority of science with a dedication to alleviating suffering that seemed inherently female. Indeed, women physicians could provide both sympathy and science to that special group of patients they suited so well: women and children (Morantz-Sanchez 1985: 184-202).[22]

The biologically based ideology of women's special place and special needs, however, also limited the role of women physicians and other women who wanted to move out of the domestic circle. The most celebrated example of the use of this ideology against women was the 1873 book written by the prominent Harvard University physician and professor Edward Clarke. *Sex in Education: A Fair Chance for Girls* argued that higher education for girls had a real potential to sap the energy needed for the proper development of the reproductive organs. Women who attempted to pursue education or a career risked producing "monstrous brains and puny bodies" and "grievous maladies which tortured a woman's earthy existence" (Morantz-Sanchez 1985:54).

Race- and Class-Based Theories of Treatment

Race, like gender, was assumed to have biological ramifications for a patient's constitution. Among American physicians of the nineteenth century, African-American patients were presumed to need distinctive treatment, although physicians could not agree on whether they needed more aggressive or less aggressive therapy. As historian Todd Savitt points out, southern physicians focused on the physical aspects of their black patients that were different from those of white patients. In particular, physicians were interested in African-Americans' immunity to malaria and their lack of resistance to respiratory infections. Savitt argues that southern physicians used these clinical observations to rationalize a special approach to African-American medical treatment and, more important, to construct a defense for enslaving blacks in the South (Savitt 1978, 1989).[23]

The term "race" as used in nineteenth-century America, however, made distinctions on the basis of national origins as well as physical characteristics, including skin color. A student's M.D. thesis from 1855 explained the prevailing wisdom. "Race, has a very great modifying influence" on the actions of remedies, he wrote. "An amputation, would be much more dangerous, in the full plethoric beer drinking Englishman, than in the very active Frenchman or Italian. It is because the former [the Englishman] is much more liable than the latter, to inflammations, on account of his peculiar mode of life. As so it is with medicines. A medicine which in the usual dose would scarcely affect the one, would produce in the other, the most inordinate effects" (Warner 1986:65).

Definitions of race in nineteenth-century America were also tied to perceptions of hierarchy based on socioeconomic class and occupational status. Doctors argued strenuously that the constitutions of working-class patients differed from those of their more affluent patients, and that therapies for each group should match their particular sensibilities. As one medical student explained in his notes: "Diseases of a purely inflammatory character are more common among the peasantry, and the labouring class of the community, than among epicures, and those who occupy a higher station in life, and live in indolence and luxury" (Warner 1986:65). Benignly interpreted, such observations implied that peasants and laborers needed more aggressive treatment than the vitiated upper classes. A critical evaluation of this therapeutic philosophy reveals that it sometimes also provided support for racism and social Darwinism, a tactic employed by both American and European physicians. Indeed, as one historian notes, the philosophy of constitutional medicine became a political ideology, one of the tools used by Europeans to advance their imperial ambitions (Nicolson 1989).

Superimposing Science on Individual Symptoms

By the early twentieth century, however, the doctor-patient relationship began to change. As early as 1880, Cincinnati medical graduates were being told: "Arm yourself with the weapons of science. . . . At the present, it takes more than gray hairs, an owl-like countenance and a gold headed cane to make a successful practitioner. It even takes more than experience" (Warner 1986:262). The successful physician at the turn of the century needed to be an expert in science, able to "trace the symptoms to the hidden cause, from a knowledge of chemistry and physiology, without which no rational system of hygiene and therapeutics is possible" (Warner 1986:262). No longer were the individual patient's symptoms crucial for treatment. As J.C. White, a Harvard University Medical School professor explained in 1870, "I would have to dispossess your minds of the too common belief that everything can be learned at the bedside; it is a fatal barrier to individual and national progress in medicine" (Warner 1986:274). By that time, physician leaders saw experimental science as the arbiter of therapeutic activity and even professional morality. This new breed of physician gained his or her professional identity not from interactions with sick patients, but from a keen knowledge of science.

What happened to change the doctor-patient relationship? In brief: the physiology laboratory replaced the "patient" laboratory. Led by the experiments of Claude Bernard and others, physicians struggled to find a relationship between the consistent and reproducible data from the physiology laboratory and the application of therapeutic agents. Experimentation in the laboratory could identify both healthy and diseased physiological processes, as well as the actions of remedies. On the basis of this information, the practitioner determined how the patient's body deviated from the norm and what adjustments were needed. Under the new epistemology that followed from this relationship, the patient was treated by a rational system derived from principles discovered in the laboratory. The laboratory data pointed to what was normal in the patient and what processes were deviant. The patient was no longer central to the understanding of disease (Warner 1986:235-84).

Though many general practitioners resisted the objectification of the patient, the reorganization of American medical education in the early twentieth century embraced this model of medical practice. Indeed, articles in many state and national medical journals during this period demonstrate the central place that the laboratory and the microscope played by then. As Alabama physician Edward Pierson Nicolson reminded his colleagues, though the country doctor might argue that he needed to "devote [himself] to the treatment of disease and the management of the sick," leaving "original research, the laboratory, the microscope, the reagent, or the test-tube" to "those who are specially trained for it," any good doctor was by then required to do microscopic investigation of the blood, the urine, and the feces (Nicolson, 1898:105).

Conclusion

The history of the doctor-patient relationship reveals its central role in defining not only medical practice but also medical theory. Historically, patients played a particularly important part in establishing the physician's professional identity and in providing a means of studying disease processes. But the working out of physiological processes in the laboratory fundamentally changed this relationship. After that, as one historian explains, it "made relatively little difference whether that process was going on in an Irish immigrant or a laboratory dog" (Warner 1986:249). The implication for the doctor-patient relationship was profound. On the positive side, physiological medicine would match the treatment to the patient's physiological processes and not to his or her "constitution" or social background. Among the negative implications of physiological medicine, the physician's presence at the bedside came to make little difference in the patient's welfare; instead, laboratory tests or X-rays made the final determination. Indeed, the ultimate example of the scientific physician might be one who, like Martin Arrowsmith, left patients altogether for the laboratory bench (Lewis 1925).[24]

But despite the temptations, we must not romanticize the historical doctor-patient relationship that preceded the physiological laboratory. As this essay demonstrates, the earlier individualized, patient-derived therapeutics was capable of upholding society's beliefs that those who differed in social class were fundamentally unequal. The results of the physiology laboratory made it clear that scientific assumptions about race, class, and gender were of little value in treating sick people. The African-American patients of the Tuskegee syphilis experiment and the gay men who were among the first victims of the AIDS epidemic might argue, however, that this ideal of scientific medicine has not yet been attained.

Notes

1. The Pythagoreans also saw music as part of a hygienic way of life.

2. Edelstein argues that new philosophical understandings about the soul in relation to the dead body allowed dissection. Longrigg claims that Edelstein cannot explain why anatomy was studied only in Alexandria. Instead, Longrigg claims that the effect of Egyptian burial practices, together with the foreign environment of Greek medicine in Egypt, fostered anatomical research.

3. Ballester also notes that, though Galen advocated typification and analogy in order to speculate about a patient's symptoms, he never advocated quantification of his findings to arrive at some "mean" as we understand it.

4. The monk was a Greek, St. Diadochus, who wrote "On Spiritual Knowledge" about 480 A.D. Amundsen (1982) has also argued that Christianity was not hostile to secular medicine.

5. Nutton notes that Christian hospitals probably didn't pioneer teaching; this was an innovation of Islamic hospitals.

6. Gourvitch suggests that ancient physicians may even have assisted with suicides.

7. Demaitre argues that medieval universities changed the emphasis from physicians as servants of nature to physicians as masters of nature.

8. Bullough notes that surgeons in England and France developed a hierarchy that attempted to imitate the hierarchy of the physicians. In these two countries, surgeons refused to do certain operations on the grounds that they would degrade the surgeon. Thus, treatment of boils, tumors, bruises, and minor wounds were left to the less prestigious, but more numerous, barber surgeons. The true hands-on skills of the barber-surgeon sentenced him to the lowest status of any medieval practitioner at the same time that it gave him most of the patients, particularly in rural areas.

9. For an extended discussion of Paracelsus, see Pagel 1958, 141-50.

10. Webster (1979b:330) makes a stronger case for the effect of Paracelsian medicine.

11. Brockliss finds that by the eighteenth century, the University of Paris was teaching iatrochemicalism and iatrophysics.

12. Shryock mentions that Robert Boyle was criticized by his Oxford colleagues for his research into the composition of the air and its relation to respiration.

13. Risse (1979) also demonstrates this relationship. Risse shows that contemporary physicians such as Rush linked disease conditions with prevalent medical ideas and practice, and he argues that several medical historians

have demonstrated this effect. See, for example, Ackerknecht (1948), who argued for a link between the epidemic diseases and the development of environmental views concerning their origins; also Rosenberg's (1962) now-classic study of cholera in the United States.

14. Rosenkrantz has also stressed that nineteenth-century physicians derived their professional status from the status of their patients or from their own family's status, and not from medicine.

15. Rosenberg's classic essay on nineteenth-century therapeutics points out that doctors and patients in the nineteenth century shared an antireductionist worldview that incorporated every aspect of a person's life in explaining a physical condition. Part of the therapeutic effectiveness lay in the doctor's understanding of the patient's constitutional idiosyncracies.

16. The quotations are from the notes of three medical students who attended Hosack's lectures.

17. Quoted by Warner, *Therapeutic Perspective*, p. 77. Warner explores the issue of regional popularity in medical practice in two articles: "The Idea of Southern Medical Distinctiveness" (1989) and "Southern Medical Reform" (1983).

18. Temkin notes that the Galenic doctrine of temperaments was widely used into the nineteenth century, but that its Galenic origin was mixed with mechanical and chemical ideas.

19. Lloyd points out that women healers were considered outside the realm of medical craft or philosophy.

20. Leavitt points out that women who called physicians in to deliver their babies mediated the authority of the physician by having women friends remain in the room. She argues that as long as birth remained in the home, women were able to retain some power in the doctor-patient relationship.

21. Morantz-Sanchez argues that female physicians were both ideological innovators and conservators of the past. She points out that most of the arguments used to buttress the right of women to receive a medical education depended on the tenets of the cult of domesticity.

22. Morantz-Sanchez argues that this ideology proved to be extremely limiting to the cause of women physicians by the end of the nineteenth century.

23. Savitt develops these themes in greater detail.

24. Some feminist historians have pointed out that women in particular suffered from this move away from the bedside. When birth moved to the hospital, for example, women lost any control over decisions about how they wanted their babies to be born. See Leavitt (1986:171-95). Russell C. Maulitz (1979), develops these themes and their subsequent impact on twentieth-century American medicine in "Physician vs Bacteriologist."

5

High Tech vs "High Touch": The Impact of Medical Technology on Patient Care

H. Hughes Evans

Technology is inextricably entwined in American medical care. Behind the scenes, in hospitals and doctors' offices, computers keep track of patient records, laboratory results, and costs. Hundreds of machines operate, analyzing body fluids, developing X-rays, and responding to the numerous demands of patient care. Ventilators enable diseased and fatigued lungs to breathe. Pacemakers sense abnormal cardiac rhythms and trigger the heart to beat normally. Ultrasound enables parents to see the movements of the fetal heart just weeks after conception. In a routine visit to the doctor, the typical patient is bombarded with medical technology; the stethoscope, thermometer, and sphygmomanometer occupy even the simplest office.

And yet, as much as American society is enthralled by the progress that medical technology embodies, it is outraged by the cost and depersonalization of modern medicine (Illich 1976; Nelkin and Tancredi 1989). Calls for "user-friendly" medical care highlight the degree to which medicine and technology are bound together, as well as the perception that technology has stripped medicine of its humanistic qualities.[1] Many chroniclers claim that high-tech medicine has evolved at the expense of the doctor-patient relationship, that machines have created a cold and impersonal chasm between the healer and the patient. In their minds the doctor has become a mere technician, a "body mechanic," who can treat the disease but not the person (Bayles 1981). These critics mourn the loss of spiritual and emotional qualities important to healing and claim that the science of medicine has advanced at the expense of the art of medicine. Such criticism, however, ignores the fact that patients often demand technical skills in their doctors and that the doctor-patient relationship has changed at least in part in response to patients' demands. Many observers believe that the only way to bridge the distance between treating the disease and treating the patient is to balance the high tech of medicine with an equal commitment to recognizing and appreciating the personal impact and meaning of disease, what might be called "high touch."[2]

A common misconception in the contemporary debate is that the tension between medical technology and patient care is a modern one, that just a generation or two ago doctors were kindly Marcus Welbys, whose very touch healed and who rarely needed more than the help of a simple stethoscope to make the correct diagnosis and calm the distracted patient (Davis 1981; Reiser 1978). With the advent of extremely sophisticated technology like intensive-care units, dialysis machines, and cardiac pumps, this position argues, the doctor lost sight of the patient, becoming more interested in the disease itself, the surgical technique, the procedure, even the instrument. An example of this technical-prowess-gone-berserk position is the highly specialized surgeon who never sees his or her patients except when they are anesthetized. The recent movie *The Doctor* depicts this widening gulf between doctor and patient and calls for physicians to narrow the chasm by paying more attention to the "high touch" aspects of medicine.

These recent examples of the conflict between medical technology and medical care rest on a long and interesting history. During the late nineteenth century, when many instruments entered the doctor's armamentarium, this tension surfaced and became part of an active debate about the future of medicine. This paper examines the historical precedents for the tension between high tech and "high touch" and argues that the issues are not new. Furthermore, it shows that even commonplace medical instruments like the stethoscope, thermometer, and the blood pressure machine have had profound effects on medical practice and patient care. These relatively uncomplicated instruments act as historical case studies of modern issues. In addition, this paper argues that the instruments are not the villains who demolished a cherished and idealized doctor-patient relationship. Instead, the ways in which the technology was received and used by *both* health personnel and patients fundamentally altered the doctor-patient relationship.

Case Studies of Medical Instruments

In 1819 French physician René-Théophile-Hyacinthe Laénnec published *On Mediate Auscultation,* a detailed treatise correlating the internal anatomy of the lung with the sounds heard when the doctor listened to the chest (Laénnec 1827). In this monograph Laénnec introduced the stethoscope (Davis 1981; Reiser 1978, 1979). Prior to the stethoscope, the doctor had occasionally listened to the patient's heart and lungs by placing his ear directly on the chest. Such an intimate act was felt to compromise the delicate modesty of female patients. In addition, immediate auscultation, as the direct method was called, did not work very well and was particularly problematic in obese and buxom patients. Recalling that sound traveling through solid bodies is augmented, Laénnec constructed a wooden cylinder and named his invention the stethoscope, from the Greek words for *chest* and *observe*.

The name Laénnec chose for his creation illustrates its symbolic and practical significance. Even though the stethoscope actually allowed the doctor to *hear* the sounds of the chest better, Laénnec felt that he could now metaphorically *see* into the chest. By correlating the sounds heard on auscultation with the symptoms a patient reported and, more important, with the gross and microscopic findings at autopsy, Laénnec found clues to the pathology inside his patients. If specific sounds corresponded to particular pathological processes, then the doctor could use sound to envision disease. As one doctor exclaimed, the stethoscope is "a window in the breast through which we can see the precise state of things within" (Reiser 1978:30). This instrument symbolically opened the internal pathological anatomy of the lungs and heart to the doctor, enabling him to associate internal evidence of disease with the signs and symptoms it produced. Laénnec's instrument thus did far more than merely augment the sounds of the chest; it epitomized a new way of conceptualizing disease, of seeing anatomy in the living patient, and hence of understanding how disease evolves.

The stethoscope not only altered the ways doctors thought about disease but also changed the techniques they used to gather information from their patients. Prior to Laénnec's time, the physical examination of the patient had held a relatively subordinate place in the diagnostic process compared with the patient's presentation of his or her symptoms (King 1982); a doctor would first take a long history from his or her patient and then devise a highly individualized conceptualization of the patient's sickness. This formulation stressed the uniqueness of each patient's illness, instead of how the patient fit into a typical disease pattern. The new methods of physical diagnosis, however, gave the doctor improved access to the disease process. By correlating signs and symptoms of disease with anatomical and pathological information, the doctor gained clues about how disease worked. In the process the importance of individual idiosyncrasies was diluted. Thus disease took on an autonomy that it had not previously held. Doctors slowly began to distinguish the disease from the patient, focusing on elements common to all patients with a particular complaint instead of on the uniqueness of the patient's presentation.

Laénnec believed that mediate auscultation (the use of the stetho-scope), in conjunction with older techniques of physical diagnosis, like percussion, pulse taking, and palpation, made these heretofore vague and imprecise standbys of the physician more reliable.[3] As a result, physical diagnosis provided the doctor with more complete informa-tion and became a more important part of the diagnostic and thera-peutic process.

In 1868, almost 50 years after Laénnec introduced the stethoscope, came the publication of German physician Carl Wunderlich's *On the Temperature in Diseases,* a book describing the clinical uses of the thermometer in almost 25,000 patients (Wunderlich 1871). Like Laén-nec, Wunderlich correlated the information gathered from an instru-ment with specific disease processes. Unlike the stethoscope, which provided qualitative information, the thermometer yielded quantita-tive data. Numbers, Wunderlich found, could record the ebb and flow of disease with a precision that words simply could not. Prior to Wunderlich's work, few physicians had employed the thermometer in patient care, relying instead on the sense of touch.[4] A physician's highly revered "trained sense of touch" was supposed to be able to dis-tinguish different degrees of temperature, but critics increasingly questioned the accuracy of the senses.

The reliability of the thermometer and the certainty and exactness of the numbers it generated struck Wunderlich as powerful ways to monitor disease. Numbers had a precision that the phrases doctors used to describe temperature simply did not. Believing that diseases had predictable fever patterns, Wunderlich presented temperature in graphical form so that trends over time could be pictorially presented. On his graphic fever curves, he correlated temperature with symp-toms and pathology. Not only did the different shapes of temperature curves suggest certain diagnoses, but they also aided in therapy and prognosis. By monitoring temperature, the physician could determine the optimum time to treat and to assess the worsening or improve-ment of disease. Like the stethoscope, the thermometer, through the temperature curves it generated, allowed the doctor to focus on the disease instead of a subjective description of the disease.

Wunderlich's temperature curves also served a didactic purpose. Temperature charts visibly reminded doctors of the clinical uses of graphic representation of disease symptoms (Warner 1986:155).[5] These charts impressed upon doctors the idea that diseases were pathological *processes* that produced evidence of their activity that could be measured and followed. The evidence, portrayed in graphic form, was more concrete than the vague impression gained from feel-ing a patient's forehead, and it seemed more immutable, more exact, more irrefutable (Marey 1878; Borell 1986; Frank 1988).[6]

In spite of these advantages, the thermometer was not immediately accepted by the medical profession (Evans 1993; Lawrence 1985a, 1985b). Technical problems, especially its fragility, made it impractical to carry on house calls. Early thermometers required frequent calibration, an added burden for the busy or skeptical physician. In addition, physicians complained that the instruments were too expensive for general use. Doctors needed to be convinced that the device was superior to their trained sense of touch.

For centuries, estimating pulse pressure had been the most revered of the physician's trained senses, but, like estimating temperature by placing the hand on the forehead, assessing pressure by feeling the force of the pulse was unreliable and subject to the interpretation and experience of the doctor. Starting with German physiologist Karl Ludwig in 1846, physiologists designed instruments to measure and monitor bodily processes (Cranefield 1957, 1966). Ludwig's kymograph, which graphically recorded a dog's blood pressure, required the insertion of a manometer inside an artery, a technique too severe for routine human use (Borell 1985). However, the promise of clinical applications of blood pressure monitoring lured physiologically minded physicians to adapt laboratory devices for clinical use (Borell 1987; Keele 1963).[7]

Among the most important of these devices were instruments like the sphygmograph and the sphygmomanometer, which aided in pulse diagnosis (Lawrence 1978, 1979 & 1979a). Early pulse-reading devices mimicked the action of fingers, with levers that rested on the pulse transmitting the arterial throbbing to a piece of moving paper or a revolving drum. Subsequent instruments sought to measure pressure by occluding the pulse and recording the pressure at which the pulse returned. These devices culminated in Scipione Riva-Rocci's (1896) sphygmomanometer, which served as the prototype for the modern blood pressure machine.

The term sphygmomanometer, from the Greek words for *pulse* and *measure,* reflects the importance of measurement in late-nineteenth century scientific medicine. While "seeing" disease had been a technological innovation of the early and mid-nineteenth-century, "measuring" physiology and pathophysiology was the product of the latter part of the century. Instruments like the sphygmomanometer exemplified the ideological movement toward a belief in quantification and objectivity that was transforming science and medicine.[8] Ultimately, these so-called instruments of precision contributed to a growing faith that disease was an entity having an essence that could be seen and measured. This belief reshaped the concept of disease, and in so doing fundamentally altered the doctor-patient relationship.

Instruments and the Doctor-Patient Relationship

As instruments gained popularity, doctors began to believe that the devices were more reliable than their patients. Physicians felt that with instruments they obtained information from the disease itself and that they no longer had to trust the patient's description of the disease. The sounds heard through the stethoscope were, as one doctor claimed, "independent of the caprice or ignorance of the patient" (Reiser 1978:31). Proponents of thermometry agreed that the instrument was more dependable than the patient: "The sensations of the patient with respect to temperature, as every one knows, are extremely fallacious; he may suffer from a feeling of heat when, to the touch of another, the surface is cold, and vice versa" (Flint 1866:82). Just as they had doubts about a patient's subjective impression of symptoms, surgeons often found it difficult to rely on the anesthetist's tactile interpretation of blood pressure. As Harvey Cushing, a proponent of sphygmomanometers, stated, "During a critical operation the hearsay dependence which the surgeon must place on the palpating finger of the anesthetist for a knowledge of the cardiac strength of his patient may oftentimes be one of his most trying responsibilities" (Cushing 1903:250). Thus the mere existence of instruments heightened the perceived inaccuracy of humans, be they patients or medical personnel.[9]

Instruments, then, enabled doctors to delegate duties without fear of compromising patient care. Wunderlich noted that properly trained nurses could take the temperature at scheduled intervals and then plot the results on temperature charts, thereby freeing the doctor to do other work. The charts could be interpreted later and could serve as tangible and permanent evidence of the disease and treatment. One of Cushing's house officers noted that blood pressure measurements also could be taken by nurses and suggested that this be done at night, when house officers were busy in other parts of the hospital. This resident

found it practicable to leave orders for stimulants of one sort or another, to be administered in accordance with the blood-pressure observations, which the nurse herself regularly made on the cases that were seriously ill. Thus without waiting for the personal advice of the attendant, oftentimes occasioning serious delay, or a fall of blood pressure to a certain subnormal level, a saline infusion or a given dose of digitaline was to be administered, to be followed, if the pressure did not shortly return to and remain at a safe level, by a certain amount of strychnia, for example. [Cushing 1903:254]

Prior to the advent of these instruments, doctors were not inclined to delegate such duties. The physician's "trained senses" were part of his revered set of talents. To ask a nurse to estimate pulse tension would have suggested that his or her senses were as finely honed as the doctor's, an insinuation that undermined a doctor's prestige. Physicians could teach underlings how to use the instruments and reserve the interpretation of the data collected to the doctor's domain. Ultimately, many of the monitoring duties would be performed by machines (Geddes 1976).

In spite of the obvious advantages, doctors worried about the emotional impact that instruments would have on patients. Proponents of the stethoscope argued that while it diagnosed disease earlier and more accurately, it also might increase patients' anxiety. "Is it nothing to foretell, and thus in some measure take from, the approaching calamity?" wrote English physician William Corrigan. "Is it nothing, instead of giving delusive hope, to prepare the individual himself for his last great change, and that, in all probability, to be sudden?" (Reiser 1978:33-34). Other physicians noted the sadness of a certain diagnosis, and felt that instruments might rob a patient of hope of improvement or cure.

While some patients were wary of the new instruments, others shared the doctor's faith in their accuracy. In fact, both doctor and patient often attributed important powers to instruments. Dr. C. Heitzmann reported to the New York County Medical Society in 1878 an example of the faith he and his patients shared in the powers of the microscope:

In fact, the microscope reveals so much of the general health of a person, that more can be told by it in many instances than by the naked eye, or by physical examination. . . . Marriages should be allowed in doubtful cases, only upon the permit of a reliable microscopist. Last season a young physician asked me whether I believed in the marriage among kindred? He fell in love with his cousin, and so did the cousin with him. I examined his blood, and told him that he is a 'nervous' man, passes sleepless nights, and has a moderately good constitution. The condition being suspected in the kindred lady, marriage was not advisable for fear that the offspring might degenerate. So great was his faith in my assertions, that he gave up the idea of marrying his cousin, offering her the last chance, viz., the examination of her blood. This beautiful girl came to my laboratory, and, very much to my surprise, I found upon examination of her blood a first-class constitution. The next day I told the gentleman, "You had better marry her." [Heitzmann 1879; Howell 1988]

Using technology to regulate socially unacceptable behavior was often legitimated by laws as well as by social mores. For instance, the Wasserman blood test for syphilis, developed in 1906, became the basis for several laws governing who could obtain a marriage license, even though the test was known to have a false positive rate as high as 20% (Brandt 1985).

Although patients often requested that their doctors employ instruments in diagnosis and treatment, the devices did not always inspire confidence in the doctor's intellect.[10] Some general practitioners worried that being seen using an instrument would suggest to their patients a similarity to surgeons, who also relied on instruments. Nineteenth-century surgeons were considered less scholarly, more like craftsmen, a designation that many doctors wished to avoid (Reiser 1978). Austin Flint (1866:6-7) stated, "In this country, the thermometer has been but little used in medical investigations, owing, probably, to a prudential reserve with regard to novelties." Dr. Daniel Cathell (1900:93), in his popular turn-of-the-century manual on how to become successful, warned physicians that to be seen doing any manual labor would take away from the doctor's respectability. Dr. S. Weir Mitchell (1891:164), an avid proponent of "instruments of precision," recognized the potentially demeaning consequences of using medical instruments when he wrote, "Alas, we now use as many machines as a mechanic!"[11] Lewis Thomas (1983:17) related a story about his own father, a general practitioner in Flushing, New York, who in 1912 bought a device that was falsely claimed to regulate the bowels—a very heavy leather-covered sphere the size of a bowling ball. Presumably, rolling the 'bowling ball' over the abdomen in specific ways would facilitate digestion by helping to move food through the alimentary tract.

My father tried it for a short while on a few patients, with discouraging results, and one day placed it atop a cigar box which he had equipped with wheels and a long string, and presented it to my eldest sister, who tugged it with pleasure around the corner to a neighbor's house. That was the last he saw of the ball until twelve years later, when the local newspaper announced in banner headlines that a Revolutionary War cannon ball had been discovered in the excavated garden behind our neighbor's yard. . . . My father claimed privately to his family, swearing us to secrecy, that he had, in an indirect sense anyway, made medical history.

Thus the fear of being misled, and embarrassed, by new and unproven instruments underlay many a doctor's wariness to adopt medical instruments (Cushing 1903).[12]

Doctors debated the best design of instruments (Janeway 1901, 1904). Convenience and durability were desirable since devices had to accompany them on their house calls, for in the nineteenth century doctors often traveled to their patients; only the most destitute patient went to the hospital. The instrument then had to withstand bumpy rides down dirt roads. It had to be convenient to use, small,

sturdy, reliable, and affordable. One of Laénnec's stethoscopes un-
screwed into two pieces to make it more portable and convenient
(Reiser 1978:25-26). An expert on sphygmomanometers withheld his
recommendation from one early model that was so bulky that it "required two men to carry it and operate it from bed to bed" (Cook
1903a:1200). Others lauded the convenience of another brand of sphygmomanometer that fit into the waistcoat pocket (Williams 1907-8). Patient comfort also was an important consideration in choosing an
instrument. One sphygmomanometer was not recommended for routine clinical use because "the procedure is so severe and the technique
so difficult as to render its use almost prohibitive" (Erlanger 1904:56).

How Instruments Transformed Medicine

With medical instruments, doctors could subject patients and their
symptoms to objective scrutiny. As doctors gained more data from instruments, the quality of the information related by the patient
seemed less important. Doctor and patient shared less knowledge;
there was less common ground between them. A medical instrument
acted as a lens through which the doctor could see disease unfiltered
by the patient's interpretations. Instruments thus altered the doctor-
patient relationship, making the patient's experience of illness less
important (Kleinman, Eisenberg, and Good 1978).

Merely saying that instruments distanced doctors from patients,
however, overlooks more subtle and substantive changes in the doctor-
patient relationship. Doctors felt so empowered that they believed the
new instruments actually put them in "closer touch" with their patients, and such claims commonly punctuate the medical literature
(Cook 1903b:37). The information that instruments provided, and the
knowledge accrued as a result of data they produced, increased the
body of biomedical knowledge about disease. By exploring the physical
and numerical evidence of disease, doctors believed that they advanced medical knowledge. As William Lee, professor of physiology at
Columbia University, optimistically explained to the graduating class
in 1878:

To measure thoughts seems now but child's play. With this simple little instrument [the sphygmograph], a simple lever pressing so lightly upon the pulse
that the slightest movement gives wide play to its free extremity, there remains a record teaching faithfully every movement of the heart, the tension of
the blood vessel, the degree of nerve force and, within certain bounds, the
character of the blood stream itself, revealing, as I said before, secrets that
were never whispered in the consultation room of earlier days. [Brim 1930:72]

The instrument also replaced time-honored methods of physical diagnosis that doctors had relied on for centuries and that had, in many ways, defined their realm of expertise (Evans 1993). The subjective arts of palpating a pulse and feeling a feverish brow were replaced by more accurate, numerical methods of determining pathology. The reliability of technology, especially when compared with other, more subjective methods available to the doctor, was very alluring. Indeed, accuracy, certainty, objectivity, and reliability became code words for medical reform and advancement (Borell et al. 1988; Warner 1985). These phrases became emblematic of efforts aimed to make medicine more rational. In the process, the healing power of the simple "laying on of hands" became less important to the physician. Doctors shifted their alliances from their own sensations, and those of their patients, to the impersonal, objective arbiter of the instrument. Feelings, be they the physician's belief in his or her own "trained sense of touch" or the patient's more ephemeral faith in a doctor's healing touch, became less important in the wake of the massive wave of interest in objectivity and accuracy.

The appeal of efficiency, accuracy, and precision was felt by all Americans—not just doctors. Patients, too, shared a faith in these qualities as symbols of progress (Haber 1964; Wiebe 1967). "Instruments of precision," a phrase with lofty overtones often found in doctors' articles, was not limited to medical literature. All over the country, artistry was yielding to machinery as Americans embraced this new ethic.

Because instruments were heralded as objective, reliable, and accurate, they subtly underscored the potential unreliability of patients. Doctors had long questioned the veracity of their patients, but prior to the introduction of instruments the stories patients told had to suffice. Instruments could objectify a patient's story, checking the facts and filtering through the emotional aspects of disease. Austin Flint noted this when he remarked that the thermometer could help distinguish between the "real disease" of inflammation of the brain and the fabricated disease of hysteria, both of which could present identical symptoms (Flint 1866:86-87). The physician had gained tools that could help distinguish disease from fabrication. If instruments became the judges used to distinguish real from fictive disease, then the patient's experience of illness lost credibility.

Instruments also freed doctors from time-consuming patient care. Physicians taught nurses and medical students how to take temperatures and blood pressures using instruments, leaving instructions about treatment should the temperature rise or the blood pressure fall. In the time saved by relinquishing some of their patient care responsibilities and following their patients from a distance, doctors could see more patients. The interpretation of data became an important duty of the doctor. The doctor-patient relationship became a less personal encounter. Patients, in turn, began to feel that they should be monitored—that numbers such as their weight, heart rate, blood pressure, and cholesterol level are synonymous with health or disease.

Instrumental recordings changed the way doctors interacted and learned. Increasingly doctors valued objective data—be it graphic or numerical—over subjective descriptions. This behavior fed the burgeoning faith in "rational science" and the "exact method." Doctors could send the information to a consulting physician, who would interpret the data. Indeed, today it is the nurse or even the nurse's assistant who takes the temperature and blood pressure.

While instruments might be a liability when it came to making house calls, they were ideal for hospital-based medical practice. In fact, hospitals became a locus for instruments in medicine (Vogel 1980). Sometimes, as in the case of X-ray machines and early electrocardiographs, the devices were too large and delicate to be transported.[13] The string galvanometer, the predecessor to the electrocardiograph, filled an entire room. The patient had to come to it, not vice versa. The sheer numbers of patients concentrated within hospitals made it possible to study the applications of instruments.[14] As doctors began to rely more on data produced by instruments, proximity to hospitals became an advantage for both patient and doctor. In this way instruments contributed to the shift of patient care from the home and dispensary to the hospital.

Instruments also contributed to the specialization of medical care, enabling doctors to "see" new parts of the body and the diseases particular to them. Many specialties got their impetus from technological advances. For instance, the discovery of the X-ray in the mid-1890s spawned the field of radiology (Brecher and Brecher 1969; Grigg 1965). Ophthalmology grew out of the invention of the ophthalmoscope earlier in the nineteenth century (Rosen 1944; Rucker 1971). More recent instrumentation has contributed to the subspecialization of internal medicine, pediatrics, and surgery. Subspecialization of medicine compartmentalized the body, and specialists, highly trained in a single organ system, began to focus on how disease affected that specific system, often losing touch with the overall illness and the patient as a whole.

Medical instruments are the visible evidence of the transformation in medicine from what one doctor called "subjective to objective, thinking to knowing" (Cook 1903c:106). Instruments helped to shape a new approach to medical problems—one that valued deductive reasoning, accuracy, and scientific, physiological approaches to disease. In the process the doctor's understanding of disease and the patient's experience of sickness changed. The high tech of modern medicine has increased the doctor's understanding of disease, but often at the expense of his understanding of the person who has the disease.

Initially ambivalent about the effects of technology on patient care and professional status, doctors ultimately accepted new instrumentation when the risks seemed minimal. Acceptance of new technology required a reprioritization of time-honored methods of diagnosis, treatment, and prognosis. For instance, feeling the pulse (and all the subtle expertise behind that action) became less important as the sphygmomanometer gained a foothold in the diagnostic armamentarium. Similarly, doctors today complain that all too often the use of the stethoscope to auscultate heart murmurs has yielded to a more sophisticated and expensive technology, the echocardiogram.

The doctor's healing touch, be it feeling the feverish brow, palpating the pulse, or a more ephemeral conglomeration of actions and responses, has yielded to more accurate and reliable methods of monitoring the patient. High-tech medicine has opened the doors for a more detailed understanding of disease. As part of this process, physicians have focused on what can be measured and objectified and have deemphasized the more mercurial and personal aspects of illness. While technology has increased knowledge about disease itself, knowledge about how disease affects its sufferers has lagged behind. But just as doctors, persuaded by a technological imperative to conquer disease, behave like "body mechanics," patients—equally under the spell of the promise of technology—often see their ill bodies as pumps and pipes gone awry. John Kendrick Bangs (1924:95) humorously summed up this feeling in his poem "A Man and His Car":

> You know the model of your car,
> You know just what its powers are.
> You treat it with a deal of care
> Nor tax it more than it will bear.
> But as to self—that's different;
> Your mechanism may be bent,
> Your carburetor gone to grass,
> Your engine just a rusty mass.
>
> Your wheels may wobble and your cogs
> Be handed over to the dogs.
> And you skip and skid and slide
> Without a thought of things inside.
> What fools, indeed, we mortals are
> To lavish care upon a car
> With ne'er a bit of time to see
> About our own machinery.

Influenced by the desire to reduce disease to that which can be seen and measured, doctors, like the patient who took care of his car but ignored his "own machinery," all too often take care of the body without attending to the aspects of disease that are felt and experienced. While there is little dispute that technological innovation has made possible great strides in medical care, medical instrumentation has fundamentally changed the way of thinking about disease. Doctors and patients alike look to medical instruments to uncover disease, guide therapy, and even wield cure, yet disease challenges people in ways that are not tangible or measurable. It is these aspects of disease and the doctor-patient relationship that the high tech of medicine does not touch.

Notes

1. See John Durant's comments in the foreword to this book.

2. I first heard this dichotomy expressed by Clarke Taylor, administrator, University Hospital, University of Alabama at Birmingham.

3. For the discussion on Laénnec, see Reiser (1978:25-27).

4. Wunderlich did not invent the clinical thermometer, nor was he the first physician to explore its clinical applications. His contribution lay in the scope of his research, as well as in the way he organized and presented his data. Wunderlich acknowledged the influence of Ludwig Traub (1871-78), who did thermometric research in the clinic without graphically displaying his results. For an overview of pre-Wunderlich clinical thermometry, see Estes (1991).

5. On the uses of temperature charts in hospitals, see John Harley Warner (1986); on the development of other types of clinical graphical charts, see Henry K. Beecher, "The First Anesthesia Records (Codman, Cushing)," *Surgery, Gynecology, and Obstetrics* 71 (1940): 689-93.

6. The original popularizer of the term *graphic method* was French physiologist Etienne J. Marey (1878). A considerable historical literature is accruing on the graphic method (Borell 1986; Frank 1988).

7. On specific instruments, see Fleckenstein (1984a, 1984b).

8. On the philosophical background and scientific and intellectual ramifications of this movement in science, see Mendelsohn (1964).

9. Most nineteenth-century anesthetists were medical students. The instrumental measurement of blood pressure in the operating room, then, bridged the gap between novice student and seasoned doctor.

10. Ironically, while instruments physically distanced doctor from patient, they eventually led to an increased emphasis on the physical exam.

11. The wish to avoid the confusion of "thinkers" with "tinkers" was not limited to medicine. The dichotomy between intellectual endeavors and manual labor helped form social and class distinctions and has been an important research agenda in the history of technology.

12. Harvey Cushing acknowledged this fear: "The belief is more or less prevalent that the powers of observation so markedly developed in our predecessors have, to a large extent, become blunted in us, owing to the employment of instrumental aids to exactness, and the art of medicine consequently has always adopted them with considerable reluctance." His article also may be found in Howell (1988:47-53).

13. For more on how X-rays and electrocardiographs, as well as other early medical instruments, became routine features of American and British hospital medicine, see Joel D. Howell (1986, 1987).

14. Wunderlich's work on thermometry had been done in a hospital. Theodore Janeway's research on essential hypertension, however, is an exception to this rule. Janeway studied patients from the private practice he shared with his father because he believed their histories were better known than those of hospital patients and because follow-up was easier.

6

Contractual Arrangements, Financial Incentives, and Physician-Patient Relationships

Robert L. Ohsfeldt

The relationships between physicians and their patients are quite complex. In theory, at least, the patient seeks advice from a physician concerning the most appropriate course of medical treatment or other actions to ameliorate the effects of a particular malady or maladies. The patient consults a physician because the physician's knowledge about the diagnosis of disease and the effects of treatments is generally superior to the patient's, and the physician has greater ability to provide treatments. Ideally, the physician would recommend the course of action that the patient would rationally select if given the information known to the physician.

The chapters in this book present a variety of perspectives on physician-patient relationships. Whatever the perspective, one of the most fundamental aspects of the physician-patient relationship is that patients pay physicians for the advice they give and the other services they render. Patients may pay physicians directly or indirectly, through a third party.[1] Thus, contractual arrangements for payment affecting the patient involve the terms of coverage by third-party payers and personal financial obligations for payments directly to physicians. Physicians' contractual arrangements include the conditions of payment directly by the patient or the patient's insurer to the physician, for compensation within physicians' practices, and for compensation by means of a physician's shares of ownership in facilities to which the physician refers patients. These often complex contractual arrangements may foster conflict rather than consensus between patients and physicians (Ellis and McGuire 1990). In other words, the course of action that is in the best interests of the patient may be in conflict with the best interest of the physician. This conflict has the potential to affect physician-patient relationships in terms of both physicians' recommendations to patients and the patient's compliance.

This chapter focuses on the financial aspects of physician-patient relationships, providing an overview of physician-patient relationships within the broader context of the economic theory of agency relationships. It discusses specific types of contractual arrangements and the nature of financial incentives implicit in these arrangements, as well as institutional and regulatory structures designed to reinforce ethical constraints on physician behavior. Empirical studies are reviewed to shed light on the extent to which financial incentives affect the physician-patient relationship. The chapter concludes with an assessment of the impact of various types of contractual arrangements and the prospects for the future.

Principal-Agent Relationships

The physician-patient relationship often has been regarded as an example of an arrangement between an agent (the physician) and a principal (the patient).[2] Agency relationships are quite common, owing to the general economic benefits of specialization and exchange among individuals. In general, the principal may acquire some type of information or service though an agent at a much lower cost than without an agent. The agent receives compensation for the effort required to obtain information and provide services for the principal. Principals generally delegate some decision-making authority to their agents, given the principals' inferior base of knowledge for decision making. Examples of agency relationships include arrangements between lawyers and clients, corporate management and shareholders, employers and employees, and so on. Ideally, the agent selects for the principal the course of action that the principal would select if given access to the same skills or knowledge.

The basic problem in any principal-agent relationship is that the objective of the agent and that of the principal generally will not be congruent. One approach to this problem is to structure compensation to an agent in such a way as to give financial incentives for actions compatible with the objectives of the principal. Unfortunately, it is generally impossible to design a financial incentive scheme that would induce the agent to behave in a manner that maximizes the well-being of the principal.[3] The difference between the ideal outcome and the outcome attained by the agent is referred to as agency cost. The principal may reduce agency costs by directly observing the behavior of the agent, but must bear the cost of the monitoring activity. The goal, then, in the design of compensation arrangements is to choose financial incentives and a level of monitoring effort that minimizes the sum of agency and monitoring costs and that is acceptable to both the agent and the principal (Spremann 1987).

The type of incentive structure that minimizes agency costs depends upon the nature of the agency problem. For example, suppose the outcome of interest to the principal depends upon the agent's level of effort (which the principal cannot observe directly) and upon factors outside the control of agent. In this case, some form of risk-sharing contract will be the most efficient compensation arrangement (Spremann 1987). Examples of risk-sharing contracts include contingent fees for plaintiffs' attorneys in torts and sharecropping for tenant farmers. If a principal has many agents and if outcomes across agents are related to external risk factors correlated across agents, then compensation based (at least in part) on the rank-order of performance of agents may be most efficient (Nalebuff and Stiglitz 1983). An example of this incentive arrangement is compensation and promotion for corporate executives. Competition among agents for the relationship with a principal generally serves to minimize agency costs by identifying the best agent for that principal (Sappington 1991).

Regarding physician-patient relationships, some have questioned the validity of an agency model, given a physician's imperfect ability to diagnose disease and the uncertainty regarding the outcome of treatment (e.g., Wennberg et al. 1982). However, exchange through agency relationships may be mutually beneficial as long as the agent has greater knowledge than the principal. If agents have misperceptions, they tend to receive payments consistent with their misperceptions and the financial incentives within the contract (Gaynor and Kleindorfer 1987). For example, those physicians who perceive a particular treatment as having substantial clinical benefit for a patient will use that treatment more intensively, whereas those physicians who perceive the treatment as having little clinical benefit will use it less intensively, when practicing under identical contractual arrangements for compensation. Thus, the physician who perceives substantial clinical benefits would receive greater payment if the contract rewards the provision of the treatment, and lower payment if the contract penalizes provision of the treatment, compared to the physician who perceives that the treatment has little clinical benefit (when paid under the same contract terms). Clearly, either or both of these physicians' perceptions of the clinical benefits of the treatment could be incorrect, but the payment each physician receives is affected by his (mis)perception of the clinical value of the treatment. Even if physicians had perfect knowledge of the probability distributions for treatments and outcomes, ideally they would make different clinical decisions for clinically identical patients because of differences in patients' preferences and environmental factors (Eisenberg 1986).

In the context of an agency model, the ideal behavior of physicians is to "make the choice the patient would have made" if given the same information.[4] This implies that the physician is responsive to the explicit costs and implicit costs (time, inconvenience) to the patient of treatment alternatives, selecting, among treatments perceived to provide approximately equivalent clinical benefits, the treatment that minimizes these costs. Choices among risky alternatives are to be determined by the patient's willingness to accept risk and the patient's—not the physician's—(informed) valuation of possible treatment outcomes. If the patient demands a treatment or test regarded as useless by the physician, the physician's role is to attempt to persuade the patient that the treatment is not necessary or useful. Nonetheless, physicians often may provide services they regard to be of limited clinical value to patients who adamantly demand such services, particularly if the iatrogenic risk is low (Harvey and Shubat 1989). They also may refer such patients to a physician whose practice style is more compatible with the patient's demands. The temptation to give the patient what the patient wants usually is attributed at least partly to fear of liability risk, but it also may indicate the degree to which the patient's demand affects the physician's perceptions of the patient's values (Eisenberg 1986). Physicians' decisions also may be affected by their role as agent for the patient's payer (Blomqvist 1991).

Given the extreme complexity of the physician's role, it should not be surprising that physicians fail to make ideal decisions as agents for their patients. In part, this may be due to poor communication between physicians and patients; physicians often do not know which treatment alternative their patients would prefer (Eisenberg 1986), or they attribute any divergence between the patient's treatment preferences and their own to patient irrationality (Brock and Wartman 1990). Even with better communication, some agency cost is inevitable. That is, "it is impossible to set up a truly incentive-neutral system in the context of the physician's role as agent and provider" (Begley 1987:119). This fact is occasionally lost in the debate over eliminating a particular type of financial conflict of interest in physician payment (Relman 1988). Of course, as an empirical matter, some types of financial conflicts may have more significant effects on physician-patient relationships than others.

Contractual Arrangements and Incentives

Physicians receive payment for their services in a myriad of forms. Each of these compensation arrangements entails financial incentives that may influence clinical decisions. Most physicians in group

Figure 6.1.   Primary Methods of Compensation among Non-Solo
Physicians, 1983

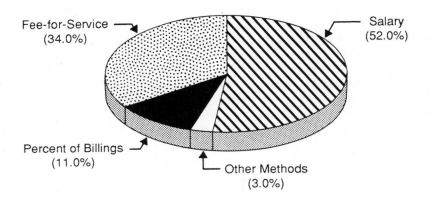

Source: American Medical Association, Socioeconomic Characteristics
of Medical Practice, 1984.

practices receive their primary compensation in the form of a salary
(fig.6.1). However, many receiving a salary also receive some compensation related to their individual level of effort or to the overall financial performance of the practice. The literature generally has focused
on two types of financial incentives: 1) broad compensation arrangements, such as fee-for-service, or capitation; and 2) financial incentives for ancillary services, such as laboratory or other diagnostic tests.

Many studies have addressed the issue of "supplier-induced demand" in the context of fee-for-service compensation. The potential financial conflict of interest inherent in fee-for-service compensation
relates to the incentive to provide excess services to obtain additional
income. No one doubts that physicians can influence the choices patients make—that is their job as the patients' agents. The issue is
whether physicians exploit the ignorance of their patients to induce
treatment "above and beyond what the patient would have been willing to pay for if the patient knew as much as the physician" (Wilensky
and Rossiter 1983:259). Early studies using aggregate data found apparently resounding support for the supplier-induced demand phenomenon (Evans 1974; Feldstein 1970; Fuchs 1978). However, these
early studies had numerous methodological flaws (Auster and Oaxaca
1981; Ramsey and Wasow 1986), which cast significant doubt on the
validity of their conclusions.

More recent studies have used better (though still very imperfect) methods to address the issue of demand inducement. Looking at the issue from the perspective of physicians' earnings, Headen (1990) concludes that increases in the supply of physicians lower physicians' hourly practice earnings, controlling for other factors, just as predicted by standard economic theory. Wilensky and Rossiter (1983) find that physician-initiated office visits (as distinguished from patient-initiated visits) increase with the physician-to-population ratio, controlling for other factors, but the effect is small in magnitude. In contrast to some of the earlier studies, they find no positive association between the physician-to-population ratio and prevailing physician fees. Cromwell and Mitchell (1986) conclude that some demand inducement occurs for surgical procedures, but the overall effect is quite small (a 1% increase in the physician-to-population ratio is associated with a 0.08% increase in the rate of surgery). As might be expected, the effect is driven by "elective" surgical procedures; there is no apparent effect for nonelective surgical procedures. Their results also suggest that competition among physicians limits demand-inducing behavior, as Stano's (1987) model predicts. Thus, despite some remaining methodological flaws (Phelps 1986), these studies suggest that some demand inducement occurs as a result of fee-for-service incentives. The effects, however, appear to be generally quite small.

If physicians can induce some demand for their services as posited in the supplier-induced demand hypothesis, a question that arises is, Why don't they induce demand to the maximum extent possible? Early studies posited an "ethical" constraint: a physician's well-being increased with income but decreased as a result of providing excessive services to patients, because of the "disutility" of an inappropriate level of services. In these models, the disutility of doing "wrong" may derive from personal pangs of conscience or from the disapproval of peers, but there is no direct financial penalty to the physician.

Early demand inducement models in effect assumed a very passive role for the patient. Dranove (1988) provides a model with a more active role for the patient, where inducement is constrained by the patient's perceived likelihood of illness.[5] The patient will doubt a physician's assessment that diverges from the patient's self-diagnosis of illness. If the divergence is sufficient, the patient will refuse a recommended treatment. As the patient's confidence in the self-diagnosis increases, demand inducement becomes less likely. Another factor in the model is the physician's reputation for apparent demand-inducing behavior. A physician with a "good" reputation is less likely to be doubted than one with a "bad" reputation. Competition may serve to reduce demand inducement if patients avoid physicians with bad reputations in favor of those with good reputations. The significant role of reputation and trust ties Dranove's model more closely to the general theory of agency relationships (Schanze 1987) than do the early demand inducement models.

Dranove's model has a clear implication for the demand inducement hypothesis: relatively uninformed patients are more likely to be induced to use services than better-informed patients. However, medically informed patients use more services than other patients. For example, physicians and their dependents use more services than other patients, controlling for other factors including the price to the patient of services (Bunker and Brown 1974; Hay and Leahy 1982). Using direct measures of the quality of a patient's health information, Kenkel (1990) finds that better information is associated with a greater, not lesser, likelihood of a physician visit and a greater intensity of service use among those who make such visits (though the latter effect is not statistically significant). The model controls for the patient's age, gender, insurance coverage, and beliefs about the benefits of medical care, as well as accounting for the health information production process.[6] Kenkel concludes that uninformed patients are not more likely to be induced into using services. Indeed, if it has any effect, patient ignorance reduces compliance and thus reduces the use of services among uninformed patients.

Another vexing conceptual issue involved in measuring the extent of physician-induced demand empirically is separating the effects of health insurance coverage on patients' demand for care (moral hazard) from the effects of financial incentives to physicians on the level of services that patients receive (Pauly 1986). Ellis and McGuire (1990) posit a model that merges the demand-side effects of health insurance (moral hazard) and the supply-side effects of payment systems with imperfect agency (demand inducement). The model contrasts, on the one hand, the quantity of services desired by the patient (desired demand), which is influenced by the coinsurance rate determining the price of services to the patient, with, on the other hand, the physician's desired supply of services, which is influenced by conditions of provider payment and the extent of imperfect agency (i.e., the degree to which financial incentives rather than the physician's perception of health benefits for the patient affect the physician's desired supply). If patients are risk-averse and physicians are imperfect agents, desired demand and desired supply generally are not equal; instead, the level of services provided is determined by "bargaining" between patients and physicians.[7] Ellis and McGuire point out that the traditional system of full cost-based fee-for-service payment to providers in no case maximizes patient welfare, even if physicians are perfect agents, regardless of the patient's copayment level. Thus, patient welfare is always improved by imposing some level of "supply-side" cost sharing. Although they provide no formal empirical analysis, Ellis and McGuire note that provider payment has increasingly incorporated elements of provider risk or cost sharing over the past two decades, representing movement toward their optimal payment system.

The relative bargaining power of patients and physicians in Ellis and McGuire's model provides some insight into the demand inducement issue. If, as seems likely, the physician's bargaining power is greater than that of the patient, but not complete (i.e., patients do not always do everything physicians tell them to do), a "second-best" optimal system of patient insurance and provider payment usually calls for: (1) a low degree of cost sharing by the patient (perhaps zero), and (2) provider compensation in the form of an appropriately scaled lump sum payment (e.g., capitation), plus some additional amount per unit of service (below the full fee-for-service payment level).[8] A high degree of patient cost sharing is not needed to counteract moral hazard in this setting because the "supply-side" considerations of the physician dominate the "demand-side" in the bargaining process that determines the level of service provision. Under the optimal payment system envisioned in the model, physicians do not induce demand but rather persuade patients to use less than their moral-hazard-induced desired demand.

Alternative Forms of Compensation: Empirical Studies

The traditional demand inducement literature focuses on the financial incentives of fee-for-service payment. More generally, however, different forms of physician compensation provide various financial incentives that may affect clinical decisions in different ways. As noted, fee-for-service compensation gives physicians the financial incentive to provide more services to patients. Conversely, a fixed salary or fixed hourly wage gives incentives to provide less care (Woodward and Warren-Boulton 1984). The effect of fixed salary or wage compensation occurs because payment per period of time is not determined by the intensity of work effort. The financial incentive thus is to work less intensively.

The relationship between compensation arrangements and treatment intensity has been the subject of several empirical studies. These studies have consistently indicated that compensation arrangements were associated with physicians' decisions in the predicted direction. However, many of the studies used a nonexperimental research design to assess the effects of different contractual arrangements. Such studies must be interpreted cautiously because there exists an unavoidable question as to whether differences in clinical decisions reflect the "pure" influence of financial incentives or whether they reflect the tendency of physicians to sort themselves into contractual arrangements consistent with their practice style.[9] In other words, physicians who tend to use hospitalization intensively would be less likely to accept a contract specifying payment on a capitation basis than would those who use hospitalization less intensively. This will cause assessments of the effects of financial incentives on physicians' decisions to be overstated. Contracts are voluntary agreements, and a particular contract's terms will be more agreeable to some than to others. Because of this confounding factor, assessments of the impact of financial incentives on clinical decisions in a nonexperimental context are a very tricky business.

Using data from a sample of Health Maintenance Organizations (HMOs), Pauly et al. (1990) and Hillman et al. (1990) analyzed the apparent ways in which different types of contractual arrangements for physician payment affected the use of services by HMO enrollees. The contractual arrangements between physicians and HMOs varied widely, reflecting differing degrees of risk sharing. Relative to fee-for-service compensation (i.e., no risk sharing), patients of physicians compensated by a fixed salary or by a per-enrollee capitation payment had lower rates of hospitalization. Regarding physician visits per-enrollee, again relative to fee-for-service, physicians subject to individual risk for the overall performance of the HMO had fewer visits, whereas those at risk for overall use of ancillary services had more visits. For both hospitalization and visits, no other compensation method (e.g., individual productivity bonuses, withholds subject to deficits in referral funds, etc.) was associated with usage substantially different from fee-for-service payment. These contractual incentives had greater effects for physicians in for-profit HMOs than for those in not-for-profit HMOs.

In a study of hospital-based physicians, Shaffert et al. (1980) found that those paid a percentage of the billings they generated received payments two to three times higher than those paid a flat salary, controlling for several other factors. As the authors note, however, they failed to account for differences in employer-paid practice expenses, which may have resulted in an overstatement of the payment differential. More important, as noted above, the variety of contract terms may be the result of (rather than the cause for) multiple practice styles. Still, despite these limitations, the differential is too large to be ignored.

To examine the role of financial incentives, Hemenway et al. (1990) made use of a natural experiment resulting from a change in compensation arrangements in a clinic, from a flat hourly wage to a bonus system based on a percentage of billings generated. After the change in compensation arrangements, the use of X-rays and laboratory tests increased substantially (by 16% and 23%, respectively), and the number of patient visits and total billings also increased (12% and 20%, respectively). However, only about half of the physicians received the bonus (the remainder failed to attain the bonus threshold and were paid a flat hourly wage). Those physicians receiving the bonus had higher billings than those who did not receive a bonus (a rather obvious outcome, since the bonus was conditional on higher billings). However, the bonus-earning physicians had higher billings even before the change in compensation arrangements. Indeed, billings for the bonus-earning and non-bonus-earning physicians increased by about the same percentage after the change in the compensation terms. It is possible that the increase in clinic billings resulted from changes in market conditions unrelated to the change in compensation terms. For these reasons, it is unclear whether the change in compensation terms fundamentally altered physicians' behavior in the clinic, or whether it simply changed the rewards for their previous pattern of behavior.

Murray et al. (1992) compared utilization among patients with hypertension treated at primary care clinics at a major teaching hospital. Every physician practicing at the clinics treated some capitated patients and some fee-for-service patients. Murray et al. found that capitated patients received fewer laboratory tests and had lower overall treatment costs than fee-for-service patients (controlling for patient age, hypertension severity, and comorbidity factors). It is unlikely that these differences resulted from differences in physicians' practice styles because the same physicians treated both types of patients. The results of this study suggest that physicians may alter their treatment decisions for individual patients in a manner consistent with differences in contractual terms of payment.

Using a purely experimental design, Hickson et al. (1987) compared the clinical behavior of pediatrics residents randomly assigned to two groups, one paid a flat salary and the other paid on a fee-for-service basis. The fee-for-service physicians missed fewer recommended well-visits than the salaried physicians, and scheduled more excess visits. This divergence in clinical behavior is consistent with the incentives to the physicians. Although the possibility of generalizing from this study is limited by its focus on the behavior of residents, because of the experimental design the findings cannot be dismissed as an artifact of physician self-sorting into contract modes. Thus, payment arrangements appear to affect some types of treatment recommendations for some physicians.

Physicians' Ownership Interests

Aside from the overall incentives imbedded in payment systems, more specific financial incentives associated with physicians' ownership interests in health facilities have generated considerable attention (Iglehart 1989; Johnson 1991; McDowell 1989; Rodwin 1989). These ownership interests usually provide indirect compensation to the physician for making certain clinical recommendations to patients. Examples include physician-hospital joint ventures (Rublee and Rosenfield 1987), physician investment in laboratory or diagnostic testing facilities (Iglehart 1989, 1990), and physician dispensing of drugs (Uzych 1988). Different forms of ownership interest entail varying degrees of association between an individual physician's clinical recommendations and the return on his or her investment.

Much of the concern over physician ownership is an outgrowth of the issue of physicians' receiving payment for referrals (McDowell 1989). Direct payment by specialists to primary care physicians for referrals (labeled "fee splitting") was a common practice in the United States in the early part of the twentieth century. The American College of Surgeons from its inception regarded fee splitting as unethical (Starr 1982), although the urge to punish unethical surgeons could be more directly related to the desire to limit competition among physicians for patients than to the desire to uphold professional ethics. At present, organized medicine tends to regard explicit fee splitting as unethical. Medicare has prohibited direct payment for referrals since 1972 (Iglehart 1990). Because such a prohibition removes one of the incentives for referral, however, a physician may withhold a referral that is potentially beneficial for the patient rather than risk "losing" the patient to the physician who receives the referral. More fundamentally, some level of "fee splitting" is inevitable in any form of multiphysician practice (Freidson 1989). Such practices differ in organizational form: different organizational forms entail different levels of implicit fee splitting and hence different financial incentives for referrals (Gaynor and Pauly 1990). Again, the issue is not elimination of financial conflict of interest but rather the form that it takes.

Physicians' ownership interests in health facilities other than their practices, and their propensity to refer patients to such facilities, have evoked considerable regulatory scrutiny. However, relatively few physicians (less than 10%) in 1989 had such ownership interests (AMA 1989). Among those with an ownership interest in an external facility, self-referring physicians indicated that their recommendations were motivated primarily by concerns about patient convenience or quality of care, but a surprisingly nontrivial number readily indicated that their *primary* reason for a self-referral was to assure a return on their investment (fig.6.2). Physicians with ownership interests in lab facilities order about 45% more tests than other physicians (Iglehart 1990). Hillman et al.(1990) found that physicians who referred patients to their own imaging facilities used imaging four to five times more intensively than those who referred patients to radiologists, controlling for case complexity (fig.6.3). Mitchell and Sass (1992) found that physicians who were indirectly "paid" for referrals through joint ventures were much more likely to refer patients than physicians without joint venture interests.

Again, these findings must be interpreted cautiously. Physicians who tend to use imaging intensively have a greater incentive to acquire imaging facilities. In other words, physicians with differing perceptions of the clinical benefits of tests have incentives to sort themselves into different types of practice arrangements. This self-selection of physicians into different contractual arrangements may cause the apparent effects of financial incentives on clinical decisions to be overstated. Nonetheless, the magnitude of the differences are striking. Intuitively, the potential for successful demand inducement (to the extent that it occurs) is greatest for services for which both patient and physician perceive no significant iatrogenic risk, which entail little or no physical pain or monetary cost to the patient, and which generate significant rewards to physicians.[10] It seems likely that at least some portion of the large differential in the use of ancillary services is caused by the financial incentives inherent in physician ownership of such facilities.

The magnitude of the differential in use has led to proposals that would ban self-referrals or require disclosure of investment interests to patients (Iglehart 1990; Rodwin 1989). Medicare has already implemented a partial ban on self-referrals to lab facilities (Iglehart 1990). Ownership interests are permitted if the individual physician's decisions have a minor impact on the return on the physician's investment. However, these regulations also generally exempt referrals to facilities within the physician's practice, an exemption that facilitates large group practices and HMOs. In this context, it is worth noting that the "self-referring" physicians in Hillman et al. (1990) include those with imaging facilities within their own medical practices. Thus, the practical effect of these regulations may be simply to encourage physicians to form larger groups and move testing facilities within their practices.

Monitoring Effort and Peer Review

One mechanism to encourage agents to act in the interest of the principal, as noted, is financial incentives that benefit the principal as well

Figure 6.2. Stated Primary Reasons for Self-Referral, by Specialty, 1989

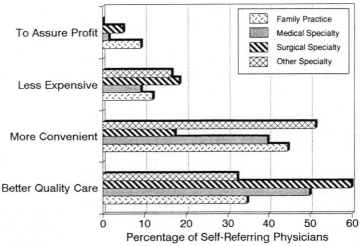

Source: American Medical Association, *Socioeconomic Characteristics of Medical Practice*, 1989.

Figure 6.3. Ratios of Self-referring to Referring Physicians, 1986-1988

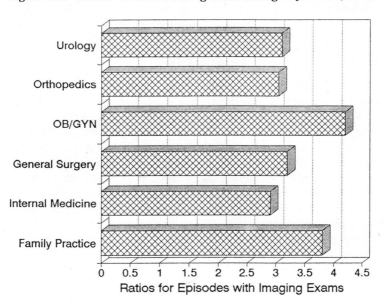

Source: Adapted from Hillman, Joseph, Mabry, et al. (1990). "Frequency and Cost of Diagnostic Imaging in Office Practice," *New England Journal of Medicine* 323:1604-08.

as the agent. Monitoring of the agent's behavior also creates incentives for performance, either as part of the payment mechanisms or in a less direct manner if the only purpose of monitoring is to determine whether the agency relationship continues. The principal may attempt to monitor the agent's behavior directly, or hire an agent (i.e., a supervisor) to monitor the agent, or provide incentives for agents to monitor each other (Arnott and Stiglitz 1991).

In physician-patient relationships, direct monitoring by the principal generally is not feasible or is quite costly, although the cost decreases as the patient's knowledge grows. Monitoring costs may be lowered if another agent monitors the physician. An example is a second-opinion program, under which a patient whose physician recommends a treatment (e.g., a surgical procedure) obtains an independent assessment of the indications for the treatment from another physician. Since the second physician is paid only for an opinion, the recommendation should not be affected by the revenue to be derived from performing the procedure.

However, the physician offering the second opinion has no financial incentive to reveal his or her true opinion (Scotchmer 1990) nor to consider the issue intensively. If payment is based in part on a tendency to disagree with the first physician's recommendation, there is a financial incentive to disagree.[11] The apparently limited usefulness of second opinions for patient welfare may in part explain why voluntary second-opinion programs are rarely used by patients (Wennberg et al. 1980). McCarthy et al. (1981) attributed reductions in elective surgery rates to mandatory second-opinion programs. In this case, however, mandatory second opinions may function as an implicit rationing mechanism by payers, rather than as a mechanism to educate patients. More recently, Jensen and Morrisey (1990) found that second-surgical-opinion programs *increased* group health insurance premiums, implying that any reduction in claims costs associated with reduced surgery rates was offset by the cost of the second-surgical-opinion program.

Peer monitoring among agents is most effective when the payment to agents for monitoring activity is linked to a jointly determined outcome. An example is a group model HMO in which physicians bear some individual risk for the overall performance of the HMO. Inappropriate decisions by one physician affect others through the effect on the HMO's financial performance and its reputation for quality of care. Each physician has incentives to monitor the behavior of the others. However, peer monitoring in this case encourages physicians to act in the best interests of the organization as a whole. Competition among organizations for patients is necessary to ensure that organizations act in the interests of patients.

Utilization management is another form of monitoring, generally employed by third-party payers to address both demand-side (moral hazard) and supply-side (imperfect physician agency) effects of financial incentives. Under utilization management, the care received by patients is monitored to determine whether a particular service or set of services is indicated by the patient's conditions, as determined by a prespecified set of criteria or process for review (Hall and Anderson 1992). Examples of utilization management tools include precertification of medical necessity for hospital admissions, mandatory second opinions for nonemergency surgery, concurrent utilization review (appropriateness of treatment reviewed at the time it is provided), and retrospective utilization review (Gray and Field 1989).

A number of studies suggest that utilization management can reduce the use of medical services deemed medically unnecessary. The best survey of the literature before 1989 is provided by Wickizer (1990). Most of this past research focused on public-sector programs for cost containment. The studies indicated that utilization review reduced costs, although the magnitude of the estimated cost savings varied across studies. Several studies have concluded that utilization review through Peer Review Organizations (PROs) was responsible for avoiding the expected increased in Medicare admissions following the adoption of its per-case prospective payment system in 1983 (Russell 1989; Sloan et al.1988). On the other hand, Nyman et al.(1990) found that review of Medicare Part B (physician) claims for medical appropriateness resulted in a very modest number of claim denials, though some unmeasured reduction in unnecessary claims could have resulted from a "sentinel" effect.

Regarding private programs of utilization management, studies using data for the mid-1980s indicated that utilization review reduced hospital admissions by 12.3%, inpatient days by 8.0%, hospital ancillary expenditures by 14.8%, and total inpatient and outpatient expenditures by 8.3% (Wickizer 1990:355). As might be expected, these studies indicated that utilization management reduced costs more in geographic areas where use rates are relatively high. Scheffler et al.(1991) estimated that precertification and concurrent review during hospitalization reduced hospitalizations by 5.3% and reduced inpatient days by 4.2% per year in Blue Cross–Blue Shield plans nationally over 1980-88. Scheffler et al. also found that retrospective denial of payment alone reduced admissions by 2.2% per year and reduced inpatient days by 4.4% per year. Comprehensive utilization management (preadmission certification, concurrent review, and retrospective review with denial of payment) was associated with a reduction in claims costs of about 5% (about $4.5 billion per year) in the Blue Cross–Blue Shield plans studied. Khandker and Manning (1991) found that a utilization review program used by a major commercial insurer reduced inpatient claims cost by 8%.

Utilization management programs thus appear to have some effect in limiting the growth of health care costs within the U.S. health care system. However, the magnitude of the reduction in unnecessary care brought about by utilization management is in many cases disappointingly small relative to the apparent incidence of unnecessary services (e.g., Sui et al. 1986; Chassin et al. 1987). One problem with utilization review is that medicine is not a exact science; often a wide range of treatment modalities may be acceptable (e.g., Wennberg et al. 1982). Review criteria are more likely to be accepted by physicians if they are designed and controlled by physicians (Hillman 1991). In practice, the review process often is structured to give maximum latitude to the patient's physician. Generally, a treatment is classified as inappropriate only in cases when the physician reviewers regard the treatment as being clearly out of line. For most questionable cases, the physician treating a patient usually is given the benefit of the doubt. For this reason, given the current state of medical knowledge, utilization management cannot eliminate all (or even most) unnecessary or inappropriate care.

Conclusion

An overarching element in physician-patient relationships is the process through which physicians are compensated by patients or their intermediaries. Contractual arrangements entail incentives to physicians for selecting different types of treatments for patients. Different arrangements imply different types of incentives, but no contract can be devised that can induce a self-interested physician to behave in the best interest of a patient. The best empirical evidence available suggests that broad financial incentives to physicians have some effect on the level of services received by patients. Patients of physicians paid on a fee-for-service basis receive more services than those whose physicians are paid a salary, but the magnitude of the effect often is small. In making some types of clinical decisions physicians seem to exhibit a more pronounced response to more specific financial incentives, such as profit derived from referrals of patients to physician-owned ancillary services. Direct monitoring of physicians' clinical decisions (typified by third-party payers' programs of utilization management) appears to reduce the use of services deemed inappropriate, although the magnitude of the effect often seems rather modest.

Physician payment in the United States still is dominated by the fee-for-service arrangement. Although "managed care" has grown dramatically in recent years (Hoy et al. 1991), most physicians bear little financial risk for the overuse of services by their patients. Considerable attention has been given to the implications of Medicare's physician payment reform based on a resource-based relative value scale (RBRVS) for the future (e.g., Frech 1991). However, in many respects RBRVS is a very modest reform that merely substitutes a government-administered fee schedule for a historical fee profile. Aside from changing the relative rewards for different types of treatment, RBRVS does not fundamentally alter financial incentives (each physician's influence over total Part B expenditures is too trivial for the Part B expenditure ceiling to have a significant direct incentive effect). The studies reviewed in this chapter suggest that a more fundamental change in provider payment—in the direction of greater risk-sharing arrangements—would be more effective in improving patient well-being.

Notes

1. Examples of third-party payment are private health insurance and taxpayer-financed or (in a broad sense) government provision of health services. In the U.S. health care system, private employment–related health insurance and taxpayer-financed insurance are the dominant mechanisms for third-party payment.

2. An excellent overview of the theory of agency relationships is provided in Sappington (1991).

3. Of course, in the context of physician-patient relationships, it should be emphasized that neither patients nor physicians are motivated solely by incentives definable purely in terms of pecuniary rewards or penalties. Patients may wish to avoid inconvenient, painful, or risky medical treatments even if available at no direct monetary cost to them. Physicians' treatment decisions may be motivated by clinical curiosity, personal pride in their professionalism, or personal concern for the welfare of their patients. The point is that, taking these nonpecuniary incentives as given, pecuniary incentives implicit in contractual arrangements affect the interests of patients and physicians in different ways.

4. An alternative view is that the physician should act to preserve the health of the patient with little regard to the patient's preferences. This paternalistic view has fallen out of favor over the past several decades (Brock and Wartman 1990). Still another (more quixotic) view is that an "ideal" physician acts in the best interest of society to attain a just allocation of resources (Glover and Povar 1991).

5. There is no direct "disutility" effect of demand inducement for the physician in Dranove's model, but if present it would simply reinforce the patient information constraint. Dranove's model also abstracts from health insurance. If present in the model, insurance would reduce the (pecuniary) cost of care to

the patient, thereby enhancing the potential use of services because of moral hazard.

6. He finds that patient information increases with age, education, and income, and that information is greater for females than males, and greater for those in health-related occupations than those in other occupations. The patient's race, after controlling for other factors, does not affect patient information.

7. This is consistent with the notion of "shared decision making" (Brock and Wartman 1990).

8. In a purely prospective payment scheme, the lump sum payment would be full payment with no per-service compensation. In a mixed scheme, the prospectively determined lump sum payment becomes smaller as the per-service payment rate increases. The optimal per-service compensation to physicians is zero in all cases when physicians are perfect agents.

9. The term *practice style* as used here refers to a physician's tendency to recommend particular treatment modes, based on medical training, knowledge, and experience, as they affect perceived clinical benefits of treatments to the patient (independent of financial considerations).

10. The word *rewards* in this context includes both direct financial benefits and other benefits of treatment to the physician (e.g., perceived reduction in liability exposure).

11. Of course, strong nonfinancial incentives are likely to exist in this setting, such as pride of profession, a sense of duty, the approval (or disapproval) of peers, and so on. The point is that there exists no set of financial incentives that can assure that reviewing physicians reveal their true opinions.

7

Fear of Malpractice Litigation, the Risk Management Industry, and the Clinical Encounter

Ferris J. Ritchey

A malpractice claim asserts two things: 1) that a physician has injured a patient, and 2) that the injury was the result of negligence, a failure of the physician to follow acceptable standards of practice. In the United States, the number of malpractice claims has increased immensely since 1970, and physicians currently spend considerable sums on liability insurance premiums.[1] This financial emergency has created what is often called "the malpractice crisis." At a systems level, it has intensified cost inflation and reduced accessibility to care—for instance, by forcing obstetrician/gynecologists (OB/GYNs) out of rural areas where hospitals are insufficient to handle problem births (Edwards 1985; Zuckerman 1984). At an individual level, if current trends continue, nearly one in three physicians can expect to be sued at some time in a career (*Medical Economics* 1986). The economic strains of this crisis have not abated over the last two decades (U.S. General Accounting Office 1986).

By this point, a critical mass of physicians has been sued, and a collective consciousness has developed about liability issues. This collective awareness has lead to the institutionalization of "defensive medicine," under which physicians order medical tests not because medical judgment calls for testing, but because medical records may one day be scrutinized in court. The malpractice crisis also has led to a reduction in the scopes of medical specialties, more frequent refusals and referrals of patients, and early retirement of physicians. Such restrictions reflect institutional forces both inside and outside medicine that now impinge on a physician's interactions with patients, greatly reducing professional autonomy (Ritchey 1981). In addition to a greater degree of peer review, more involvement of lawyers, and increased skepticism of patients and their families, other vested interests now look in on the physician's actions. For instance, malpractice liability insurance companies retain experts in loss prevention and risk management who may scrutinize hospital records as a criterion for insurability.

The purpose of this paper is to focus on how both macro- and microlevel elements of this malpractice crisis influence the physician-patient relationship generally and the nontechnical aspects of the patient encounter in particular. Specifically: What shapes a practitioner's frame of mind about potential liability? How does the risk management industry influence the patient encounter? To what extent do physicians fear litigation, and how do they react to these fears? Are some patients more likely to be perceived as suit-prone? What physician behaviors are likely to be affected in encounters with patients? Are the malpractice avoidance strategies proposed by the risk management industry truly effective in reducing the incidence of claims? The answers to these questions reveal a number of ethical dilemmas for physicians as well as society in general.

The Risk Management Industry

To ameliorate (and perhaps to financially exploit) physicians' fears of litigation over claims of malpractice, a risk management industry has developed that has a substantial influence on the autonomy of medical practice. The workers in this "industry" include malpractice liability insurance companies, their sales agents, and their experts in loss prevention, risk reduction, and quality assurance. To minimize the number of lawsuits and encourage physicians to reduce risks, liability insurance carriers do things such as sending physicians monthly newsletters with information on recent suits and verdicts and advice on record keeping. A company may provide obstetricians with videotapes for pregnant women to view to inform them that there are "normal" risks in giving birth. These companies hold loss prevention seminars and give attending physicians discounts on insurance premiums. Teams of inspectors analyze hospital records to establish loss prevention guidelines and to identify physicians with unusual medical occurrences or high injury rates. These companies may conduct alcohol or drug screenings as a prerequisite to insurability. The influence of these risk managers on physician autonomy is great. They may deny a physician the right to practice surgery, for example, and may humiliate an older surgeon by examining his or her hands for steadiness.[2] The motivation is minimization of claims and settlement costs and maximization of company profits. In fact, these companies often are accused of exploitative profit taking (*Consumer Reports* 1986). While this charge is debatable, insurance companies clearly must seek to maintain profits through aggressive loss prevention strategies.[3]

Other workers in the risk management industry include entrepreneurs who, for substantial fees, enthusiastically counsel physicians on better patient management, and authors of such books as *Malpractice: A Guide to Avoidance and Treatment* (Brooten and Chapman 1987) and *Medical Risk Management: Preventive Legal Strategies for Health Care Providers* (Richards and Rathbun 1983). Even Melvin M. Belli, in his *Belli: For Your Malpractice Defense,* (1989) uses his experience as an attorney for plaintiff patients to advise doctors on how to avoid suits. This is a somewhat ironic role for Belli, who has fought doctors in court for decades and is notorious among them as the "King of Torts" (Belli 1989:xi).

Physicians themselves participate in collective counseling through articles published in medical journals and magazines that render common sense solutions for avoiding malpractice suits (e.g., *Ohio Medicine* 1990). The American Medical Association's Special Task Force on Liability Action attempts via office pamphlets to inform patients that results are not always as expected (Montgomery 1987). The unstated premises of the risk management industry (which is heavily populated with attorneys) are (1) that litigation, not injury, is the thing to be avoided, and (2) that lawsuits arise primarily because patients have unrealistic expectations as a result of a failure of communication (Green 1988).

Such unstated premises about the cause of litigation foster an in-group–out-group mentality among physicians toward the legal profession, as revealed in Brooten and Chapman's avoidance manual (1987:147-61). In the chapter "The Plaintiff's Attorney," the subheadings include "first salvo," "tricky phone calls," "related preliminary games," "the let's-settle-it-now ploy," "psychological warfare," "convoluted questions," "the excess [monetary] judgement threat," "personal attack," and "courtroom antics and skullduggery." Risk management counselors also foster a we-they mentality toward malcontent, "suit-prone" patients (Curran 1981). As Brooten and Chapman (1987:28) assert:

No one can predict with certainty which patients are most likely to sue for medical malpractice, but in selected patients, you can identify early signs and symptoms. There is a "malpractice prodrome," a series of telltale warning signs that should alert you that a claim may be brewing as reliably as clinical signs can foreshadow the deterioration of a condition. If you can spot them soon enough when they occur—an unexplained lack of payment, a chronic lack of compliance or poor communication—you can nip a claim before it reaches the stage where you need to notify your carrier or personal attorney.

Although there is a paucity of sound empirical evidence to substantiate the effectiveness of the risk management industry, its activities
most assuredly contribute to the collective consciousness about, and
fear of, litigation. One message it sends is that medicine must now be
practiced with legal principles in mind. This state of affairs reduces
the autonomy of physicians (Ritchey 1981) and contributes to their deprofessionalization (Haug 1988). For instance, physicians who are not
board-certified for a given type of surgery are now less likely to perform it because their liability insurance carrier will charge significantly more for such infrequent procedures. Loss of autonomy is
implied in the need for extra tests, second opinions, and referrals,
which are now often motivated by social or legal rather than medical
reasons (Ritchey 1980). A second message is that every patient is a potential legal adversary and some are especially suit-prone. That this
message is given credence implies a state of affairs that strikes at the
heart of the physician-patient relationship.

Malpractice, Medical Uncertainty, and Professional Esteem

Among the various types of liability claims, medical malpractice
claims are distinctive. When someone sues because of product liability,
the object of the suit is a large bureaucracy. The product, not a person,
is allegedly at fault. In contrast, a medical malpractice claim challenges a personal sense of competence and self-esteem, making professional life less rewarding (Shapiro et al. 1989:2193). It turns the
Hippocratic oath on its head, as the physician can no longer look to
serve the patient but must play the part of a legal adversary. At a time
when there is great distrust of institutions in American society and
growing pressures to rationalize medicine (Ritchey 1981; Ritzer and
Walczak 1988), this crisis brings to bear the most formally rational institution in society—the judicial system. Here justice is negotiated in
an adversarial context within the vagaries of tort law, the branch of
civil law that deals with disputes where contracts and consensual relations are absent (Green 1988). Within this game of strict rules but
ambiguous evidence, the goal of the patient-plaintiff's attorney will be
to manipulate evidence in such a way as to portray the physician-
defendant as incompetent, noncaring, and negligent. A generation ago
the literature on the medical profession referred to a halo effect (Simpson 1956). A malpractice claim replaces the halo with horns and as-
saults the core of a practitioner's identity by asserting a lack of
professionalism in the extreme.

Underlying the liability crisis is medical uncertainty (Weisman et
al. 1989:17). In their review of the concept of uncertainty, Gerrity et al.

(1992:1022-30) discuss several aspects of this phenomenon that inform its place in the malpractice crisis. First, they note that in preindustrial societies, witchcraft addresses the uncertainties of life through a ritual system that precisely resolves mysteries (Evans-Pritchard 1937). In reviewing the works of Douglas (1966) and Fox (1976), they describe the relationship of uncertainty to the social order and how industrialization shifts our treatment of uncertainty:

Uncertainty does not exist in the absolute but only in relation to order. The more differentiated the order, the more uncertainty appears. Conversely, uncertainty defines what is ordered and known. Elaborate rules and rituals are developed to prevent uncertainty, to minimize it, to attribute responsibility for it, and to eliminate it. In particular, we have replaced symbolic spiritualism with scientific materialism and therefore no longer "see" the symbolic role of our ideas about it. We are not even aware of our own rituals, which frame, aid, and ultimately formulate and modify experience. . . . Scientific medicine is itself a symbolic system for coping with the fears and uncertainties of medicine. [Gerrity et al. 1992:1024-25]

Thus, the symbolic system for minimizing uncertainty becomes more complex as knowledge, technology, and organization do so. The malpractice crisis complicates uncertainty further. It represents the interjection of a fundamentally different symbolic system—the legal system—with its adversarial nature. This system has its own practitioners (i.e., lawyers), whose ethical and client obligations are distinct in both ends and means. Lawyers now play a hand in the practice of medicine by influencing standards of care. Yet, significantly, lawyers can demand ideal standards, medical precision, even though they are not responsible for producing the results. From the standpoint of the physicians who must deal with uncertainty on a daily basis, the interjection of legal symbols simply adds elements of uncertainty that physicians are not trained to control. Therefore, the threat of litigation— ironically in the name of exact standards, rational science, law, and justice—inserts irrationality and ambiguity into a practice environment already saturated with uncertainty. From a practitioner's view, the process of attempting to reduce uncertainty within medicine from without simply compounds the difficulties of an already demanding job.

Regardless of the quality of treatment, a certain number of patients will in fact have adverse outcomes that raise questions of negligence. The *res ipsa loquitur* cases—those that speak for themselves, such as amputation of the wrong limb or surgery on the wrong patient—account for only a small proportion of claims however. For the majority of medical liability claims, what occurs by chance, what occurs because of patient negligence, and what is attributable to the physician's negligence are difficult to disentangle.

Figure 7.1. Medical Injuries, Negligence, and Malpractice Claims

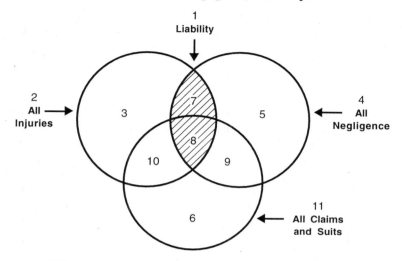

1. Liability—injuries due to negligence
2. All injuries, whether or not caused by negligence
3. Nonnegligent injuries resulting from standard procedures
4. All negligent conduct, whether or not injury occurred
5. Negligence not resulting in injury
6. Malpractice claims and suits not justified by injury or negligence
7. Negligent injuries for which no claims are filed
8. Negligent injuries for which claims are filed
9. Claims filed for negligence in the absence of injury
10. Claims filed for injuries in the absence of   negligence
11. All malpractice claims and suits

Source: U.S. Department of Health, Education, and Welfare, *Medical Malpractice,* 1973.

Note: This figure cannot be reasonably drawn to scale because what constitute injury, negligence, and negligent injury are uncertain and normative (i.e., dependent on cultural context, time, and place). For instance, for hundreds of years "bleeding" was not considered negligent but rather the "best technology" of the time. Furthermore, as Meyers (1987) shows, the lack of strong correspondence between "objective" assessments of injury and patients' subjective assessments reveal many injuries go unreported and many foreseeable, nonnegligent injuries to be perceived by patients as caused by negligence.

Relationship of Injuries to Claims

The relationship between liability, injury, negligence, and malpractice claims and suits is quite complex and reflects the uncertainty of medical practice (fig.7.1). True liability is negligent injury (area 1, fig.7.1). But not all iatrogenic injuries (circle 2) are due to negligence; nonnegligent injuries (area 3) are a normal part of medical practice, most evident in the scars and pain that accompany surgery. Arguably, negligence (circle 4) is quite common, although it often goes undetected (area 5) when adverse effects cannot be distinguished from the normal course of disease (Annandale 1989:9). The uncertainty of medical treatments and the legal and social components of the malpractice

claims process result in many claims that lack true injury or true negligence (area 6) and in much negligent injury for which no claims are
made (area 7) (see Meyers 1987:1546). Area 8 represents a claim of
malpractice liability for the situation of true injury and true negligence. But a claim may be filed also in the absence of injury (area 9),
or in the absence of negligence (area 10).

Whether or not to file a claim is itself a complex decision. Meyers
(1987:1546) shows that many patients who perceive themselves to
have been injured may not discuss this with a lawyer because the
event is not serious, the harm is seen as unintentional, the patient
does not like or cannot afford lawyers, the prospects of winning a suit
are seen as dim, or the patient is simply not the suing type. He found
that only 3% of patients discuss their injuries with a lawyer, and that
the likelihood of doing so is not strongly related to the seriousness of
the injury. In other words, social-emotional and financial conditions
equal or exceed biomedical conditions in their influence on whether a
claim is filed.

If an injured party consults an attorney and the attorney sees
merit in pursuing a claim, other factors—social, financial, judicial,
ethical—come into play and make the determination of true injury,
true negligence, and just compensation an even more complicated issue. Danzon (1985:33-37) shows that the disposition of a claim depends on assessments of the probability of plaintiff verdict, the
monetary size of the claim, and the costs of litigation, and that these
factors are not always determined by the severity and permanence of
injury. Danzon (1985:19-32) examined the relationship of injuries,
claims, and settlements using 1974 data from 23 California hospitals,
supplemented by matching aggregate claims data from the National
Association of Insurance Commissioners. Danzon's analysis provides
estimates of iatrogenic injuries occurring in hospitals, the proportion
due to negligence, the share of such injuries resulting in claims, and
the dispositions of claims. Extrapolating from Danzon's proportions,
figure 7.2 portrays the relationship among these events. Her most
striking findings are: (1) there is less than a 1% chance that a patient
admitted to a hospital will suffer iatrogenic injury due to physician
negligence, and only about 10% of such injuries will result in a malpractice claim; (2) of these claims, nearly half will be settled in the
physician's favor (i.e., dropped without payment or favorable trial verdict); (3) fewer than one in 10 claims (7.5%) reach a trial verdict, and
only about one-fourth (28%) of these are settled in the patient's favor.
Noting that her data did not account for undetected iatrogenic injuries
and those outside the hospital, Danzon (1985:24) concludes that "at
most one in 25 negligent injuries resulted in compensation through
the malpractice system." She also estimated that 15% of all malprac-

Figure 7.2. Disposition of Malpractice Claims

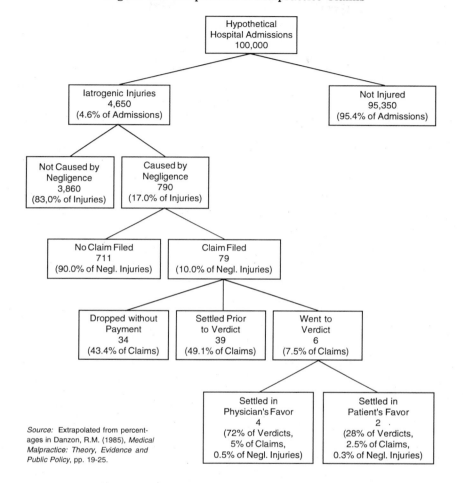

Source: Extrapolated from percentages in Danzon, R.M. (1985), *Medical Malpractice: Theory, Evidence and Public Policy*, pp. 19-25.

tice claims involved emotional injury only, but she lacked data on the dispositions of these cases.

An Epidemic of Injuries or of Litigation?

Irrespective of Danzon's evidence that only a small fraction of negligent injuries result in litigation, data from physician surveys and anecdotal accounts reveal that physicians see the legal system, not negligence, as the problem (Shapiro et al. 1989:2192). They fear that in a trial setting the patient-plaintiff's lawyer will present expert testimony as though medicine were an exact science. The jury will be comprised not of professional peers, but of ordinary citizens who, rightly so, are influenced by societal and human values. Physicians perceive that in court an act of God may be misconstrued as an act of negligence, and this possibility is a major consideration in deciding whether a malpractice claim should be settled out of court.

It is in this atmosphere, where uncertainty of law compounds the effects of medical uncertainty, that physicians now practice. In the mid-1960s, medical journals began reporting testaments (editorials, letters to the editor), and studies about the trauma of going through the protracted, two- to five-year legal process of malpractice claims. For example, after 1960 there was a tremendous increase in the number of articles from the *Journal of the American Medical Association* that were indexed under the heading "malpractice." The malpractice claims process clearly takes a toll on affected physicians. It has been compared to Kübler-Ross's (1969) five stages of grief over death (Lavery 1988). Research on a Chicago sample of 154 physicians who had been sued found that over half experienced anger, depressed mood, frustration, and irritability, and 40% experienced insomnia and fatigue (Charles et al. 1984, 1985). Yet the anger of these physicians tended to be aimed at lawyers and the legal process rather than at patients.

How Risk Management Affects the Patient Encounter

Assuming that most physicians become sensitive to the threat of litigation because of increases in liability insurance premiums, or because of the consciousness-raising activities of risk management counselors and colleagues, what is it that the risk managers recommend? Using physician role-task dimensions popularized by Freidson (1970a), table 7.1 summarizes risk management techniques from a number of sources, sorted along the analytical dimensions of the physician-patient encounter.

First, when one considers the cognitive, technical-therapy aspects of the physician's role, the practice of defensive medicine stands out. The significance of the great increase in defensive medicine is that once a critical mass of physicians adopts such procedures, they are accepted as standards. Furthermore, during the malpractice crisis the basis for establishing whether a physician-defendant fails to follow acceptable standards of practice has shifted from the individual locality to the national level (DHEW 1973:36). This change means that the patient-plaintiff's attorney can hire expert witnesses from outside the local community—witnesses not likely to be friends or acquaintances of the physician-defendant. Such nationwide standardization

7.1. Behavior Modifications Advised by the Risk Management Industry to Avoid Malpractice Suits

Physician's role	Physician's behavior modifications

I. Cognitive, technical-therapy tasks

Physician's role	Physician's behavior modifications
A. Observation, testing, therapy decisions	1. Practice defensive medicine: order tests for legal, not medical, reasons. 2. Limit physician assistants' and nurses' roles in diagnostic and treatment decisions.

B. Information transfer ("what is said")	1. Physician-patient orientation
	  a. Fully inform patient (mutual participation model often recommended).
	  b. Avoid creating unrealistic expectations.
	2. Quantity
	  a. Provide sufficient information.
	  b. Allow plenty of time for discussion.
	3. Mode of transfer
	  a. Use written and audiovisual methods in addition to verbal.
	  b. Use open-ended questions.
	  c. Be very specific in stating expectations of patient health behavior.
	  d. Summarize at end of encounter.
	  e. Provide patient with written diagnosis and a list of treatment instructions.

C. Obtaining informed consent	1. Rely on hospital's legal department for general consent forms, but also verbally inform patient of detailed plan of treatment, alternatives, potential risks, and complications. 2. In office practice, do not leave informed-consent responsibilities to nonphysicians. 3. Inform patient even when risk is statistically low but untoward results might be extremely severe. 4. Make consent process more detailed as procedures become more elective.
D. Solicitation of patient input on treatment alternatives	1. Use the mutual participation model. 2. Use open-ended questions. 3. Listen patiently and carefully.

7.1. Continued

II. Patient-management tasks ("how things are said")	

E. Affect: dealing with patient feelings, emotions, and evaluations of care; physician affability	1. Personalization: *caring* about the patient
	  a. Spend plenty of time with the patient and family; do not appear hurried.
	  b. Focus comments on patient, not disease; touch the place that hurts.
	  c. Provide patient with reassurance and positive feedback.
	  d. Give patient psychological support, a sense of accomplishment or satisfaction.
	  e. Show remorse for any negative outcome.
	  f. Use social statements and questions to establish rapport.
	  g. Involve the patient's family.
	2. Style of communication
	  a. Communicate caring and concern in nonverbal ways.
	  b. Avoid interruptions.
	  c. Avoid long silence.
	3. Staff
	  a. Employ a compassionate and friendly staff.
	  b. Train staff to recognize and anticipate problems.

F. Dominance: asserting physician authority to encourage patient compliance	1. Avoid medical jargon. Use appropriate level of vocabulary. 2. Do not appear too businesslike. 3. Avoid threatening the patient's self-esteem or sense of control when questioning. 4. In the event of unanticipated treatment complications, immediately tell the patient the facts, but do not say, "I made a mistake." 5. React to hostile patients with calm; offer to refer them. 6. If patient refuses treatment, obtain a signed release from liability for self and staff.
G. Convenience	1. Avoid delays in consultation. 2. Follow up on broken appointments.
H. Coordination of care from other physicians	1. Maintain contact with patients who have been referred. 2. Give patient notice if colleague is to substitute for you.

3. Do not refer a patient to a doctor rumored to be incompetent because of age or alcoholism.

4. Document differences of opinion with consulting physician.

5. Avoid showing support for patients who disparage a previously seen physician.

III. Clerical tasks

I. Maintenance of patient's technical record	1. Document a thorough history, physical exam, and any clinical problems encountered.
	2. Provide a written treatment plan.
	3. Specify and document medication doses and possible side effects.
	4. Record not only information given, but also patient response.
	5. Never alter record once a malpractice claim is made.
	6. Do not allow staff to record abnormalities in the patient record.
J. Maintenance of business and patient health insurance forms	1. Staff should assist patient with insurance forms even if fee already has been paid.
	2. Take side of patient in fee disputes with health insurance companies.
	3. Offer patients scheduled fee payment plans.
	4. Do not press overdue bill collections for "angry" patients without reviewing results of treatment with personal malpractice defense attorney to assess potential liability.
	5. Do not sue a patient for fees owed until the statute of limitations for malpractice has expired.

IV. Special circumstances and cases requiring extensive risk management techniques

1. The hospital emergency room

2. Writing "do not resuscitate " orders for terminally ill patients

3. Prescribing medication, especially for critical care patients

4. Discharging patients under pressure of diagnostic-related-groups payment plans

5. Hospital transfers

6. Informed consent for surgical procedures

7. Medical experimentation

8. High-risk cases such as birth delivery and neurological surgery

Sources: Brooten and Chapman 1987; Valente et al. 1988; Adamson et al. 1989; Applegate 1986; Bartlett 1990; Belli 1989; Geyman 1985; Green 1988; Griffith 1985; Hirsch et al. 1987; Richards and Rathbun 1983; Rubin 1978; Sommers 1985.

constitutes informal regulation and significantly reduces physician autonomy (Ritchey 1981).

Defensive medicine also includes making sure that patients receive full and accurate information so that they will not develop unrealistic expectations (Green 1988). Much of the emphasis here is on informed consent. Harrison et al. (1985) propose that this concept is central to malpractice law, and interaction in the patient encounter thus becomes a starting point for malpractice prevention. The literature stresses that physicians should become oriented to the mutual participation model of Szasz and Hollander (1956), which emphasizes an egalitarian relationship, and that they should view medicine as a process of mutual discovery (Applegate 1986). Much of this advice has to do with proper attention to formal consent documents, as well as modes of soliciting and providing information. The mere quantity of information conveyed to the patient is seen as critical, and sufficient time spent with the patient is thus important (Adamson et al. 1989; Waitzkin 1990). Issues of informed consent present special problems since, as Gutheil et al. (1984:51) advise, physicians must "wean the patient from the fantasy of certainty," yet avoid making him or her feel helpless by doing so. Obtaining patient input on treatment alternatives after informing patients of variable risks of injuries is seen as a way to share liability for adverse outcomes of treatment.

The second dimension of the physician's role is the task of case management. Part of this has to do with affect—feelings and emotion. Modern medicine has long been criticized for its focus on the disease instead of the patient (Reiser 1978). Caring and effective communication are purported to be the key factors here. The implied theory is that an affable, trusting relationship and effective communication will intervene between poor medical outcome and a patient's decision to file a malpractice claim. The quality of the relationship prior to any injury may be the key factor in what happens after an injury.

Physicians accept even avoidable injuries as having a certain probability of occurrence because of human limitations (Bosk 1979). The literature of risk management suggests what to do when patients are dissatisfied with outcomes. One suggestion is that the physician show remorse, but there is an interesting contradiction in this recommendation. As Danzon shows (1985:22), only one of twenty-five injuries results in claims. This is partly because about 60 percent of all injuries heal within a month and do not cause long-term disabilities—the evidence disappears. Unless negligence is extremely obvious, it would behoove the physician to portray such injuries as the normal course of events. Would not a "premature" show of remorse possibly be interpreted as an admission of guilt (i.e., negligence) and encourage the patient to consider filing a malpractice claim? How physicians deal with these situations raises potentially ethical problems (which are discussed later).

Patient management also has to do with social distance and education differences between physician and patient and how such gaps affect the authority and dominance of the physician. A physician may appear too dominant by letting technical language make the patient feel inadequate—reputedly a common communication failure. Risk managers also advise the full participation of the patient's family and informal caregivers. Patient management in modern American society also must consider convenience and factors such as ease of obtaining appointments, time spent in waiting rooms, and facilitation of health insurance claims.

The fragmented nature of medical care delivery today, one of the elements that results in an impersonal client relationship, leads risk managers to offer plenty of advice on coordinating patient care among diverse specialist-consultants. Their advice includes cautions about how consultant actions may lead to malpractice lawsuits, thus implying that there is yet another category of people of whom to be wary.

The third dimension of medical practice is clerical. Much attention has been paid to this area because written records make for good evidence in a trial. Recommendations include keeping thorough records of patient behaviors and comments as well as detailed records of consultant behavior. Recommendations abound also on how to avoid angering patients over the matter of fee payment, and such advice often implies that patients' greed and fiscal irresponsibility are at the root of the malpractice problem. Finally, the risk management literature is replete with advice on statistically risky cases ("Special circumstances," table 7.1).

A focus on the patient encounter raises several questions: Which physicians are more fearful of litigation? Which patients are more likely to be perceived as suit-prone? How do physicians react to them?

The physicians expected to be more fearful of litigation include those in medical specialties that incur more injury, or in which adverse outcomes are endemic to treatment (Langwell and Werner 1981:235). Neurosurgeons and OB/GYNs are cases in point. Social and circumstantial factors related to status may also determine whether a physician is fearful of being sued.

Stereotypes of the Suit-Prone Patient

The risk-management industry tends to focus on avoiding litigation rather than on preventing injury, and then proceeds to search out potential malpractice litigants (Annandale 1989). This hunt for "the enemy" encourages the formation of stereotypes for the "suit-prone" patient. Even in a publication as astute as the *New England Journal of Medicine,* one finds explicit references to patient stereotypes. For instance, in a discussion of stressors that affect physician practice, McCue (1982) seems to take stereotypes for granted and attributes the "problem" behavior of patients to mental illness: "The stereotypes of 'clingers,' 'demanders,' 'help-rejectors,' and 'deniers' are familiar to all physicians. They elicit anger, avoidance, fear, and despair. The biomedical model fits these patients poorly, since they cannot or will not get better. Most problem patients have important psychiatric disorders, which are at the basis of their frustrating interactions with physicians" (McCue 1982:460).

Similarly, malpractice counselors use vague terms that denote shared stereotypes, presumably to better communicate risk avoidance instructions by appealing to physicians' fears and angers concerning the malpractice crisis. For example, Brooten and Chapman (1987:29-32, 115) cite a list of problem patients: "the shopper," "the reluctant payer," "the expert . . . inspired no doubt by Ralph Nader . . . [who] will even try to set traps for [the physician]" (p.31), "the patient who fails to comply," "the nester . . . perhaps the most litigation-prone bird of the species," and "the emotionally disturbed patient." Melvin Belli (1989:19-57) has his own list of problem patients, which he derives from his experience as attorney for both plaintiffs and defendants: "the secret grumbler," who complains to the staff but not directly to the doctor; "the complainer"; "the malingerers"; "the cynics"; "the grievers"; and "the consumerists."

If there is any circumstance that would lead a person to rely on stereotypes, the fear of litigation fits the bill. In 1976, at the height of the original malpractice crisis, I conducted a mailed survey of general and family practitioners in Austin, Texas, to identify physicians who were at the extremes of possible attitudes toward the prospects of being sued for malpractice—feeling either highly threatened or not threatened at all (Ritchey 1979, 1980; Annandale 1989). Subsequently I conducted in-depth interviews among these two groups to determine what distinguished them. All respondents tended to have stereotypes about the "suit-proneness" of patients (which, incidentally, did not correspond to their actual claims experience):

(1) Unfamiliar patients were suspect until the physician felt that a trusting relationship had developed. The physician's age and its relationship to the stability of the practice clientele was an important aspect of developing trust; thus, young physicians with open-door practices were especially fearful. Nonthreatened physicians asserted that their main reason for lack of fear was that they either took no new patients or took only those with familial relations to existing clientele.

(2) Patients with legal connections were suspect: lawyers, their families, patients with pending automobile insurance claims or workers' compensation claims. The reasoning was: If this person will sue someone else, what's to stop them from suing me?

(3) Patients who joked about malpractice set off alarms.

(4) Another category of suit-prone patient included those with personality quirks. Physicians expressed deep concern about dealing with patients who appeared to be looking for something other than a stable relationship with a physician, especially "doctor shoppers," who go from one doctor to another in search of a diagnosis for nondescript symptoms.

(5) When the physicians were asked to stipulate demographic correlates with suit proneness, some political and social class biases were evident. Blue-collar, high school–educated patients were described as more likely to sue. As one respondent put it: "These guys always want something for nothing and are educated just enough to know how to manipulate the legal system." Political ideology was evident when respondents were asked what they thought had caused the malpractice crisis. They made references to liberalism, Naderism, a "gimme" society, the Democratic party, and Massachusetts Senator Ted Kennedy, a long-time proponent of greater government involvement in health care. In general, they saw the malpractice crisis as merely one of a large number of social and political processes that diminish the physician's control over medical practice.

Notwithstanding the physicians' expressions of worry about suit-prone patients, when asked what percentage of their patients fit this category the responses ranged from zero to 5%. At the time of that study, in other words, a collective fear by the medical profession was stoked by a perceptibly small proportion of patients. The proportion of patients perceived as suit-prone today must surely have increased.

Inaccuracy of Stereotypes

How accurate are these stereotypes? The ideological link between stereotypes of suit-prone patients and the perceived cause of the malpractice crisis (Ritchey 1979) suggests that responses to fear may be arbitrary and thus a form of misplaced discrimination. In fact, in contrast to my finding that physicians believe young, male, blue-collar workers are more suit-prone, Doherty and Haven's (1977) analysis of claims data of the same period found the facts to be the opposite. It was older, white-collar workers who actually filed more claims. Similarly, Langwell and Werner (1981), in comparing geographic incidence of suits and defensive medicine, found no relationship between physicians' likelihood of being sued and the ordering of extra tests. Brook and Williams (1978:847), in summarizing the evidence from National Association of Insurance Commissioners data, note: "The word 'malpractice' has come to be emotionally charged. Nonetheless, if the issue is approached scientifically, certain important facts emerge. For example, malpractice claims are almost always rooted in medical injury and poor practice; they are not often produced by the whim of an hysterical person. No more than about 5% of all incidents that would result in favorable legal decision to the person are actually brought to litigation."

Differential Treatment Based on Fear of Lawsuits

To explore the specifics of how the patient encounter might be affected by fear of litigation, I asked my sample of general practitioners whether they treated suit-prone patients differently from others. A typical response was risk avoidance behavior—screening out those patients perceived as suit-prone, or quickly referring them to specialists. Unknown prospective patients who "sounded squirrelly over the phone," as one doctor put it, would be told that the doctor does not take new patients. Another physician turned away what he called the "gimme society" types and "cedar choppers" by requiring an expensive initial examination. (He explained that cedar choppers were people so ignorant that the only way they could make a living was by cedar tree timbering). Another typical reaction of Austin physicians was to be reticent with threatening patients. This behavior contradicts all of the literature on nurturing effective communication. A further reaction was to keep more thorough patient records. (This corresponded to Zuckerman's (1984) finding that 57% of physicians were augmenting patient records in response to the threat of litigation). Finally, nurses were often called in to witness visits with threatening patients.

Studies conducted since my own are consistent with my findings. Weisman et al. (1989) surveyed family and/or general practitioners, internal medicine specialists, and OB/GYNs to ascertain whether they had made changes in their medical practices and procedures because of the "malpractice climate." These authors identified both risk reduction and risk avoidance behaviors. The risk reduction behavior took two forms: 1) provision of additional services and 2) improvements in communication and record keeping. Risk avoidance behavior involved cutting back on certain services and avoiding high-risk patients and circumstances. Risk reduction strategies were more common than risk avoidance strategies among the three specialty groups, but the findings for patient screening (risk avoidance) by OB/GYNs were striking:

49.3% "cut back on the number of high-risk patients treated." Similarly, Langwell and Werner (1981) found that upwards of 30% of physicians in a national sample refused certain medical cases. A risk reduction strategy akin to avoidance was referral to, and more frequent consultations with, other physicians. Weisman et al. (1989) found that 55.2% of OB/GYNs used more consultations, and Zuckerman (1984) found that 44.8% of his sample made more referrals.

Walker, Broyles, and Furrow (1990) found evidence that once a patient files a malpractice claim, the patient is likely to be viewed as an adversary, worthy only of abandonment. In a survey, they presented physicians with a hypothetical case study of an elderly patient who had a malpractice claim pending against a physician but who nonetheless was requesting further care. More than 80% of respondents would refuse such a patient further treatment, and the majority of the refusers (61.3%) saw no obligation to even refer to another physician. The authors point out that such situations have great bearing on accessibility to medical care, especially in rural areas.

Malpractice Claims: The View from Both Sides

Another approach to understanding the dynamics of fear of litigation in the patient encounter is to look at the disparate views physician-defendants and patient-plaintiffs have about their relationships prior to a lawsuit as Shapiro et al. (1989) did; their study included a comparison group of nonsued physicians. Table 7.2 lists some of the differences they found in the perceived reasons for litigation. Perhaps too predictably, sued physicians tend to blame the patients and vice versa, and nonsued physicians spread the blame around. For example, suing patients attribute malpractice claims to physician error and negligence, while sued physicians blame patients' desires for financial compensation and poor patient health behavior. Nonsued physicians tend to have a more abstract notion of reasons for litigation. For example, 75% of them assume personal conflicts must cause litigation, but only 11% of sued physicians and their patients cited this factor.

Shapiro et al. (1989) also found differences in physicians' and patients' suggestions for reducing litigation (table 7.3). Patients see the solution in terms of professional accountability. In sharp contrast, a majority of physicians suggested changing the legal (tort) system. A substantial percentage of both groups see better physician-patient communication as important in reducing litigation.

Shapiro et al. (1989:2192) found additional disparities in the views of sued physicians and their suing patients about the affective dimension—trust and honesty in their relationship—prior to the malpractice

Table 7.2. Perceived Reasons for Malpractice Action

Cause	% of suing patients	% of sued physicians	% of nonsued physicians
Physician blamed			
1. Physician error	96	20	66
2. Physician negligence	97	10	51
3. Physician's failure to pursue pertinent health history	22	8	29
Patient blamed			
4. Patient's desire for financial compensation	22	83	85
5. Need to place responsibility for injury	41	66	85
6. People expect too much from medical technology and/or the physician	3	44	95
7. Physician's directions were not followed	0	23	44
8. Patient withholds pertinent health information	3	16	20
Other			
9. Unanticipated complications	64	52	86
10. Unavoidable consequences of medical treatment	34	39	66
11. Physician/patient personal conflicts	11	11	75

Source: Shapiro, Robin S., et al. 1989, "A Survey of Sued and Nonsued Physicians and Suing Patients," *Archives of Internal Medicine* 149: 2192.

claim. Around 70% of the physicians felt that their relationships with patients were honest and open, while only 40% of their patients felt so. And while 70% of both groups agreed that patients hold physicians in high respect, only 45% of patients agreed that physicians held them in high respect. These findings reveal the stark differences in professional and lay cultures regarding medicine, physician competence, and patient satisfaction.

Are Risk Managers on the Mark?

This analysis of the risk management industry suggests that its advice is not based on scientific or even rough statistical evidence. Thus, the industry may not be providing useful information and may, in fact,

Table 7.3. Evaluations of Proposals to Reduce Malpractice Litigation

Proposals	"Very effective"		
	% of suing patients	% of sued physicians	% of nonsued physicians
Physician accountability			
1. Enhance peer review	61	15	10
2. Give more disciplinary power to state medical examining board	79	19	38
3. Increase government involvement	28	2	3
Changes in tort system			
4. Eliminate the contingency fee arrangement	32	79	70
5. Limit noneconomic damages	15	58	76
6. Encourage alternative dispute resolution mechanisms	35	35	30
Other			
7. Improve doctor/patient communication	65	63	62

Source: Shapiro, Robin S., et al. 1989, "A Survey of Sued and Nonsued Physicians and Suing Patients," *Archives of Internal Medicine* 149: 2194.

exacerbate fear and prejudices that could lead to poorer patient care. For instance, stereotypes of the suit-prone patient appear not to be referenced to true risk, but rather to prejudices and fear. Additional skepticism comes from the pervasive notion that a breakdown in communication, not the quality of technical care, is the cause of liability claims. While this recurring theme is an underlying assumption of most editorials about the malpractice crisis and most case studies of sued physicians, the evidence is not conclusive.

The question arises, then: Why do both physicians and patients see better communication as important in reducing litigation? Perhaps it is because it is at this level of direct contact that human beings believe that they can influence the course of one another's behaviors. But when cooperation fails in direct interaction, the result is extremely painful and stressful. It is no surprise then that risk managers emphasize communication. Their advice may not ultimately reduce litigation, especially when anticipated severe injuries occur. But the risk management industry's advice is aimed at reducing physician anxiety and restoring the practitioner's sense of control over the prospects of malpractice claims. Although the ultimate interest of risk managers is loss prevention, and not expressly to encourage physicians to emphasize the "caring" aspects of practice, an unintended consequence may be higher patient satisfaction and perhaps better medical care (Annandale 1989:7-10), two empirical questions that offer researchers a challenge.

Future Research

There is a scarcity of sound research on how the nature of the physician-patient relationship, including communication, averts litigation. Moreover, the existing research has many limitations that call for further investigation. First, studies of communication fail to utilize data (such as Danzon's 1985) that control for the severity of injury. The filing, pursuit, and termination of a malpractice claim is susceptible to a type of triage based on severity of injury, cost of litigation, and assessed risk of a finding of negligence (Danzon 1985:31). For example, blatant-negligence suits, the *res ipsa loquitur* cases, are much more likely to be settled prior to verdict, as are cases in which the cost of damages is low relative to the cost of litigation. The most troublesome litigation involves high-cost severe injury or death in which the issue of negligence is disputable. Similarly, it is reasonable to hypothesize that physicians' fears of litigation vary according to perceptions of the likelihood of medical mistakes and patient injury. Perhaps the relationship between risk and reactions to fear of litigation is nonlinear: those physicians with little risk of incurred injury or establishable negligence may see no point in adjusting their practices. Likewise, those who face extreme likelihood of patient injury, adverse outcomes, and lawsuits because of the nature of their practice—e.g., neurosurgeons—may have limited options in adjusting their practices to reduce the fear of litigation. Physicians between these extremes may be more likely to practice defensively because they experience greater uncertainty. In any case, future research on fear of litigation needs greater control of these factors.

A second limitation in research is that studies of communication fail to precisely distinguish affect from information transfer. On the one hand, physicians and patients alike agree that communication is important for reducing lawsuits, yet sued physicians and their suing patients do not see personal conflict as a reason for litigation (Shapiro et al. 1989). In fact, the research in this area does not take advantage of sociological and communications theory and conceptualization (Northouse and Northouse 1985; Waitzkin 1990). The existing data appear most valid for the information transfer dimension of medical practice; they provide little precise advice on patient management, and much of the advice is contradictory.

A third shortcoming of research is its narrow focus on physicians and patients. As the population ages, family members increasingly assume caregiver roles. Meyers (1987) shows, however, that most patient communications about perceived injuries take place within the informal network of the family; less than half of his sample mentioned their concerns to a health care provider at any time. The effectiveness of physicians' communication with informal care providers and the influence of these elements on the likelihood of litigation need further investigation.

Similarly, more research is needed on the interpersonal relationships of lawyers, the formal and informal aspects of the claims settlement process, and how the intentionally adversarial relationship of litigation bleeds over into the more informal physician-patient relationship. Lawyers tend to bring legal solutions that are merely ideal and that fall short in practice. For instance, some legal advisers in the area of risk management have gone so far as to propose a transition from tort to contract law, as though the uncertainties of medical practice may indeed be accurately appraised (Green 1988).

Another question that has not been substantially researched but that has implications of ultimate importance is: What effects do physicians' adjustments to litigation anxiety have on the quality and accessibility of medical care? This ethical issue has been raised many times in the past (Somers 1977; Danzon 1985; Annandale 1989), yet it is obscured in the literature by the view that the malpractice crisis is merely a legal and economic issue.

Finally, in the past two decades, the tremendous changes in health care have greatly reduced professional control and autonomy (Haug 1988; Light and Levine 1988; McKinlay 1988; Ritzer 1988; Starr 1982; Stoeckle 1988; Wolinsky 1988). There is increased government involvement (Ruggie 1992), new elites have entered the arena (Imershein et al. 1992), and boundary disputes have divided health professionals (Abbott 1988; Halpern 1992). While research in such areas is abundant, very little of it has focused on how increased litigation has played a role in change. Looking at social change in medicine over the past two centuries, it may be argued that a key process is the formal rationalization of its organization in response to technological change and the legitimation of science; yet this process was retarded by medicine's professional power (Ritchey 1981). In the 1960s, the increase in malpractice litigation, along with Medicare and Medicaid legislation, signaled a "baby boomer" cohort effect that was particularly powerful in accelerating change in all arenas of medical practice. These changes undermined professional autonomy in fundamental ways. More recent changes, such as corporate management and cost containment, would not have been conceivable in an earlier cultural context. It is this author's belief that the effects of the malpractice crisis have been grossly underestimated because they are not the result of overt policies. More research in the "sociology of medicine" vein is needed on the consequences of this crisis for professionalism at both micro and macro levels.

Ethical Dilemmas

The malpractice crisis and its impact on the physician-patient relationship raise a number of ethical questions. First, the crisis clearly poses special problems for the healer-patient relationship. This particularly personal alliance, believed to be most efficacious for healing when there is strong agreement between parties, can turn into an anxiety-producing adversarial relationship. La Puma and Schiedermayer (1989:414) note that "perceived legal obligations can distort a physicians's clinical judgement." In their adjustments to the threat of litigation and the uncertainty it adds to medical practice, physicians often appear to assess the suit-proneness of patients using stereotypical criteria (Hershey 1982). Annandale (1989:13) observes the contradictions in the risk prevention literature. On the one hand, taxonomies of problem patients portray medical clientele as an out-group. On the other, recommendations abound about how to better include the patient in the care process, an in-group notion. Annandale notes that, in addition to the ethical implications of social discrimination, stereotypes are "problematic for physicians because they violate the very reforms that they are attempting to make in the doctor-patient relationship." Should physicians, then, be educated to avoid stereotyping patients? One is, of course, inclined to say yes, but can physicians ultimately be expected to behave differently from the rest of us when encountering a perceived threat?

Second, an ethical dilemma ensues when a physician makes "an honest mistake" that results in mild injury. It would behoove the physician to portray such injuries as the normal course of events by not fully informing the patient. Aside from the obvious matter of honesty, such actions fly in the face of the advice of most risk managers. Moreover, if the injury worsens, lack of disclosure could encourage the patient to consider a claim when otherwise no such possibility would have arisen. Such a dilemma highlights the complexities with which physicians must deal—making decisions while attempting to resolve often contradictory sociolegal and professional norms with the realities of medical uncertainty.

Third, given the complexity and uncertainty of medicine, can we expect physicians to police themselves by removing any but the most obviously incompetent of their number? Practicing physicians who must deal daily with medical uncertainty are likely to believe in the ethic of "forgive and remember"—overlook the occasional technical failure with the proviso that every effort will be made to prevent a reoccurrence. Errors in technique, often due merely to limitations in the state of knowledge, are seen as less culpable than are errors in moral conduct (Bosk 1979). On the other hand, if medicine fails to police itself, is the tort system the solution to compensation and is it an effective deterrent to negligence? What are the unintended consequences of technical medicine being constrained by legal as well as medical ethics and norms? The great influence of external agencies on professional practice is a sign of deprofessionalization and a loss of autonomy, requiring practitioners to adhere to externally created norms that demand idealistic certainties. Deprofessionalization potentially leads to deethicalization. That is to say, as physicians lose professional privileges, can we not expect them to forsake professional obligations by placing self-interests ahead of those of the patient? Put another way, since it is the state of the larger culture and its value system that defines ethics, how can we expect the ethics of these role players to be different from ours? The malpractice crisis may cause physician-patient relations to become even more impersonal. In so doing, the crisis may simply be a reflection of just how impersonal and formal relationships tend to be in a modern industrial society.

Fourth, given that the malpractice issue seems to be perceived as a crisis only when high insurance premiums create financial problems for physicians or insurance companies (Somers 1977), some have questioned whether we have missed the true crisis—a high incidence of perceived or real iatrogenic injuries and an insufficient and inefficient system of compensation. As Meyers (1987:1548) notes: "Medical malpractice litigation is the expression of deep and highly complicated problems, which cannot be solved or even significantly alleviated by false solutions motivated only by concerns of costs and cost containment." Annandale (1989:15) observes that the risk prevention industry's focus on manipulating patient interaction is a reductivist approach, and a rather covert way for the profession to protect its power, authority, and interests by shifting attention away from the need for financial and organizational reform of the health care system. But can reform of the system occur within the private sector?

Given that the liability crisis aggravates cost and accessibility problems in our health care system, should government get more involved in reducing its effects? Put in concrete terms, what of justice in a system of compensation that, irrespective of liability, leaves much iatrogenic injury uncompensated, while some plaintiffs receive exorbitant monetary awards? Danzon (1987:7) questions the underlying assumptions of American society's approach to medical injury by noting: "A negligence-based form of liability makes sense only if it is performing some additional function in terms of reducing the incidence of negligent injuries. It cannot be justified as a system of compensation." And Schwartz (1976) raised this issue in proposing a no-fault compensation system in conjunction with a national health insurance program.

Notwithstanding the deficiencies of the American system of dealing with medical malpractice, there are no easy solutions. In a pluralistic, capitalist society, it is difficult to challenge the legitimacy of profit taking in health care as evidenced, for example, in the increasing "corporatization" of medical services (Stoeckle 1988). In these days of frequent litigation, is it not reasonable to expect lawyers and insurance companies to maximize their profits, and physicians to pass along the costs? These ethical dilemmas reveal that the malpractice crisis is pure Americana. It involves competing individual interests that often strain the collective welfare. Like so many of our social problems, it defies easy solution.

Notes

1. The focus of this paper is on the United States. Other industrialized countries are also experiencing increases in patient complaints making the findings of this research somewhat generalizable to Western industrial countries. However, in the United States, medical complaints are much more likely to be handled through formal mechanisms involving third parties, especially within the legal torts system. Many other countries utilize alternative mechanisms that reflect greater government control over medical services, greater cooperation between health providers and the government, and relatively fewer lawyers. For example, in Great Britain patient complaints are successfully dealt with through professional regulatory mechanisms, and in Sweden, through no-fault insurance (Rosenthal 1988). An underlying assumption of this paper is that the U.S. experience is quite distinct.

2. This information was provided by Paul Lawrence, a former agent of the liability insurance company that insures 65% of Alabama physicians.

3. Insurance carriers' profits are determined by gains on investment as well as premium charges, with poor gains often leading to higher premium charges. Thus, the health of the industry is influenced by economic cycles. (See Danzon 1987.)

Communicating with
Patients and Caregivers

8

Incomplete Narratives of Aging and Social Problems in Routine Medical Encounters

Howard Waitzkin, Theron Britt, and Constance Williams

When older people talk with doctors, their conversations often touch on social problems. Bereavement, financial insecurity, isolation, dependency, inadequate housing, lack of transportation, and similar issues cause difficulties for the elderly. In some cases, patients or doctors raise these issues directly. Alternatively, such problems may surface indirectly, in passing, or marginally, as doctors and patients focus on technical concerns.

The appearance of social problems within medical encounters poses a challenge for researchers and practitioners. Certain geriatric programs use multidisciplinary teams, including social workers, to help resolve problems that derive from the social context of medicine; to some extent, these interventions can improve conditions that seniors face. Meanwhile, many older people continue to consult practitioners who feel that the social context is not relevant to the medical task or that their ability to grapple with contextual problems is limited.

Although physicians' responses to patients' psychosocial needs previously have generated criticism of the medical profession, little is known about how these troubles of communication emerge in the language of actual medical encounters. Research on patient-doctor encounters seldom has focused on the ways that contextual problems arise and get processed (Waitzkin 1984; Kleinman 1988; Mishler 1984; Roter and Hall 1989), and this gap in research appears also in the sparse literature on communication with older patients (Greene et al. 1986, 1987, 1989; Haug and Ory 1987; Rost and Roter 1987; Rost et al. 1989). The present study asked how patients and doctors deal with social problems in the discourse of routine medical encounters.

Conceptual Approach, Definitions, and Method

Our research developed from a long-term, quantitative study of patient-doctor communication, which has been described previously (Waitzkin 1984, 1985, 1986). Although that project led to new information about communication processes in medical encounters, it also revealed new questions, on both conceptual and methodologic levels. Conceptually, some of the most interesting and seemingly important features of recorded encounters involved concerns about contextual matters that appeared marginal or peripheral to the technical goals of clinical medicine. Such contextual concerns, which emerged in approximately two-thirds of the encounters that we studied, typically included comments about work, family, financial matters, or other issues outside the traditional categories that describe the content of medical visits (history taking, physical examination, discussion of diagnostic studies and treatment, patient education, and so forth). We had initially designated most of these concerns within a residual category of "miscellaneous comments." Methodologically, these apparently marginal phenomena in medical encounters proved difficult to analyze quantitatively or even to describe in convincing qualitative terms with the research techniques previously in use.

In our conceptual work, we have adapted several theoretical strands from literary criticism, critical theory, and narrative analysis in the humanities and social sciences to study the nonliterary texts of medical encounters. Our theoretical analysis has emphasized elements of ideology, underlying structure, and superficially marginal features of medical discourse. This approach focuses on attempts at story telling about contextual issues and on structural features of medical language that interrupt or marginalize the full expression of these issues, thus leaving them incompletely discussed or resolved (Waitzkin 1989; Waitzkin and Britt 1989b; and Waitzkin 1991). A brief summary and definitions follow.

Ideology, although difficult to define simply, comprises the ideas and doctrines that form the distinctive perspective of a social group. Subtle ideologic features of medical discourse illustrate what Lukács has termed "reification"—the transformation of social relations into things or "thing-like" beings that take on their own separate reality in human consciousness. Through reification, according to Lukács, consciousness focuses on the concrete problems and objects of everyday life, while the "totality" of social relations that lie behind these routine concerns escapes conscious attention (Lukács 1971a, 1971b; Taussig 1980). From this perspective, we have argued that ideology in medical encounters tends to remove from critical scrutiny those broader issues that are rooted in medicine's social context.

Medical discourse often contains an *underlying structure*—a consistent pattern of verbal elements that emerges in a similar way across medical encounters whose surface characteristics initially appear quite diverse. Predictably, such a structure seldom reaches the conscious awareness of patients and doctors as they interact (cf. Jakobson 1985). In this structure, superficially *marginal elements of discourse* can become crucial, especially as these elements convey contextual concerns. Such marginal elements typically appear in inconsistencies, breaks in logic, interruptions, silences, and absence of pertinent details (Jameson 1981).

After a critical appraisal of our own and others' prior research on patient-doctor communication, including both quantitative and qualitative studies, we have set forth several methodologic criteria that offer reasonable compromises in dealing with the weaknesses of earlier methods (Waitzkin 1990). These criteria guide the sampling of encounters, transcription of recordings, interpretation of transcripts, and presentation of transcripts and interpretations for publication. Although interpretation of spoken narratives necessarily remains a qualitative method, it permits in-depth analysis of contextual issues in spoken discourse. By emphasizing interpretation of contextual issues in specific, illustrative encounters, our approach takes a perspective somewhat different from those traditionally adopted in the fields of sociolinguistics, conversation analysis, and discourse analysis. Our criteria also attempt to create more systemic research standards that guide the sampling of encounters, transcription of recordings, interpretation of transcripts, and presentation of transcripts and interpretations. Our criteria are:

(1) The discourse under study should be selected through a random sampling procedure to increase the degree to which it is representative of discourse in similar settings and under similar conditions.

(2) The sampled discourse should be recorded so that the primary recordings can be heard by other observers.

(3) Standardized rules of transcription should be applied to the recorded discourse in producing texts for subsequent analysis.

(4) The reliability of transcription should be assessed by multiple observers.

(5) Inductive procedures for interpreting the prepared texts should be decided in advance, should be assessed for validity in relation to theory, should address both the content and structure of texts, and should allow for alternative interpretations of similar textual material.

(6) The reliability of applying these interpretive procedures should be ascertained by the participation of multiple observers.

(7) If an interpretation is published, a summary of the transcript should precede its interpretation; within the interpretation, excerpts from the transcript should help substantiate the interpretive arguments; and the full transcript should be made available, for instance as an appendix, on microfilm, or on computer diskette, for the reader's review.

(8) If published, the texts and their interpretations should convey accurately the observed variability of content and structure across sampled texts.

We have implemented these methodologic criteria in our recent research, based on a sample of audiotaped encounters involving patients and general internists. Methodologic details about the sample, transcription conventions, selection of transcripts for analysis, and interpretive techniques appear in other articles (Waitzkin 1985, 1990). In brief, a large ($N = 336$) stratified random sample of doctor-patient encounters in internal medicine practices was selected. After encounters were recorded on audiotapes, questionnaires were administered to doctors and patients to obtain demographic, diagnostic, and attitudinal data, as well as information about the social context. A smaller sample ($N = 50$) was selected randomly from the larger sample of tapes for more intensive study. Our research group adhered to the cited criteria of an appropriate interpretive method in transcribing the tapes, carrying out interpretations, and presenting transcripts and interpretive conclusions for publication. The study was approved by the institutional review committees at the University of California, Irvine, and at other institutions where data were gathered. Informed consent was obtained from patients and physicians who participated in the study.

The following samples of physician-patient encounters convey the variability observed in discourse involving older patients and illustrate our interpretive approach. An interpretive analysis of textual material requires space that inevitably restricts the number of encounters that can be presented, or even summarized, in an article of this scope. Because of space limitations, we have chosen here to apply the interpretive approach to two illustrative encounters. Although these encounters do not reflect the entire spectrum of encounters that we observed or that occur in clinical practice, they show patterns that we have found to recur frequently. For each encounter, a summary and pertinent demographic information appear first, followed by an interpretation that refers to excerpts from transcripts of audiotaped recordings.

In interpreting these encounters, we do not intend to criticize the doctors or patients involved but rather to reveal patterns of discourse that emerge under the constraints of modern medical practice. Both encounters, as well as others we have studied, inevitably raise the question of change. That is, how might the structure and process of medical discourse be modified to improve on the conditions revealed here? While this question is not an easy one to answer, we speculate in the concluding section on this study's implications for change.

Encounter A: Independence and Physical Decline

Summary: An elderly woman visits her doctor for follow-up of her heart disease. During the encounter she expresses concerns about decreased vision, her ability to continue driving, lack of stamina and strength, weight loss and diet, and financial problems. She discusses her recent move to a new home and her relationships with family and friends. Her physician assures her that her health is improving; he recommends that she continue her current medical regimen and that she see an eye doctor.

Vision, mobility, autonomy. From the questionnaires that the patient and doctor completed after their interaction, we learn that the patient is an 80-year-old white high school graduate. She is Protestant, Scottish-American, and widowed, with five living children whose ages range from 45 to 59 years; she describes her occupation as "homemaker." Her doctor is a 44-year-old white male, a general internist. The doctor has known the patient for about one year and believes that her primary diagnoses are atherosclerotic heart disease and prior congestive heart failure. The encounter takes place in a suburban private practice near Boston.

From the start of the encounter, the patient complains about her vision and its implications. Although her cardiac symptoms have improved, she still feels "rocky," by which she means visual symptoms:

P: But I:: feel kind of rocky.   10
D: You are (word).
P: My eyes are bothering me. I can see perfectly, read signs,
     but R——[friend] said she wondered if I was eating right, and if I,
     a little vitamin A or something would, ah, when I go back, turn
     back from a bright lights, it looks dark to me, although I can see.   15

The patient attaches importance to eyesight as a critical aid for mobility and autonomy. At age 80, she still drives a car and wants to continue. She emphasizes the link between vision and transportation immediately after the doctor refers her to an ophthalmologist:

P: I drove my car yesterday, down Arlington Heights
    [
D: Oh, dear. Eighty miles an hour again.   50
P: No, I didn't. I went thirty.
D: Thirty.
P: Yeah, down Mass Avenue.
D: Well, that's the first time in years you've ever slowed
    down to thirty.   55
        [
P: Nope
    Hm hmm.
      [
D: Yeah. Ha haa.

The negotiation that follows expresses several themes, which objectify and—to use Lukács's term (1971a, 1971b)—reify the complex social conditions facing this older person by converting them into a concrete professional decision about physical capacity to use a car. First, the patient depends on her car for a variety of functional necessities and social contacts. She indicates these concerns later:

P: It's all right for me to drive a little bit if I feel like it?   365
D: I guess we're not gonna stop you.
P: Well, no, that isn't the question. It's whether you feel my-
              [
D: I, I think it's all right, yes.
P: Like going (words)
    shopping center on Baker Street.   370
              * * *
P: (word) driving, I went to a funeral (words)   381
D: Yeah. Well, I don't if you use your judgment that way, sure.

The patient requests the doctor's approval for continuing to drive. His response proves less than enthusiastic, as he uses the royal "we" to note that he will not invoke his legal responsibility, as a doctor, to prohibit driving when physical incapacity predictably might interfere with safety. As the patient begins to reply that the doctor's stopping her "isn't the question," she begins to clarify the question, but the doctor interrupts (line 367). After the doctor gives tentative approval, the patient alludes to the importance of using the car to go shopping and also for social responsibilities like a recent funeral. Her car thus becomes her means to buy the necessities of independent living, as well as a way to fulfill social obligations—among which the funerals of friends and relatives figure prominently at her age.

The mobility that the patient's car provides then becomes part of
a story about functional capacity that the patient spontaneously narrates. As she lives alone, long after her husband has died and her children have departed, autonomy in activities of daily living has become
an increasing struggle. For instance, she expresses pleasure in her
ability to do housework, to cook, and to feed herself:

P: Now I'll tell you what I did yesterday. Uhm,   120
    I did all my own work, and I've been, been doing a fair amount
    of vegetable cooking, getting better meals for myself.
D: Mm hmm.
P: I managed to get a whole tomato down this week.
D: There you are.   125
P: And a whole banana. Ha! Kidding. Well,..ah, I took the
    car out, then I came home, and I said, "Well I've got (word),"
    so I ironed.

Later she alludes to gratification in buying groceries on her own:

P: Still I'm getting better, I can, I can move around pretty well.   215
    I went ramblin', picked a (word), oh I have two, three weeks
    ago, all my groceries myself.

While the patient uses a humorous and ironic tone, she takes such accomplishments seriously. The doctor punctuates the narrative with
brief conversational fillers ("Mm hmm," "There you are," and so forth),
which convey tolerance and support for the patient's efforts to preserve autonomous function.

   Social support, family life, and the meaning of home. Although the
patient values her independence, she also tries to maintain a social
support network, which she describes without prompting in an incomplete narrative. Allusions to a support network usually arise within
this medical encounter as marginal features, which the patient mentions in passing and which the doctor does not pursue in depth. Among
her social contacts, R——, a friend, appears the most central. The patient tries to see R—— regularly for lunch and other get-togethers. So-
cializing with R—— brings her pleasure, advice, and support. For
instance, when she describes her current nutritional status and medications, she says:

P: And I'm trying hard to eat a banana once in a while, trying
    to eat some tomatoes, and
D: uh
P: I ate a R—— took me to lunch and I had an elegant lobster   340
    salad sandwich.

As a source of advice, R—— has raised a question about vitamin A as a factor in the patient's complaints about her vision (lines 13-15). The patient also mentions that R—— has helped her to move and to buy clothing.

Family members figure less prominently as sources of support, and they create some rather burdensome obligations. Most of the family have moved to other geographical areas. The patient keeps in touch by telephone and mail, especially on birthdays, but she finds herself unable to do as much as she might like, partly because of the number of people involved:

```
P:  Well I should- now I've got birthday cards to buy.
    I've got seven or eight birthdays this week—month. Instead
    of that, I'm just gonna write 'em and wish them a happy
    birthday. Just a little note, my grandchildren.                100
D:  Mm hmm.
P:  But I'm not gonna bother. I just can't do it all, Dr. ——.
D:  Well,
P:  I called my daughters, her birthday was just, today's the third.
D:  Yeah.                                                          105
P:  My daughter's birthday in Princeton was the uh first, and I
    called her up and talked with her. I don't know what time
    it'll cost me, but then, my telephone is my only indiscretion.
```

At no other time in the encounter does the patient refer to her own family, nor does the doctor ask. The patient does her best to maintain contact, even though she does not mention anything that she receives in the way of day-to-day support.

Compounding these problems of social support and incipient isolation, the patient recently has moved from a home that she occupied for 59 years. The reasons for giving up her home remain unclear, but they seem to involve a combination of financial factors and difficulties in maintaining it. She first mentions the move quickly but then moves on to a visit with R—— and her shopping accomplishments:

```
P:  And of course I'd been awful busy changing addresses, 'n-
D:  Yeah.
P:  And today, I've been to lunch with R——. And I've done all      80
    my week's shopping. And here I am.
```

During silent periods in the physical exam, the patient spontaneously narrates more details about the loss of possessions and relationships with previous neighbors, along with satisfaction about certain conveniences of her new living situation. Further, as the patient speaks, the

doctor asks clarifying questions about the move and gives several of
his usual pleasant fillers, before he cuts off this discussion by helping
the patient from the examination table:

P: Yeah. . . . .((moving around noises)) Well, I sold a lot of my   225
     stuff.
D: Yeah, how did the moving go, as long as (word)
                              * * *
P: And y'know take forty ni- fifty nine years' accumulation. Boy,
     and I've got cartons in my closet it'll take me till doomsday   235
     to, ouch.
D: Gotcha.
P: But I've been kept out of mischief by doing it. But I've got
     a lot to do, I sold my rugs 'cause they wouldn't fit where I
     am. I just got a piece of plain cloth at home.   240
D: Mm hmm.
P: Sometimes I think I'm foolish at 81. I don't know
     how long I'll live. Isn't much point in putting money into
     stuff, and then, why not enjoy a little bit of life?
     [
D: Mm hmm, (words).   245
P: And I've got to have draperies made.
D: Now, then, you're (words).
P: But that'll come. I'm not worrying. I got an awfully cute
     place. It's very very comfortable. All-electric kitchen.
     It's got a better bathroom than I ever had in my life.   250
D: Great. . . . Met any of your neighbors there yet?
P: Oh, I met two or three.
D: Mm hmm.
P: And my, some of my neighbors from Belmont here, there's Mrs.
     F—— and her two sisters are up to see me, spent the afternoon   255
     with me day before yesterday. And all my neighbors um holler
     down the hall (words) . . . years ago. They're comin',
     so they say. So, I'm hopin' they will. I hated to move,
     cause I loved, um I liked my neighbors very much.
D: Now, we'll let you down. You watch your step.   260

After this passage, the doctor mentions briefly that the patient's heart
"sounds good," and he and the patient go on to other topics. The doctor's cutoff and a return to technical assessment of cardiac function
have the effect of marginalizing a contextual problem that involves
loss of home and community.

For the patient, the move holds several meanings. First, in the
realm of inanimate objects, her new living situation, an apartment
(line 257 mentions a hallway), contains several physical features that
she views as more convenient, or at least "cute." On the other hand,

she apparently has sold many of her possessions, which carry the memories of 59 years in the same house. Further, she feels the need to decorate her new home but doubts the wisdom of investing financial resources in such items as rugs and draperies at her advanced age.

Aside from physical objects, the patient confronts a loss of community. In response to the doctor's question about meeting new neighbors, the patient says that she has met "two or three." Yet she "hated" to move, because of the affection that she held for her prior neighbors. Describing her attachment, she says first that she "loved" them but then modulates her feelings by saying that she "liked them very much." Whatever the pain that this loss has created, the full impact remains unexplored, as the doctor cuts off the line of discussion by terminating the physical exam and returning to a technical comment about her heart.

Throughout these passages, the doctor supportively listens. He offers no specific suggestions to help the patient in the areas discussed, nor does he guide the dialogue toward deeper exploration of her feelings. Despite his supportive demeanor, the doctor here functions within the traditional constraints of the medical role. When tension mounts with the patient's mourning a much-loved community, the doctor returns to the realm of medical technique.

Financial problems. Worries about money come up at several points in the encounter. As already noted, economic considerations are constraining the patient's decisions about decorating her new home. Further, desire to maintain mobility and autonomy by driving a car also creates financial stress:

P: So, uh, I sha'n't do anything about buying something for myself
    until I get my bills paid. So, and I suppose I was awfully
    foolish to put my car on the road this year.   313

Driving thus increases financial pressures, despite helping her to maintain autonomy.

The costs of medical care also have become a burden. Noting that her insurance coverage remains incomplete, the patient describes a hospital bill that has affected her ability to make needed purchases— for instance, of clothes:

P: So I told R——, I said I'll go and get a dress at a time. I
    got a nice bill from ——Hospital yesterday. Two hundred
    and forty-one dollars. ((sniff))   300

                              * * *

D: How about Medicare?   305
P: I::ve got, you see I didn't have Medicare D [*sic*], Doctor.
    A—— didn't think we needed it. And I was so, well, negligent I
    should have had it. But I am registered for it the first of July.

Like many seniors, she regrets that she had underestimated the need
for insurance. Consistently the patient initiates consideration of financial problems. While the doctor seldom interrupts the contextual
narrative, his style remains nondirective. The patient's financial difficulties thus remain unengaged and ultimately marginal elements of
the discourse.

   Physical decline and approaching death. The patient knows the
implications of her age. She wonders about the wisdom of decorating
her new home when she may not be able to enjoy it for very long (lines
242-44). Further, after mentioning her difficulty in keeping up with
birthdays in her family, she assumes a pessimistic tone:

P: I don't care, I never go to the movies, and I very seldom watch
     movies on television even. So, ... uh (word) oh, if I could
     only (word) with my own self
                              [
D: ((cough))
     [
P: and go like I used to. But what can you expect when I'm,   115
     when I'm, when you're almost, when you're gonna, going toward 81?

A scenario of deterioration also appears in a discussion about weight
loss and its impact on the patient's wardrobe:

P: So I ironed. I had three dresses, which I'll never wear because
     they're about that wide and I'm about that wide. If you want
     to see something, come here, look at me.   130
D: Uh huh.
P: Look, look at that.
D: Well, you've lost a little weight, huh?
P: A little? I've lost about 20 pounds.

After the doctor questions her about her diet and performs a brief
physical exam, the patient alludes to her continuing attempts to sew
clothing for herself:

P: Oh, the dress, good Lord, I've made my clothes for years.
     And I'm heart broken because I had a couple of nice summer   295
     dresses that I made myself, and, they're miles too big.

In short, the patient is experiencing distress about changes in her
body and her image of it. As her body shrinks, she no longer is able to
clothe it as she once could. The loss of clothes that she has sewn for
herself then blends with the effects of her other losses.

   The technical meaning of weight loss remains ambiguous, as the patient never questions the doctor explicitly about it, nor does he offer an explanation. A possible association between cancer and weight loss remains absent from the conversation, although this explanation may have occurred to this intelligent patient. Further, while she has experienced a series of losses and verbalizes a few depressed emotions, the patient does not mention the word "depression"; likewise, the doctor neither asks about depression nor lists it as a possible diagnosis.

Throughout the encounter, death waits in the background. When the patient obliquely refers to the end of her life, the discourse does not encourage exploration of her feelings or plans about dying. In all this, the patient stoically observes her own physical deterioration, and the doctor listens supportively as she describes her attempts to transcend the sadness of physical aging.

Context, ideology, and structure. Dialogue concerning the socioemotional context of aging predominates in this encounter. Typically, the patient initiates such topics; the doctor listens and enunciates brief verbal fillers that convey interest and support. Technical content gives way in most instances to extensive conversation about the experiences of aging. Patient and doctor engage in warm and mutually respectful dialogue, as they both confront troubling issues that presumably remain beyond medicine's reach.

Several ideologic assumptions become apparent. For this patient, coping with the vicissitudes of aging remains a matter of individual responsibility. This ideologic orientation emphasizing individual responsibility is consistent with a dominant ideologic pattern in U.S. society (Sennett and Cobb 1972). Further, preserving her functional capacity to carry out activities that are typical of women's social role—homemaking, shopping, cooking, feeding, sewing, and so forth—remains a high priority. In the face of physical deterioration and impending death, the dialogue objectifies and reifies the totality of the patient's contextual difficulties, even as it reinforces her stoical attempts to cope.

This encounter shows structural elements that appear beneath the surface details of doctor-patient communication, shown schematically in figure 8.1. Contextual issues affecting the patient include social isolation; loss of home, possessions, family, and community; limited resources with which to preserve independent function; financial insecurity; and physical deterioration associated with the process of dying (A). Because of these contextual difficulties, the patient experiences loneliness, frustration, and anxiety, in addition to the physical troubles of heart disease, problems with vision, and weight loss (B). In a visit with her doctor (C), she expresses concerns about contextual problems at great length. The doctor listens supportively, allowing the patient to describe her situation in detail and to emote about it (D).

Figure 8.1. Structural Elements of Medical Encounter A with an Elderly Woman Trying to Maintain Independence in the Face of Physical Decline

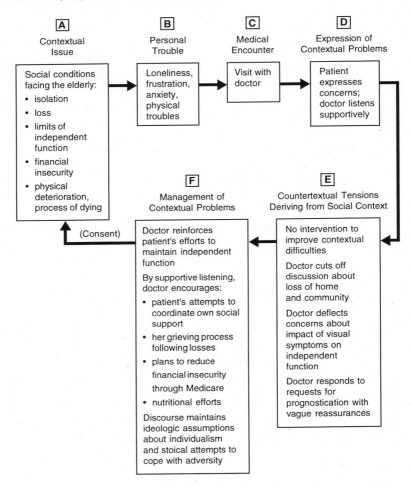

There is no intervention to improve any of the contextual difficulties that the patient presents. Nevertheless, tensions in the discourse arise that reflect medicine's presumed inability to affect the contextual issues that most trouble the patient.

Facing these tensions, the doctor cuts off a discussion about loss of home and community and deflects concerns about the impact of visual symptoms on independent function by referring the patient to another specialist (E). To manage the patient's contextual problems, the doctor reinforces her efforts to maintain independent function, despite some questions about her ability to drive safely. Through supportive listening, he also encourages her efforts to coordinate a social support network, her grieving process following the loss of a home and community, her plan to reduce financial insecurity by registering for Medicare insurance coverage, and her nutritional efforts to resist physical deterioration. In these ways, the discourse maintains ideologic assumptions that value individualism and stoical attempts to cope with adversity. Critical exploration of alternative arrangements to enhance her social support does not occur (F). After the medical encounter, the patient returns to the contextual problems that have troubled her, consenting to social conditions that confront the elderly in this society.

That such structural features should characterize an encounter like this one becomes rather disconcerting, since the communication otherwise seems so admirable. At an advanced age, the patient has retained a keen intellect and takes initiative to lead her life with independence and dignity. She shows no hesitation in voicing whatever questions and emotions seem pertinent. Likewise, the doctor manifests patience and compassion, as he encourages a wide-ranging discussion of socioemotional concerns that extend far beyond the technical details of the patient's physical disorders. Yet the discourse does nothing to improve the most troubling features of the patient's situation. To expect differently would require redefining much of what medicine aims to do.

Encounter B: Retirement and Death of a Spouse

Summary: A man comes to his doctor for a routine semiannual appointment. During a short encounter, the patient reports that he is feeling good and has no problems. Doctor and patient review two psychotropic medications and the status of the patient's diabetes mellitus. They also discuss the patient's recent trip to Florida and his son's work activities but do not mention the patient's retirement or the death of his spouse.

The questionnaires completed by patient and doctor after the visit indicate that the patient is a 66-year-old white male, who lists his occupation as "retired" and his marital status as "widowed." A high school graduate who also has taken some college courses, the patient reports that his religious preference is Protestant and that his ethnic background is English. The doctor is 38 years old and specializes in internal medicine and gastroenterology. Practicing in a Boston suburb, the doctor has known the patient for about three years and gives the following diagnostic impressions of the patient: "mature onset diabetes mellitus" and "mild depression secondary to death of wife from cancer."

An absence of problems. Why did the patient come? In his questionnaire, the patient states that the reason for the visit is a routine, "semiannual visit." During the entire encounter, the patient indeed mentions no specific physical or psychosocial difficulties. As the encounter begins, in response to the doctor's general questions, the patient says that, as far as problems are concerned, he experiences none. The doctor reconfirms this lack through sequential questioning:

D: How are you feeling?
P: Good, thank you.
D: Are you?   15
P: Yes.
D: No problems?
P: No.

Yet, based on changes that he knows have occurred in the patient's life, the doctor may expect problems to be present.

Although the recorded dialogue does not at any time mention contextual issues affecting this aging patient, information from the patient's and doctor's questionnaires indicates that at least two major life transitions have taken place. Since the patient is 66 years old and states his occupation as "retired," retirement from work has occurred in the not-too-distant past. Further, as the doctor notes in his diagnostic impression, the patient has become depressed since his wife recently died of cancer. Such transitions comprise substantial sources of stress. Yet in the discourse of this medical encounter, the contextual issues of retirement and loss of spouse remain absent.

Psychotropic medications and the achievement of normalcy. The lack of verbalized problems contrasts with the psychotropic medications that the patient is taking at the doctor's instruction. These drugs include thioridazine (Mellaril), a major tranquilizer, and a second pill which, based on its description, probably is amitriptyline (Elavil), an antidepressant.

As the encounter begins, just after the patient denies active problems, the doctor reviews his medications and inquires about his "nerves":

D: What are you taking
     for medication now, Mr. ——?
P: Ah, Mellaril, Mellaril, those little green pills,
                                 [
D: Yeah
     [
P: Doctor, and then the uh the large . . . white and blue pill.   25
                              * * *
P: I find that the uh Mellaril, if that's the name of it, Doctor, . . .

D: [
                              yeah, uh mm
        [
P: they make me a little bit loggy, so I just take one before I
      go to bed and it uh has me pretty well, you know
        [
D: yeah. How're your nerves?   35
P: Well, they're (words), yeah, yeah. Uh, I
          [
D: (words) huh? How's the
      eyes doin'?

Because the patient has experienced uncomfortable sedation with
Mellaril, he has reduced the dose. On the other hand, he here expresses no desire to terminate either the tranquilizer or the antidepressant. Further, when the doctor asks the first direct question about
"nerves," the patient responds with a brief (and largely inaudible) account of psychologic status. Then, when he asks about the patient's
eyes, the doctor for the moment cuts off the quick consideration of
emotional life and moves to other medical problems.

In the midst of the physical exam, as he listens to the patient's
lungs, the doctor resumes the prior discussion of psychotropic medications, and the patient responds by expressing a self-image of normalcy.
The doctor then negotiates with the patient about adjustments in one
of these medications, before he turns quickly to another technical observation concerning blood sugar:

D: Now breathe, breathe. In, breathe out, in. Take a real
      deep breath. OK. OK. OK. Uh, I think what you could do. Take   65
      your shirt off, but you could just take the Mellaril when you
      think you need it
              [
P: Sure.
        [
D: don't take it on a regular basis. You know when you think you feel
      off (words) OK   70
        [
P: at night time. See, I'm a (word) normal man, I don't
      normally, nothing normally bothers me
        [
D: Yeah, right.
                              * * *
      As I think the less we have you on the better.   80
P: Yeah, I'd rather not
          [
D: Your blood sugar is doin' fine.

Here the patient makes a claim about his emotional stability. Since
"nothing normally bothers" him, he as a "normal" man usually would
not need medications like Mellaril. His comment about normalcy implies that his present condition is abnormal in some way. In this as in
all other parts of the discourse, however, the contextual issues imping-
ing on this patient remain absent.

    Just before the encounter concludes, the doctor introduces an im-
age of control as he reviews the patient's prescriptions:

P: By the way, I did drop it down. They were giving me a
     hundred of the Mellaril, the little green pill   95
     [
D: Yeah, sure.
P: And that would last me three months
     [
D: Sure, I get fifty at a whack. I think as long as that's
     holding it, you look good and you say you feel good, so
P: Yeah, thank God.   100

Here both parties talk around the psychologic problem without mentioning specifics other than medication. By expressing hope that the
concrete, technical intervention provided by medication will continue
to "hold" the problem, the discourse values technical control of emotional reactions, in the face of stressful life transitions associated with
aging. As doctor and patient negotiate about drug dosages, they leave
these contextual issues in the margins of their talk.

    Remaining family. While much of this encounter focuses on the
technical realm, a brief portion of the dialogue deals directly with nontechnical matters. For instance, when the doctor initiates a brief discussion of the patient's son, the conversation focuses on the son's
problems at work:

D: Is your boy out this way now?
P: Oh, yeah, he's   yeah
     [[
D: You said he was comin' back   55
P: But he just, while I was away he went out to Detroit and had
     to fire a manager he hired, which was a kick in the fanny.
     So now, he's back in Detroit trying to find another man.
D: So he's, he's stationed here with, uh with (words)
                     [
P: oh, yeah, yeah, yeah.   60
D: Your pressure's good, 110 over 70.

That the son's job proves the main topic of interest for the patient reveals the patient's concern with work and its challenges. Whether the patient misses such challenges at work since his retirement receives no attention. Further, the patient omits other aspects of his relationship with his son, including the degree to which the son serves as part of his own social support network. A return to the technical again cuts off this quick dialogue about family, as the doctor mentions a favorable blood pressure reading. At no other time do they return to the contextual situation. Instead, the conversation stays grounded in the technical details of medications and additional brief references to the patient's satisfactory blood sugar readings.

Content, ideology, and structure. While the contextual issues differ from those in the previous encounter, the discourse manifests largely similar ideologic content. In the face of stressful life transitions associated with aging, stoical acceptance proves the most appropriate response. When the emotional reaction to such transitions becomes too difficult, the technical, reified interventions that medicine offers, especially mood-altering medication, become useful options in reachieving control. A vision of normalcy diminishes the degree to which personal problems are acknowledged or discussed. As a result, an individual copes with these problems mainly in isolation, with little apparent social support.

Some structural elements of the encounter appear in figure 8.2. Again, social conditions facing the elderly comprise the chief contextual issue that affects this patient. Specifically, he has lost his wife through death and his career through retirement. Because his physical problems are limited to mild diabetes mellitus, his health has not deteriorated. On the other hand, he apparently leads his life in relative isolation, as he mentions only a son with whom he maintains regular contact (A). He suffers from depression, a personal trouble that his doctor attributes to the wife's death (B). In the medical visit (C), the patient denies the presence of any problems whatsoever. Instead, he alludes to his own normalcy, as he discusses adjustment of the psychotropic medications that he is taking (D). The absence of explicit reference to contextual issues, including retirement or the death of a spouse, introduces tensions in the discourse. Such tensions become evident as the doctor cuts off brief discussions of "nerves," the patient's feelings about medication dosage, and the patient's son. In each instance, the cutoff comprises a return to a technical matter—the patient's eyes, blood sugar, and blood pressure (E). Medical management mainly involves a continuation of psychotropic medications with an adjusted dosing schedule. In additional technical comments, the doctor also offers reassurance about diabetes mellitus. Partly through the absence of attention to social context, the discourse reinforces an

Figure 8.2. Structural Elements of Medical Encounter B with a Retired
Man Who Has Diabetes Mellitus and Depression Associated with the
Recent Death of His Spouse

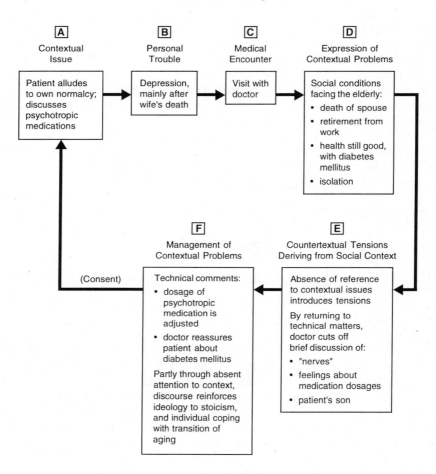

ideology of stoicism and individual coping with the transitions of the
aging process (F). With the aid of medication, the patient then continues to accept the contextual conditions that he faces.

In short, this patient and his doctor leave a narrative about the
social context mainly in the margins of their discourse. One could not
know the existence of bereavement and retirement without information supplied in the questionnaires. Medicine's technical capabilities
help doctor and patient exclude such details from their talk, and it is
not clear that either party would have it otherwise.

Conclusions: Aging and the Discourse of Medicine

Our study differs substantially from prior research on patient-doctor communication in general and communication with older patients in particular. Conceptually, we have extended perspectives from narrative analysis in the humanities and social sciences to examine ideology, underlying structure, and superficially marginal elements of medical discourse. We have focused especially on problems of social context and the incomplete processing of these problems in medical encounters. Methodologically, after appraising the limitations of both quantitative and qualitative methods in studies of patient-doctor communication, we have applied a series of systematic criteria to guide our sampling techniques, transcription of recordings, and interpretation of transcripts.

Although the encounters presented here do not reflect the entire spectrum that we observed in our study or that clinicians encounter in practice, they illustrate patterns that recur frequently. The encounters derive from a large, stratified random sample of audiotaped encounters between patients and general internists. A longitudinal subsample included observations of encounters over time, as the patient-doctor relationship evolved. In our prior evaluation of the sample, we found that its characteristics conform fairly closely to those of typical internal medicine practice situations in the United States (Waitzkin 1985). On the basis of sampled tapes and transcripts, we also believe that the two encounters presented here capture some of the variability in discourse involving doctors and older patients.

From our research we have found that several contextual issues typically arise in encounters between primary-care practitioners and older patients, to a greater extent than in encounters with younger patients: (1) bereavement; (2) retirement from work; (3) financial insecurity; (4) gender roles and sexuality; (5) isolation and loneliness; and (6) dependency in activities of daily living. We have not yet studied a large enough number of encounters with older people to speculate on the relative frequencies with which these contextual issues emerge. On the other hand, based on our observations, we recommend that practitioners view this list as a tentative inventory of contextual issues that arise in encounters with older patients and that probably should be explored at some point during the clinical history. By dealing with this list as a preliminary protocol for clinical encounters, practitioners are likely to elicit meaningful contextual information that will guide their communication with patients and that may influence interventions to improve contextual conditions.

We recognize certain limitations of our approach. Most important, the process of interpreting transcripts and selecting encounters for presentation involves intrinsically subjective elements. On the other hand, our methodologic criteria include several precautions—including a group process of interpretation and a requirement of presenting the variability of findings—that help to reduce the impact of bias in this nonquantitative work (Waitzkin 1990). The complete audiotapes and transcripts of the encounters also remain available for alternative interpretations.

Another limitation of our study involves changes that may be occurring because of geriatric medicine's widening influence in clinical practice. For instance, our sample did not include encounters within interdisciplinary geriatric assessment programs. Because such programs often include psychosocial components designed to grapple with social problems, the processing of contextual concerns may prove different from that reported here. Further, our sample of internal medicine practices did not include patients with marked perceptual or cognitive losses, despite the emphasis on such problems in prior discussions of communication difficulties with older patients (Haug and Ory 1987; Dreher 1987). We recommend further studies in programs and practices that implement principles of interdisciplinary assessment and that deal more extensively with perceptually or cognitively impaired patients.

To what extent *should* physicians intervene in the social context? The answer to this question depends partly on clarification of the practitioner's role, especially the degree to which intervention in the social context comes to be seen as appropriate and desirable. Practitioners reasonably may respond to this analysis by referring to the time constraints of current practice arrangements, the need to deal with challenging technical problems among older patients, and a lack of support facilities and personnel to improve social conditions. Further, "medicalization" of social problems, as many critics have noted, has its disadvantages (Waitzkin 1983). How doctors should involve themselves in older patients' contextual difficulties, without increasing professional control in areas where doctors claim no special expertise, therefore takes on a certain complexity.

On the other hand, this study suggests that the processing of social problems in medical encounters with older patients warrants more critical attention. Elsewhere, we and others have spelled out suggestions for improving medical discourse by dealing with contextual difficulties more directly (Waitzkin and Britt 1989b; Mishler et al. 1989; West 1984). Briefly, on the most limited level, we have argued that doctors should let patients tell their stories with far fewer interruptions, cutoffs, or returns to technical matters. Patients should have the chance to present their narratives in an open-ended way. When patients refer to personal troubles that derive from contextual issues, doctors should try not to marginalize these connections by reverting to a technical track.

Clearly, it also would be helpful if older patients and doctors could turn to more readily available forms of assistance outside the medical arena to help in the solution of social problems, but current conditions do not evoke optimism about broader changes in medicine's social context. Such changes will require time and financial resources, although not necessarily more than are now consumed in inefficient conversations that marginalize contextual issues. From our study, we are convinced that the contextual problems affecting older patients warrant social policies to address unmet needs like those expressed in these encounters—needs for companionship, housing, transportation, nutritional services, financial aid, and support services focusing on life transitions like retirement and widowhood. Of course, these suggestions are not new. Yet it is evident that meaningful improvements in medical discourse between doctors and older patients will depend partly on such wider reforms.

There is some cross-national evidence, from observations in western Europe and Latin America, that the greater availability of social support services facilitates a more explicit approach in medical discourse to contextual change for older patients. That is, in countries where services for older people are well organized and widely publicized, concrete opportunities for contextual intervention create more straightforward possibilities for dialogue (Waitzkin and Britt 1989b). In the United States, where contextual options often are limited, medical discourse confronts a narrower range of possibilities. Pending the development of more responsive social policies, older patients and their doctors will continue to face the social context of aging through narratives that remain indirect, tense, or otherwise incomplete.

9

Family-Centered Geriatric Medical Care

Rebecca A. Silliman

At the turn of the century, the average life expectancy at birth was 47 years; now it is 75 years. The ramifications of this change are many and will be felt for many years to come. For example, birth cohorts are living into old age relatively intact (almost 90% of women can be expected to live to age 70 or greater) (Fries 1990). The life expectancy at age 65 for these women is 18.57 years, 13.61 years (73%) of which, by current estimates, will likely be spent being fully functional, while 4.96 (27%) will be spent in various dependency states. Of this latter figure, the majority, 3.61 years, will be spent living in an impaired state in the community. Figures for men differ but are similar. Their life expectancy at age 65 is only 14.44 years, but for most of these years (11.87 years, or 82%) they are projected to be fully functional, with correspondingly less time spent in dependency either in nursing homes or in the community (Manton 1991).

Stated another way, data from the National Health Interview Survey's Supplement on Aging indicate that 7.3% of noninstitutionalized persons 65 years of age or older suffer from one or more dependencies in activities of daily living (ADL) and an additional 16.4% have one or more dependencies in instrumental activities of daily living (IADL) (Elston et al. 1991). (See table 9.1 for examples of ADLs and IADLs). By contrast, fewer than 1% of persons aged 18-44 years, for example, have either ADL or IADL dependencies (Nagi 1976).

With age, the prevalence of dependency increases, but the increase is nonlinear. For example, while in the age interval of 65-69 the percentage of persons with ADL dependencies is 4.06%, this increases to 7.51% in the age interval 75-79, and to 23.23% among those age 85 and older. The picture is similar for IADLs, where the corresponding percentages are 11.1%, 18.5%, and 31.5% (Elston, Koch, and Weissert 1991).

With increasing dependency, of course, comes greater need for help from others. At the extreme, recent estimates suggest that of all those

Table 9.1. Activities of Daily Living and Instrumental
Activities of Daily Living

Activities of Daily Living (ADL)	Instrumental Activities of Daily Living (IADL)
Bathing	Inside/outside mobility
Dressing	Meal preparations
Toileting	Grocery shopping
Transferring	Money management
Eating	Housework and laundry
	Taking medications

Source: Elston, J.M.; Koch, G.G.; and Weissert, W.G. (1991), "Regression-Adjusted Small Area Estimates of Functional Dependency in the Noninstitutionalized American Population Age 65 and Over," American Journal of Public Health 81:335-43.

who turned 65 years of age in 1990, 43% can expect to spend at least some portion of their remaining years in a nursing home (Kemper and Murtaugh 1991). While a more optimistic view argues that this may be an overestimate because of declining morbidity (Fries 1990), the reality is that we are faced with ever-growing absolute numbers of dependent elders. With or without institutional care, families play important roles in the lives of these dependent persons. This reality has important implications for physicians who care for dependent older patients and/or their family members.

What are the major areas of geriatric care in which families are likely to be involved? Depending on the nature of patients' dependencies, the care required ranges from (1) providing accurate information regarding symptoms of health problems, including type, duration, and severity; to (2) planning and making decisions regarding future personal and medical care, including institutionalization and the aggressiveness of medical interventions; to (3) managing medical care for both chronic and acute illness, including coordinating physician visits, facilitating the carrying out of diagnostic procedures, and monitoring compliance with medications; to (4) providing assistance with personal care, including bathing, dressing, and feeding, and with household management, including shopping, cleaning, paying bills, and arranging for household repairs. Each aspect demands different intensities of interactions with physicians, regardless of the involvement of nonphysician health care professionals. When physicians fail to engage families, misadventures in any or all of the above areas can easily occur.

To identify, organize, and solve problems in these areas optimally, what approaches can maximize the efficiency and effectiveness of physicians' efforts? At the most fundamental level, physicians need to develop a *family-centered* approach to care and problem solving (Doherty

Figure 9.1. The Doctor-Patient-Family Caregiver
Relationship

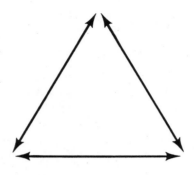

Source: Silliman, R.A. (1989). "Caring for the Frail Older Patient:
The Doctor-Patient-Family Caregiver Relationship," Journal of
General Internal Medicine 4:237-241.

and Baird 1987). This undoubtedly will be easier for many family physicians, who may have received specific training in family systems and/or family therapy. In contrast, internists may have more difficulty, since most have been trained more narrowly in a *patient-centered* approach to care. This shift in approach, at a minimum, requires thinking of the context of care as the triadic doctor–patient–family caregiver relationship (fig.9.1) rather than merely the dyadic doctor-patient relationship (Silliman 1989). This perspective is arguably simplistic since all three components of the triad are parts of overlapping larger systems, but it is a beginning point.

The remainder of this chapter will (1) characterize family caregivers and difficulties associated with their role; (2) describe the expanded clinical database required for providing care in the context of the doctor-patient-family caregiver triad; (3) illustrate the dynamic nature of the relationship over time; and (4) identify pitfalls to be anticipated when entering into this relationship. Case examples will illustrate effective functioning of the triadic relationship as well as potential problems.

Family Caregivers: What Do We Know?

Although care of dependent elders occurs, in general, within family systems, little empirical work has focused on the dynamics of family interactions in this context; they are extremely difficult to study, particularly since longitudinal studies are of greatest value (Biegel, Sales, and Schulz 1991). There is a far greater volume of empirical work that describes primary family caregivers and the problems and rewards of caregiving. But even this field is only now achieving some degree of maturity. The discussion that follows, therefore, will draw from the available literature and concentrate on what is known about primary family caregivers.

A wide range of studies have documented that older women, most frequently spouses or eldest daughters, are the major providers of care to dependent elders. Most such caregivers are married. Although one-third are working, a greater proportion report incomes below the poverty line than among age-matched peers. About three-quarters live with the disabled persons for whom they are caring (Biegel, Sales, and Schulz 1991).

In spite of methodologic weaknesses in the studies of the consequences of caregiving, it is fair to say that caregiving does have untoward consequences for many caregivers. The effects on caregivers are influenced by characteristics of the patients' illnesses (e.g., onset, trajectory, nature of disabilities, embarrassing or difficult-to-manage behaviors) and by the caregivers' circumstances (e.g., living arrangements, competing role demands, availability of social support) (Biegel, Sales, and Schulz 1991; Silliman and Sternberg 1988).

The cumulative effects of caregiving reported in the literature include institutionalization of patients, role changes of caregivers, and declining health status among caregivers. In the latter instance, the evidence is strongest and most consistent for effects on psychological well-being (Biegel, Sales, and Schulz 1991; Schulz, Visintainer, and Williamson 1990).

A logical outgrowth of research that identifies deleterious effects of caregiving is the development and evaluation of interventions designed to improve caregiver outcomes. To date, however, the documented positive effects of such interventions have been modest. Investigators have been particularly slow to study the nature of physician interactions with caregivers of chronically ill older patients, and the effects of these interactions on outcomes, for both patient and caregivers. It is clear from surveys of families, however, that many feel that physicians are doing less than an optimal job in addressing their needs for information about prognosis and for assistance with management in the home setting (Silliman 1989; Haley, Clair, and Saulsberry 1992). What can be done to change this?

The Need for a Clinical Database

The first step toward effective management of dependent elders within their family context is acquisition of a clinical database. The most efficient method of approaching complexly ill older persons is to broaden information gathering, both in scope and source. This can be accomplished in most circumstances by expanding the review-of-systems screening method to include psychological, social, and physical functioning in addition to traditional biomedical issues (Fretwell 1990). Alternatively, a nurse or aide can assist with this expanded information gathering in the office or home setting. The goal is to accurately identify the complete list of problems and to develop appropriate goals of care and strategies for attaining them within the family system of care.

The psychological dimension includes cognitive and emotional functioning and values regarding life-sustaining care and sites of care. To assist in information gathering and diagnostic precision, standardized instruments such as the Mini-mental State Examination (Folstein, Folstein, and McHugh 1975) and the Geriatric Depression Scale (Yesavage et al. 1982) may be helpful.

With respect to the social dimension, the key components for assessment include (1) financial resources, with special attention to adequacy for meeting projected care needs; and (2) patients' social skills and the composition and health of the family care system. A useful method of organizing and summarizing this latter information is to develop a genogram (McGoldrick and Gerson 1985). Instead of emphasizing patterns of diseases within families, the genogram in this instance is used to describe the relationships among family members: Who is helping out now or might be available in the future, should care needs increase? What is the nature of relationships among family members and between each and the patient? What is the process for decision making and who are the decision makers? Answers to these questions will help guide the physician in determining the best way to advocate for patients and in identifying the persons who are to receive information and by whom clinical decisions will be made. (See figure 9.2 for an example of a simple genogram.)

Finally, in the physical dimension, attention should be paid to difficulties with mobility and to problems in performing both the basic tasks of daily living (e.g., bathing, dressing, toileting) and the instrumental activities (e.g., shopping, finances, taking medications). (See table 9.1.)

This expanded focus usually requires that information be obtained from collateral sources, primarily family members but sometimes including close friends or paid attendants. This may best be termed "dual history taking." When considering this approach, however, it is important to employ measures that preserve patients' confidentiality, for the overarching goal of care is to optimize patient well-being while preserving autonomy insofar as possible. Thus the most sensitive and

Figure 9.2. Example of a Genogram

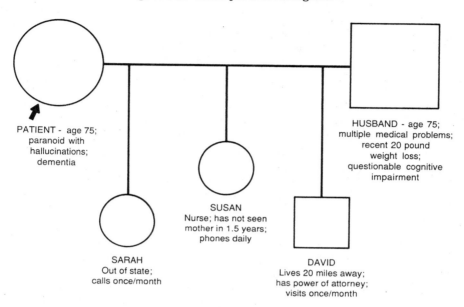

PATIENT - age 75;
paranoid with
hallucinations;
dementia

HUSBAND - age 75;
multiple medical problems;
recent 20 pound
weight loss;
questionable cognitive
impairment

SUSAN
Nurse; has not seen
mother in 1.5 years;
phones daily

SARAH
Out of state;
calls once/month

DAVID
Lives 20 miles away;
has power of attorney;
visits once/month

most efficient approach to "dual history taking" proceeds by consulting, first, the patient alone, then the family alone, then patient and family together.

The first step helps to establish and cultivate the doctor-patient side of the triangular relationship as well as to the identify and evaluate the patient's needs and concerns. Observation complements the history and the physical examination in the assessment of cognitive and physical functioning. Seeing the patient alone also provides the opportunity to seek the patient's permission for speaking with family members privately and for raising special concerns with them. Obtaining such permission is critical and only with the most paranoid or impaired patients should it be omitted. This systematic approach safeguards against violating patients' confidences. If permission is granted—and only rarely is it withheld—family caregivers can be seen alone for a few minutes to determine accurately a complete list of the problems. Listening to caregiver concerns will help create another key alliance (the doctor–family caregiver relationship), which is essential for compliance with diagnostic and therapeutic regimens. As a final step, the patient and the family members are seen together. This creates a neutral forum for open commmunication about sensitive or painful issues that must be resolved if accurate diagnosis and appropriate treatment and care planning are to take place. Everyone in such a gathering is given the same information. Although this strategy requires "front loading" of time, it saves time in the long run by identifying all needs and developing strategies for meeting them that are sensitive to both patient and family concerns. During subsequent visits, needs and responses to treatment can be monitored by inquiring of both patients and family.

What emerges, then, is a focus on the health of the family system. The physician, while primarily responsible for the well-being of the older patient, also maintains an alliance with family members. Over time, caregivers' answers to simple but important questions can be monitored: What are your concerns? How are you doing? The answers may suggest new patient problems or the need for formal services such as adult day care or referral for counseling. At the very least, the questions open a path for empathic understanding of problems for which there are no good solutions.

The Evolving Three-Way Relationship

Although the doctor-patient-family caregiver relationship can be illustrated simplistically by an equilateral triangle, in reality the relationship is best characterized as a dynamic one in which the strength and nature of relationships evolve over time. Two major factors condition each diadic component of the triangle: the stage of illness and the source and acuity of active problems. A case history illustrates these points.

Case Example: Mrs. B was 69 years old when first seen. She was originally brought for an evaluation because of her children's concern about her increasing difficulty with short-term memory, social withdrawal, and general lack of interest in life. During the year prior, a head and neck tumor had been diagnosed and successfully treated with radiation and chemotherapy. Although successful from an oncologic point of view, these treatments caused her to lose her hearing, sense of taste, and ability to produce saliva. During the month prior to the diagnosis and treatment of her cancer, her husband, with whom she had been very close, died unexpectedly of complications following a myocardial infarction. When asked about how she had managed her grief, Mrs. B replied that her husband's death had been a shock, especially since the couple had "done everything together," but because she had been ill herself at the time, she had not really had the opportunity to think about what was happening around her.

In this case, the possibilities of biomedical illness, depression, and/ or dementia were potential explanations for Mrs. B's behavior and loss of function. Unfortunately, she did not have any treatable biomedical problems, she was clinically free of cancer, and she was not depressed. The diagnosis of a primary degenerative dementia was made. Mrs. B and her six adult children needed information about the diagnosis, its prognosis and, in general, the kinds of problems they might encounter, especially problems with safety, hygiene, and behavior. They also needed to know what kinds of legal issues might arise, and "when to worry" about changes in their mother's function. The latter proved particularly prudent as Mrs. B developed herpes zoster on her face, in the area of her original tumor-related pain. Not long after the zoster infection had resolved, she became increasingly anxious and experienced a dramatic decline in cognitive and basic ADL function; she recognized the magnitude of her memory loss. An empathic physician response coupled with low-dose antidepressant therapy improved overall functioning for the short term.

As Mrs. B's dementia slowly worsened, the relationship between her physician and her middle daughter, the primary family caregiver, became increasingly important for information exchange and care management. Descriptions of new complaints came from the daughter, since Mrs. B could not remember them during visits to the doctor. This was the case when she had face pain for the second time, this time due to sinusitis. Although she had the support of six adult children who had good relationships with her and each other and who lived nearby, as Mrs. B's care needs increased and urinary incontinence not amenable to treatment developed, attention had to be given to identifying additional sources of care, including adult day care and in-home services. If Mrs. B's needs overwhelmed the abilities of her children to meet them, they might have to seek nursing home placement. This became of particular concern when Mrs. B began to experience increased nighttime confusion and restlessness.

Mrs. B never became more than "a little feisty," and this state responded to low-dose neuroleptic treatment. Fortunately also, caregiver stress was never an overwhelming problem. However, face pain recurred for the third time, in this case caused by recurrent tumor. At the time, Mrs. B was able to understand that she had recurrent untreatable disease and could outline in general terms her preferences for aggressiveness of future care.

Over the next year, Mrs. B's dementia worsened, as did the pain from her slowly growing tumor. Treatment with narcotics controlled her pain but clouded her thinking. Her family chose to care for her at home, with the help of adult day care, hospice, and additional in-home services. Nursing home placement was offered as a safety valve should the family become overwhelmed by either the extent of care required or their own reactions to her impending death, but a nursing home

Table 9.2 The Evolving Doctor-Patient-Family Caregiver Relationship

Stage of illness	Patient care issues	Family issues
Early	Evaluation/treatment of other conditions	Natural history, prognosis, and future care needs
	Treatment of anxiety and depression	Safety and legal issues, including finances
	Assessment of values/ preferences for site and aggressiveness of care	Family conflict resolution
Middle	Identification and management of new conditions	Concern about change in patient function
		Caregiver well-being
		Need for formal services
		Management of disruptive behavior
Late	Symptom control comfort	Effects of increasing dependency
		Limiting care
		Nursing home placement
		Guilt, grief

was not needed. Mrs. B died quietly at home 15 months after the diagnosis of recurrent tumor.

The issues that develop during the doctor-patient-family caregiver relationship over time, as illustrated by the case of Mrs. B, are shown in table 9.2. It should be recognized that the categorization of problems is artificial, however, and the array of problems will vary, depending on the patient, the family caregiver, and the larger family system, as well as the kinds of diseases and disabilities that the patient experiences and their rates of progression.

Pitfalls Associated with Family-Centered Care

Although the preceding example might suggest that family-centered care always works smoothly, such is not the case. The litany of pitfalls is too lengthy for thorough treatment here. However, dealing with conflicting goals and priorities of older persons and their families is common and often problematic, and this issue will thus be addressed in some detail.

A conscious awareness of differences in interaction styles forms an important foundation for the discussion. In general, older persons tend to be more passive than younger persons in the medical encounter. Older persons grew up at a time when physicians were highly regarded and their opinions and instructions were not questioned. This is less true for their children, who are much more likely to be active participants in the medical encounter (Haug and Ory 1987). These style differences, coupled with the physical, emotional, and/or cognitive impairments common in older persons, mean that three-way discussions with the physician can easily be dominated by families. A conscious effort must therefore be made to avoid this trap.

For example, consider the dominant daughters who think that their mother should not be living alone any longer because she is becoming more forgetful. A careful assessment of Mom's cognitive and functional abilities is necessary to determine whether the daughters' assertions are indeed true and to elicit Mom's values and preferences as to where she lives. The physician's recommendation may support the patient's wishes if Mom has mild cognitive impairment but can function safely in her own home, where she would like to continue living; or, in quite a different case, the recommendation may support the daughters' wishes if the patient has more marked impairment, has caused several near-fires by leaving cooking food unattended on the stove, yet still wants to continue living in her own home.

The ethical territory illustrated by this kind of problem is, for the most part, uncharted. Ackerman has used the term "modified advocacy" to refer to circumstances when family interests may override the patient's interests. He notes, "As the degree of harm to family interests increases and the degree of compromise in the patient's interests can be minimized, it becomes less plausible to assert that the patient's interests should always take precedence" (Ackerman 1988). A clinical example illustrates this point.

Case Example: Mrs. G was an 80-year-old woman whose judgment and competency were questioned by her son. She had CT scan evidence of two strokes and had consumed alcohol heavily in the past, enough to require inpatient detoxification. Clinical evaluation pointed to the diagnosis of a primary degenerative dementia, in spite of a history suggestive of other etiologies. In conversation Mrs. G frequently integrated past events into the discussion of present ones and had deficits in short-term memory, ability to perform calculations, and time orientation. At the time, she was not able to drive safely and was not cooking, cleaning, or shopping. She could not manage her medications (she had a history of delirium associated with taking over-the-counter sleeping pills) or finances (she had lost her checkbook on several occasions and could not account for nearly $3,000). Despite all this, Mrs. G was adamant about moving from an assisted living unit and buying a new home. The correct course of action in this case was clear: Mrs. G lacked judgment and insight and needed to be protected from herself and others.

When the correct course of action is less clear in advocating a patient's best interests, it is prudent to support the patient's wishes. Adherence to this can be particularly useful when families are dysfunctional or in conflict.

Comment

This chapter has outlined the importance of, and the complexities and challenges of, the doctor-patient-family caregiver relationship. They have important implications for education, policy, and research. With respect to education, it is clear that all physicians caring for older persons need to receive training in geriatrics and family systems. However, if they are to engage in the necessarily time-consuming care required by a comprehensive approach to these patients, reimbursement for care must be adequate. The current pressures to control health care costs will make achievement of this goal problematic.

Although difficult to study, the doctor-patient-family caregiver relationship is an area ripe for empirical research. Basic medical care effectiveness studies are needed that describe how often, where, and for what reasons doctors enter into triadic relationships with older patients and families, as well as the effects on patients and, secondarily, on caregivers. Of interest here is the involvement of families in managing chronic disease, in promoting patients' autonomy, in medical decision making, and in complying with medical treatment regimens. The outcomes of interest include physical, psychological, and social function; perceived health status; and satisfaction with care.

Other critical questions: (1) How does the caregiver's presence affect the doctor-patient relationship? For example, is the relationship enhanced or does the alliance between physician and caregiver overshadow it? (2) Under what circumstances is the quality of information obtained from patients improved by the presence of a family caregiver? While at first blush this question seems trivial, it is not. At times, as described earlier, a caregiver's own agenda may distort the nature and quality of information that is collected. (3) Can an interdisciplinary team for geriatric care more effectively manage the triadic relationship than a single physician? Under what circumstances is it cost-effective (e.g., for patients with specific disease entities, or patients below a specific functional level)? (4) What can be learned by comparing the roles of the family in different contexts: chronically ill children, the mentally ill?

Attention to measurement also is needed, for research purposes as well as for clinical care. For example, if physicians were able to collect information about family functioning and well-being in a succinct yet valid and reliable fashion, interventions could be designed that would use this information in concert with patient-focused functional information to improve patient and caregiver outcomes.

Investigators and clinicians alike are challenged to think critically about the roles that families play, and should play, in the management of chronically ill elders, and the ways in which health care providers can facilitate these.

10

Parenting a Disabled Child: Problems in Interacting with Health Professionals

Jan L. Wallander and Denise F. Hardy

Parenting evokes a myriad of thoughts and feelings. The content of the thoughts and the emotional tone of the feelings are noticeably varied in scope; however, parental expectations that the child will be normal and healthy do not vary. What happens, then, to an individual's perspective on parenting when confronted with the birth of a disabled child? As important, what happens when those charged with providing care for a disabled child—such as parents and health professionals—have markedly discrepant perspectives? Parents of disabled children oftentimes face impediments in dealing with such issues.

This chapter will explore the differing perspectives of parents of disabled children and the health professionals they interact with. The factors that contribute to these perspectives will be examined. Special attention will be paid to problems in information sharing by the professional. Suggestions for ways to improve the parent-professional relationship, with the ultimate goal of providing better services for the disabled child and the parents, will be presented.

Parent-Professional Encounters as Stress

Research in the area of stress and adaptation of parents of children with a chronic physical illness or disabling condition has shown that differences in children's physical or functional condition do not explain significant portions of the variance in mothers' psychological adjustment (Wallander, Pitt, and Mellins 1990, 1991a). This has led us to attempt to learn more about the stressors experienced by mothers of children with varying chronic physical conditions. We asked 120 mothers to identify the most stressful situation they encountered related to their child's handicapping condition on each of four occasions over a

15-month period. Though we are still in the process of analyzing the responses we have received, encounters with professionals charged with helping the disabled child or the family are consistently reported as one of the most common type of stressful experiences (Wallander 1991). Depending on the age of the child, the professionals in these encounters are most often school personnel or health care professionals.

These findings are consistent with our own clinical experiences. Parents of disabled children frequently share with us their frustration in relating to health care professionals. Oftentimes, they communicate significant distrust of health professionals, going back to the time when their child was diagnosed as having a disability. In our experience, the primary issue distressing parents is not the inability of the health professionals to cure the child, but rather their treatment of the parents as people. This view is supported by other studies that address the relationship between professionals and parents of children who are chronically ill, physically disabled, or mentally retarded, or who have other developmental disabilities (Darling 1983; McKay and Hensey 1990). For convenience, these children with widely varying diagnoses will be referred to as disabled throughout the remainder of this chapter. Examples from the literature of comments made by professionals and parents are used as illustrations.

By necessity, health professionals and parents have differing perspectives on any child. They play different roles in the parent-professional relationship. However, the more discrepant their perspectives, the more problems are likely to surface during their encounters. Literature and experiences shared by parents we have encountered suggest that the perspectives are often very discrepant. Consider the following comments, the first made by a pediatrician and the second by a parent of a child with Down's syndrome: "It's somebody's tragedy. I can find good things in practically everything—even dying—but birth defects are roaring tragedies. . . . There's nothing interesting about it. . . . Death doesn't bother me, but the living do" (Darling 1979:215). "They told me it would be a long, hard road with nothing but heartaches. . . . It hasn't been that way at all. . . . She's my baby, and I love her and I wouldn't trade her for another child" (Darling 1979:166,169). Where do these different perspectives come from?

The Clinical Perspective

Health professionals are first of all people and as such are exposed to the same social influences as other members of society. Much research indicates that the predominant social attitude towards those who are "different" is one of stigma, and stigmatized people are regarded as morally inferior to those who are "normal" (Darling 1983; Goffman 1963). Given that the majority of the general public's exposure to handicapping conditions is negative, this pediatrician's view of disabled children should not be surprising: "It's hard to find much happiness in this area. The subject of deformed children is depressing. Other problems I can be philosophical about. As far as having a mongoloid child, I can't come up with anything good it does. There's nothing fun or pleasant" (Darling 1979:214-15).

It is conceivable that such attitudes could be counteracted by professional training, but stigma may be reinforced by education in medical schools and other health profession training programs as a result of the *clinical perspective* emphasized in the majority of such institutions. This clinical perspective has several components (Mercer 1965).

First, there is a tendency, typically but not always unintentional, to blame the victim. Education for clinical work tends to focus on the patient in isolation, excluding the social framework within which the patient exists. Moreover, if there is exposure to a social–behavioral science perspective in medical training, concrete problem areas such as feeding, toilet training, and discipline are more commonly addressed (Breunlin et al. 1990; Glasscock et al. 1989), rather than the broader issue of the parents' perspective toward disabled children and the family dynamics. If the parents' perspective is covered, it is often based on older literature, which is replete with psychological interpretations emphasizing parental guilt over having given birth to an imperfect child (Forrer 1959; Powell 1975). There also are frequent attributions of psychopathology to such parents, an interpretation that is not supported in more recent research literature (Darling 1983; Wallander and VanBuskirk 1991). A more compelling explanation for whatever problems may be observed in parents of disabled children is that society is structured for typical families, and appropriate goods and services for handicapped children are difficult, if not impossible, to find.

Second, the medical model has several implications that may interfere with optimal care for disabled children and the development of positive relationships with their parents. The primary focus of medical education is on curing and restoring normal physical functioning (Darling 1983). Diseases that are amenable to cure provide the greatest rewards for most medical students and physicians and ultimately enhance their feelings of self-worth and success. Pediatricians, in particular, have been trained to cure the acute illnesses of childhood, and many have chosen their specialty because of an appreciation for the qualities of typical, healthy children. Consistent with this philosophy, pediatric education has traditionally neglected the area of developmental disabilities. Powers and Rickert (1979) found that only 27% of the pediatricians they surveyed felt their medical training had adequately prepared them for work with disabled children. Wolraich (1980) determined that pediatric practitioners had less knowledge of developmental disabilities than residents with only one month of special training in this area.

Third, power and subordination often characterize the professional-client relationship (Haug and Lavin 1981; Slack 1977). Medicine, in particular, has perpetuated authoritarianism as an essential component of medical care and thereby deprives the patient of the self-esteem that comes from self-reliance. Understandably, the training of physicians places strong emphasis on their taking responsibility for their patients, but too often this has translated into a need to be "in control." Wolraich (1982) has noted that "medical training often neglects to teach physicians how to say 'I don't know' in a manner that will not reflect poorly on their competence" (p. 325).

Health professionals can maintain dominance by controlling the amount of information the patient receives. When curing is not possible, the professional's dominance is threatened, and a power status is maintained only as long as the client does not recognize the professional's inability to change the ultimate outcome. One result is that information about diagnosis and prognosis of a disabled child is often withheld from parents. These techniques are often rationalized with statements about the parent's inability to handle emotion-laden information, as exemplified in these pediatricians' remarks: "Birth is a traumatic experience. For 24 to 48 hours after birth the mother has not returned to a normal psychological state, so I just say everything is O.K., even if it isn't" (Darling 1979: 205). "With cerebral palsy, I sort of lead them into it. I say, 'Wait and see.' I hedge. Usually I don't call in specialists for two or three months. It depends on parental pressure" (Darling 1979:208).

A final component of the medical model worth noting is the bureaucratic context. The professional sees many clients with similar problems. Consequently, individual clients are rarely seen as special or unique, contrary to the way the parent of a disabled child sees the child. Moreover, the professional often sees the child within the context of a medical specialty, whereas the parent sees the child in almost all relevant contexts. The advent of increasing medical specialization often results in physicians' inability to address medical problems outside their own specialties. To compound the problem, information regarding the distinctions between specialists is not always available, adding to parents' frustration and further decreasing their chance for an evaluation of the "whole" child.

The Parental Perspective

Prior to their experience of having a disabled child, the parents too have been exposed to the prevailing social attitudes that stigmatize human beings who are "different." Parental perspective is observed to change over time, but the nature and the extent of the change are not clear. A study conducted by Nursey, Rohde, and Farmer (1990) demonstrated that parents tend to have strong positive feelings toward their disabled child. The physicians in the study, however, did not expect parents to have more positive attitudes than they themselves did toward people with mental handicaps, suggesting that doctors tend not to appreciate the strength of positive parental feelings (Nursey, Rohde, and Farmer 1990).

Traditionally, stage theories have been posited to describe the process whereby parents may come to change their perspectives regarding disabilities. Although there are many specific manifestations of such change, the following commonalities are typical (Gargiulo 1985): *primary phase,* characterized by shock, then denial, and finally grief and depression; *secondary phase,* marked by ambivalence, followed by guilt, then anger, shame, and embarrassment; *tertiary phase,* beginning with bargaining, then adaptation and reorganization, and finally acceptance and adjustment.

The following description, provided by a parent of a deaf child, may illustrate the evolution of the stages: "At first I had a feeling of numbness, of unreality and expression. The 'pain' gradually overcame me during the next few days . . . an all-consuming pain. . . . I hid [the hearing aid] for about two weeks. Then, one day I remember thinking, 'I can't hide it forever.' . . . At that point I took my first steps toward adjustment. . . . The terrible pain was still present, but I was better able to cope with it. . . . Now I cry mostly because I'm so proud of Jeffrey and what he has become" (Allen and Allen 1979:280-82).

Although their viewpoint is not necessarily inconsistent with stage theory, others have argued that parents of disabled children at no point completely abandon the grief process; rather, they suggest, the normal reaction to the diagnosis of a child with a disability is chronic sorrow (Olshansky 1962). Chronic sorrow should not be viewed as pathological but possibly normative. Sorrow and acceptance of the child may coexist as part of the normal and long-term process of parental adjustment.

Most research on parents' relationships with health professionals has centered on the birth of the disabled child and the revelation of the diagnosis of a chronic disability. Parents of a child born with an obvious disability are in an especially precarious position. Although there have been some changes in recent years, obstetrical delivery is dominated by a medical model. As a result, powerlessness is commonly experienced by parents at that time, even under the best of circumstances.

To compound feelings of powerlessness, concerns by professionals about a baby are typically not revealed in the delivery room. Parents, however, often relate that they become suspicious as a result of unintentional cues given by the medical professionals involved: "I remember very vividly. The doctor did not say anything at all when the baby was born. Then he said, 'It is a boy,' and the way he hesitated, I immediately said, 'Is he all right?' And he said, 'He has ten fingers and ten toes,' so in the back of my mind I knew there was something wrong" (Darling 1979:129).

Physicians may, in fact, deliberately create powerlessness in the belief that they are protecting the parents, who are "not ready to hear the truth" so soon after birth. Yet studies show that most parents do want to know their child's diagnosis right from the beginning (Darling 1979; McKay and Hensey 1990).

Although the parents' reaction to the news that their child has a disability is likely to be negative, and the professional may have to deal with a significant degree of affective reaction, uncertainty and suspicion may be more stressful than bad news. The professional who provides this information early on shows integrity and is likely to set the stage for development of a positive future relationship with the parents. If parents are not told as soon as possible, they are deceived, and later attempts to establish a helping relationship will be hindered.

The initial negative reaction by parents may lead to some rejection of the baby during the early postpartum period. This reaction may interfere with parent-child attachment and make parents especially vulnerable to pressures by outsiders, such as the medical team, with regard to how to deal with their baby. Families have a tremendous adaptive capacity, however, as evidenced by the strong attachments to their disabled infants formed by most parents. All but the most disabled children are able to respond to their parents to some extent.

The process of attachment is usually encouraged by supportive interactions with other people, including health professionals, as illustrated by the experience of the mother of the child with Down's syndrome who was quoted earlier: "I talked to a nurse and then felt less resentment. I said I was afraid, and she helped me feed the baby. . . . Then my girlfriend came to see me. She had just lost her husband, and we sort of supported each other. . . . By the time [the baby] came home, I loved her. When I held her the first time I felt love and I worried if she'd live" (Darling 1979:136).

Irvin, Kennell, and Klaus (1982) make a number of recommendations to health professionals that may encourage parent-child bonding, including:

(1) *Initial contact:* Bring the baby to the parents as soon after birth as possible.

(2) *Positive emphasis:* Show the baby's positive features to the parents.

(3) *Special caretaking:* Assign a specific professional who has time to listen.

(4) *Prolonged contact:* Leave the child with the parents for as long as possible.

(5) *Questions:* Encourage the parents to ask questions.

(6) *Explanation of findings:* Professionals may need to repeat explanations several times.

(7) *Pace:* Progress at the parents' pace.

Problems in Information Sharing by the Professional

As repeatedly illustrated above, an essential problem in the professional-parents interaction is the provision of timely and adequate information by the professional to the parents. In many cases, however, it is not possible to make a diagnosis of a chronic disease or developmental disability immediately at birth or even shortly thereafter. In any case, studies have indicated that most parents want diagnostic information as soon as possible.

In a study of mothers of Down's syndrome infants, Carr (1970) found that 50% of those told within the first week would have preferred to be told even sooner. Similarly, Berg, Gilderdale, and Way (1969) noted that, of 44 mothers they interviewed who were dissatisfied with the timing of the information they received, 43 thought they should have been told sooner. The main reason given for their dissatisfaction was that "the grave news was all the harder to bear if they had time to build false hope for the affected child" (Berg et al. 1969:1195). Svarstad and Lipton (1977) found that parents who received specific, clear, and frank communication were better able to accept a diagnosis of mental retardation in their children than those who received vague or evasive information.

Parents' reactions to lack of information are illustrated by the story of the mother of a six-year-old child with mental retardation and cerebral palsy:

On our third visit, the neurologist said, "I think I know what's wrong with your son but I'm not going to tell you because I don't want to frighten you." . . . We didn't go back to him. . . . We insisted that [our pediatrician] refer us to [the local children's hospital]. He said, "He's little. Why don't you wait—you don't need to take him there yet." I have a feeling that he knew what the diagnosis was going to be and he didn't really think that we needed to know yet. . . . The chief of pediatrics at [the local children's hospital] told us [our child] was retarded. . . . That was the first person we talked to that we really felt we could trust. . . . Everyone was pablum-feeding us, and we wanted the truth. [Seligman and Darling 1989:229]

One would like to feel that such an approach by professionals is uncommon, but we know from our own clinical experience that it is not. We frequently encounter parents who bring their children to our agency several years after they themselves have begun suspecting something was not right with their child's development, only to have been told by their pediatricians "not to worry" and that "the child will grow out of it." Aside from the emotional toll, this wait-and-see attitude can result in the delay of needed services and early intervention, sometimes at a significant detriment to the child.

Uncertainty on the part of physicians about imparting information regarding the child's disability can be classified into two types (Davis 1960). *Clinical uncertainty* is considered to be a "real" phenomenon of questionable diagnoses, when a firm prognosis cannot reliably be issued. *Functional uncertainty,* however, is considered to be a patient management technique that is often used—even after clinical uncertainty has been resolved—in an attempt to prevent emotional confrontations with parents (Seligman and Darling 1989). Functional uncertainty is exemplified in this medical report of a severely brain-damaged child: "I have discussed the above results with [the child's] parents but have not emphasized his very poor developmental outlook. I feel it is more humane and would be easier for them to accept this child if they observe and come to understand his slow progress for themselves" (Seligman and Darling 1989:232).

Studies have suggested that four stalling strategies are commonly used by professionals to manage patients:

(1) *Avoidance* occurs when the physician makes no suggestion at all about the existence of a problem and denies any such suggestion by the parent. The following explanations for spina bifida, a serious birth defect, have been noted: "he has a piece of skin missing from his back" or "he has a small lump on the spine, nothing to worry about" (D'Arcy 1968; Walker 1971).

(2) *Hinting* is exemplified in the following pediatrician's quotes: "The first visit I make a note on the chart. Maybe I make a suggestion to the parent by listening longer to the baby's heart or whatever. By the next visit, parents start to ask" (Darling 1979:207).

(3) *Mystification* involves the use of medical jargon or euphemisms. Although the truth is told, the parent cannot equate the diagnosis with any known defect. We have found this to be common with mental retardation, which can be expressed as "developmental delay" and "slow learner," or autism, which can be expressed as "he has some autistic-like features," or cerebral palsy, which can be expressed as "motor delay" or "developmental lag."

(4) *Passing the buck* may be used by a primary-care practitioner, who can avoid a diagnostic confrontation by referring to a specialist, without sharing his or her clear initial findings.

All these techniques typically increase, rather than alleviate, parental distress and anxiety.

The need for concise information is not confined to the parent-professional interactions centering around the child's first diagnosis. Parents of a disabled child experience an ongoing need for information about the meaning of their child's condition. Studies suggest that the basic underlying factor in all expressions of parental worry is uncertainty and that the most important type of help they received from professionals was information (Baxter 1986). This help was perceived as more important than sympathy and emotional support, although this response should not imply that sympathy and support are unimportant.

Nonetheless, misconceptions about parental desire for information continue to plague the parent-professional relationship. Waitzkin (1985) found that physicians overestimate the time they spend in information giving and underestimate parents' desire for information. These findings may partially explain the oft-observed tendency in parents of disabled children to continually search for treatment. Numerous studies refer to parents "shopping around" for a professional program that would make their child "normal" (Seligman and Darling 1989). When parents are questioned about such behavior, however, most do not report that the goal is finding a cure. Rather, like parents of non-disabled children, they are simply trying to be good parents and do whatever they can to improve their child's quality of life.

Suggestions for Improvement

Surveys have reported that a very high proportion of parents are dissatisfied with services they have received related to their disabled children, including lack of information about diagnosis and treatment, vague and evasive responses, professional avoidance of labeling the condition, lack of support during critical periods, lack of help in locating community resources, and scarcity of advice about how to cope with their child's symptoms or problem behaviors (Cunningham, Morgan, and McGucken 1984; Darling 1983; McKay and Hensey 1990; Quine and Pahl 1987). Such negative indicators of professional-parent relationships should constitute a strong stimulus for professionals to reexamine how they view and treat families with disabled children.

At one level, the problem appears to be an interactive one. A theory of the interactional aspects of the clinical encounter has been advanced that may shed light on this problem. Maynard (1991) proposed that the asymmetry between professionals and parents might be manifestations of more than just institutional power and authority. He posited that clinical discourse between professionals and parents has an internal logic and orderliness that derive from interaction order and sequential organization. In ordinary conversation there are strategies for "giving" your opinion or assessment of a situation. One such strategy is "perspective display series (PDS)," whereby an individual solicits another individual's opinion and then produces a report in such a way as to take the other individual's perspective into account.

Used during clinical discourse, this mechanism provides information regarding the context in which the physician is imparting the "bad" news. During this discourse, however, clinicians and parents produce opinions and reports through contrasting displays of knowledge that enact deference and authority. Parents show an orientation to the authority of the institutional environment, thereby suppressing parental experience in favor of the clinical perspective. This asymmetry is usually presumed to represent the imposition of the physician's power and authority.

Maynard (1991) concluded, however, that although medical discourse is strongly entrenched in institutional philosophy, there is a strong interactional component that functions as well. By having prior knowledge of the recipient's (in this case, the parent's) knowledge or beliefs, a clinician may be able to deliver the news in a hospitable conversation environment, confirm the parent's understanding, coimplicate the clinician's perspective in the news delivery, and present the diagnosis in non-conflictual manner.

Although the problem is an interactive one, and parents may benefit from different approaches to interacting with professionals, professionals should learn to become better helpers. Such a goal raises the question, What makes for an effective helper?

Combs and Avila (1985) have found that effective helpers share certain attributes:

(1) A body of *knowledge:* To be effective, professionals must be personally committed to acquiring specialized knowledge, including knowledge about family dynamics, disability, and the ways in which a child's disability may affect family functioning.

(2) A view of *people:* Effective helpers view people as being able rather than unable, worthy rather than unworthy, internally rather than externally motivated, dependable rather than undependable, and helpful rather than hindering.

(3) Certain *self-concepts:* Effective helpers feel personally adequate, identify readily with others, feel trustworthy, wanted, and worthy.

(4) A *helping purpose:* Successful helpers are freeing rather than controlling, deal with larger rather than smaller issues, are more self-revealing and involved with clients, and are process-oriented in helping relationships.

(5) *Special approaches* to helping: Effective helpers are more oriented to people than things and are more likely to approach clients subjectively or phenomenologically than objectively or factually.

Many of these attributes involve empathy, the ability to put aside one's own biases and opinions as one tries to understand what is being said and felt. Many families immediately perceive the presence of an empathic helper, who makes them feel understood and who respects their point of view and values their input.

The health professions need to consider these valuable characteristics when formulating their selection criteria for membership. Additionally, they need to provide training experiences that emphasize preparing practitioners for effectively relating to parents of disabled and chronically ill children, while at the same time enabling these parents to acquire more helpful attitudes about their disabled children. Techniques that may facilitate attitudinal changes include:

(1) Writing about and discussing one's own experiences with and thoughts on disability (e.g., recall of disabled individuals, how encounters felt).

(2) Conducting in-depth interviews with disabled adolescents or adults, as well as parents of disabled children.

(3) Observing situations in which individuals with disability and their family members function (e.g., preschool programs for disabled children, a sheltered workshop, a group home, a parent group meeting).

(4) Reading personal accounts written by parents of children with disabilities or reading literature written for such parents (e.g., *Exceptional Parent*).

Adopting a Social Systems Perspective

Up to this point, suggestions for improving parent-professional relationships have focused on changes within the clinical perspective. Given the dominance of this particular perspective and the extent to which most health professions attempt to adopt it, this may be the easiest way to implement changes. However, the limited value of the clinical perspective in addressing the entire range of the child's and the family's needs raises severe questions about whether this is the most efficacious approach. Mercer (1965) and Darling (1989) and others have suggested that a social-system perspective might provide a more appropriate model for parent-professional relationships.

The social-system perspective emphasizes the need for the professional to accept the statements of parents as meaningful, regardless of whether they agree with the parents' opinions or think their statements are factual. Intervention, furthermore, must be based on what is real for the family. Finally, parents must not themselves become objects of clinical analysis simply because they happen to be the parents of children with disabilities.

Thus, the professional must work to become aware of the parents' perception of the situation and to tailor the treatment to fit their needs, as opposed to defining the problem for the parents and implementing a treatment plan based on that diagnosis. Since physicians often incorrectly perceive their clients' needs (e.g., underestimation of the parents' desire for information, overestimation of the negative impact of the disabled child on family relationships), a relationship that gives professionals a clear definition of the parents' needs has numerous advantages. Contrary to the clinical perspective, the social-system perspective suggests that the professional respect the parental point of view and share it as much as possible. This is not to imply that professionals be limited to addressing only those needs that the parents present. Their role, however, should be supportive and guiding, as opposed to subordinating and dictatorial.

This social-system perspective is receiving increased recognition and has been codified in the 1986 P.L. 99-457, the amendments to the U.S. Education of the Handicapped Act. Title I of this law recognizes a need "to enhance the capacity of families to meet the special needs of their infants and toddlers with handicaps." The law also underscores the need "to develop and implement a statewide, comprehensive, coordinated, multidisciplinary interagency program for. . . . services for handicapped infants and toddlers *and their families*" (pp. 1-2; emphasis added). When providing services, at least to this age group of children, it has become a requirement to recognize the family system and its needs explicitly in the development of an Individualized Family Service Plan. Moreover, the U.S. surgeon general, in a broad initiative, has advocated "family centered" care for children with special health needs. There clearly is a growing momentum toward achieving a better balance between professionals and parents in the care of children with chronic disability and disease.

11

Quality-of-Life and End-of-Life Decisions for Older Patients

Robert A. Pearlman

Quality of life is an increasingly popular goal of health care involving older patients. Whether the patient has heart disease and the goal of treatment is to reduce the frequency of angina or chest pressure, or the patient resides in a nursing home and the goal of care is to promote autonomy, the term "quality of life" is commonly heard. At the policy level, "quality adjusted life years" is a method of determining treatment effectiveness in social and economic calculations that attempts to consider quality of life and length of life in assessments of outcomes. In research, quality of life is becoming a standardized measure of health- and function-related well-being (Spitzer et al. 1981). However, the consideration of quality of life in some interprofessional medical discussions implies the absence of or limitations in patient quality of life (Pearlman and Speer 1983). In the practice of geriatric medicine, this viewpoint of quality of life seems to occur frequently when the patient has severely impaired physical or cognitive functioning; when the burdens or costs of treatment are great and the benefits appear limited; when the treatment is life sustaining but the prolongation of life appears merely to prolong the dying process; or when the probability of an untoward outcome is high and discussions take into account cost-effectiveness, cost-benefit analysis, or the need for cost containment in health care.

Most recently, discussion of quality of life has been introduced into debates about medical futility. Medical futility has been proposed as a professional standard for withholding or withdrawing life-sustaining treatment. Medical futility often is discussed as having two criteria: quantitative and qualitative (Schneiderman, Jecker, and Jonsen 1990). In quantitative futility there is only a very rare likelihood, or none at all, that the treatment will have a beneficial effect. Qualitative futility, or the quality-of-life component of medical futility, is a description of the treatment outcome in which the patient's quality of life after treatment is extremely poor. Examples might include being in a permanent coma or merely being kept alive for an abbreviated period of time with the constant use of life-sustaining technology.

Although at first blush discussions about "quality of life" may appear sensitive, holistic, and relevant, there is potential for misuse of the concept. To make this point, two clinical case histories are presented in this chapter. Following that, the appropriate and inappropriate roles for quality of life as a consideration in medical decision making are outlined; empirical data that support the contention that quality-of-life considerations should be used judiciously are reviewed; and new areas of applicability for the concept of quality of life are offered. The chapter finishes with several caveats for consideration.

Case Histories

Mr. R.B. was an 87-year-old married man who resided in a nursing home primarily because he was somewhat forgetful and demonstrated carelessness. His active medical problems included preleukemia, diabetes mellitus, hearing difficulties, hypertension, an argumentative personality, and a history of "noncompliance" with medical recommendations. He was admitted to the acute-care medical service because of severe left hip pain due to aseptic necrosis of the femoral head that had developed after a recent hip fracture and surgical pinning. Over the preceding two weeks, his mobility had diminished to the point where he was bedridden on admission. The medical house staff evaluated his condition and suggested at rounds a treatment of proper pain control and return to the nursing home. When queried why this seemed most appropriate for the patient, they volunteered that he had a terrible quality of life (cognitive decline, nursing home residence, shortened life expectancy, and being bedridden). These attributes seemed to justify the withholding of potentially beneficial treatment.

After discussions with the attending physician and the patient, total hip replacement surgery was offered to the patient and accepted by him. The patient successfully completed rehabilitation and returned to the nursing home as an ambulatory patient. He lived for several years without becoming bedbound or dependent on pain medications.

In a second case, J.I. was admitted to the acute-care medical service of the hospital because of a significant deterioration in his mental status. J.I. was a 67-year-old male living in a nursing home because of extensive rheumatoid arthritis with multiple flexion contractures involving his extremities. His other active problems included cognitive deficits from multiple strokes, expressive aphasia, decubitus ulcers, and urinary incontinence.

The house staff evaluated Mr. J.I. and ascertained that he had pneumonia and dehydration. He received intravenous antibiotics and hydration for several days. However, the patient was unable to receive enough fluids to reverse the significant dehydration. Several attempts at nasogastric feeding failed when the patient, in his delirium, pulled the tube out from his nose. At this point in the patient's care, the house staff queried whether the artificial delivery of food and water was medically futile. Upon questioning, the house staff did not cite a low probability that the treatment would provide a benefit (in fact, their estimate of success was 50/50 for rehydration and possible life prolongation). Their suggestion that artificial provision of food and water would be medically futile was based instead on their judgment that this patient's quality of life, past and future, was not good enough to justify treatment. Here again, after discussions with the attending physician and the patient's proxy decision maker, the decision was made to continue to provide artificial feedings. Despite treatment, the patient died two days later.

The Meaning of Quality of Life

Because quality of life may mean different things to different people, it is important to define this term as clearly as possible. The definition for medical purposes should identify the relevant attributes (e.g., Is quality of life health-related or global?), the time frame to be considered, and the person who makes the judgment.

Quality of life probably includes many of the attributes discussed in the social indicators literature. From an individual's perspective, the attributes may include health (physical, cognitive, and psychological), functional status, family and social relationships, social and religious activities, economic status, neighborhood, and life satisfaction (Campbell, Converse, and Rodgers 1976; Pearlman and Uhlmann 1988). However, the degree to which these potential attributes contribute to a person's quality of life may be quite unpredictable, differing between people and changing even within the same person, depending on whether the time frame considered is the last month or the last ten years. The time frame clearly affects the relative importance of the issues. Over the course of a lifetime, one's children may contribute significantly to quality of life, yet in any given short time period children may have little to do with quality of life; other issues such as finances, job satisfaction and health may be more important.

In current medical research, aspects of quality of life are assessed in clinical trials (Wenger et al. 1984). In this context, quality of life is often health-related and temporally related to initiation or discontinuation of treatment. For example, research addressing treatment for back pain may look at temporally related improvement in functional abilities, minimizing loss of workdays, and any change in the use of pain medications. These outcomes pertain to quality of life, but are restricted to anticipated benefits of medical care. It would be beyond the scope of medical treatment to anticipate an effect on non-health-related aspects of quality of life, such as religious activities or neighborhood.

In ordinary and clinical situations, quality of life is usually assessed in one of three ways (Jonsen, Siegler, and Winslade 1982:112-13). In the first method, one person, influenced by his or her subjective preferences and attitudes, assesses another's quality of life. This is exemplified when a young person is asked to judge an older person's quality of life; the evaluation is inevitably lower than the older person's self-assessment. Another example is an economically well-off, suburban-dwelling professional's view of an inner-city, blue-collar worker, raising the possibility of a social value judgment. An alternative method for assessing quality of life is to compare an individual with an external standard, usually a celebrity (e.g., Ronald Reagan) or a politically powerful individual (e.g., Margaret Thatcher). However, there is no consensus on the standard, and it is defined by a limited view of the celebrated person's life. The third approach to assessing quality of life is an individual's subjective evaluation of his or her own life's experiences. From an ethics perspective, this is the preferred approach to deciding who judges and what constitutes quality of life. The individual evaluates the importance of the components in his or her own life without any imposition of value judgments by others. This method demonstrates respect for the variability in interindividual, subjective assessments of what and to what degree life's experiences contribute or take away from quality of life.

Whenever a patient comes to a physician's office to receive treatment for an acute or chronic medical problem, the patient's quality of life is impaired by the disease or illness, and the physician's recommended treatment is geared to better the patient's quality of life. This is the most common, appropriate application of the concept of quality of life in the medical context. When quality of life is defined in this way, there is no ethical concern because quality of life is rooted in the patient's self-evaluation, and the physician's role and behavior honors patient autonomy and promotes well-being (beneficence).

Other common and appropriate considerations of quality of life occur during discussions of the side effects and possible outcomes of treatment. Both of these contexts illustrate the central role of quality of life in informed decision making. Patients need to be aware of the side effects if they are to provide valid consent to refusal of treatment. Moreover, depending on the likely outcome of treatment (the resultant state of health), the quality of life after treatment may be an influential factor in a patient's determination about the acceptability of treatment.

A less common but important clinical situation in which quality of life is considered occurs when mentally incapacitated patients require life-sustaining treatments to prolong biological life that is lacking in the ability to experience meaningful interaction with others or the environment (e.g., persistent vegetative state or severe dementia). In this context, family members or appointed surrogate decision makers, acting in the best interests of mentally incapacitated patients, may use quality-of-life considerations as a justification to withhold or withdraw life-sustaining therapy (Pearlman and Jonsen 1985). The basis for the acceptability of such a decision is respect for the patient's assessment of quality of life (expressed through the surrogate decision maker), the inability to identify any meaningful benefit to the patient, and the avoidance of doing harm (prolonging an unacceptable quality of life).

Inappropriate considerations of quality of life usually occur either when inter-patient judgments are made at the bedside without guidance from explicit policies on why one person should receive treatment and another be deprived of it, or when one person justifies the withholding or withdrawing of life-sustaining treatment because the patient's impaired quality of life is interpreted as having a lower value. These judgments often undermine respect for patient self-determination (when the patient or surrogate is excluded from the discussion), undermine the sanctity of human life (by suggesting that people's lives are of differing value), and create opportunities for capricious decision making by health care professionals (which translates into unjust practices).

Empirical Data Supporting Concerns about the Use of Quality of Life in Medical Decision Making

During the last 15 years, there has been an increase in literature that addresses the role of quality of life in medical decision making. The following citations raise concerns about the fairness and potential capriciousness of the judgments. They also raise the issue that quality of life often means value of life.

Early work by Crane identified the importance of cognitive functioning to health care workers (1975). These data demonstrated that physicians are likely to be much more aggressive in their treatment for patients with terminal illness than for patients with cognitive dysfunction. Other work supported this finding that cognitive dysfunction is an important consideration in limiting medical care. In another early study, Sudnow's (1967) findings demonstrated that old age and "deviancy" (e.g., prostitution and alcoholism) were associated with less aggressive treatment in emergency rooms and less comprehensive determinations of "dead on arrival" (DOA) status in emergency rooms. More recent work concerning older patients residing in nursing homes identified several factors, such as a diagnosis of cancer, bedridden or incontinent state, and requirements for pain medication, as factors associated with less aggressive treatment of febrile illnesses (and an increased likelihood of death) (Brown and Thompson 1979). Similar findings of less aggressive treatment have been documented for cancer diagnoses (after controlling for life expectancy) (Lawrence and Clark 1987). Some diagnoses such as AIDS have been associated with "do not resuscitate" (DNR) status more frequently than other diagnoses with the same prognosis, such as severe heart failure and cancer (Wachter et al. 1990). Although this may suggest biases in favor of limiting treatment, it may reflect different access for patients' involvement in medical decision making. Regardless of the interpretation, the results suggest the possibility that different approaches to health care are influenced by quality-of-life issues.

In another investigation, more than 200 physicians reviewed the identical case history of a patient with a life-threatening exacerbation of his chronic obstructive pulmonary disease. These physicians had widely divergent interpretations of the patient's quality of life (Pearlman, Inui, and Carter 1982). The variations were clinically significant because these determinations were significantly associated with the physicians' inclinations about treatment: physicians who interpreted the patient's quality of life as good were inclined to treat and prolong life, whereas the physicians who interpreted the patient's quality of life as poor were inclined to withhold treatment and to allow death.

Subsequent research identified that physicians have a more health-related orientation about patient quality of life than do the patients themselves (Starr, Pearlman, and Uhlmann 1986; Pearlman et al. 1988). Repeatedly, physicians assessed their patients' quality of life to be lower than did the patients themselves. With greater scrutiny of the data, it became apparent that patients considered a host of attributes, which included, but were not limited to, physical health, mental health, relationships, and finances. Patients' subjective assessments of their quality of life were significantly more important to them than objective attributes such as education, income, and use of health care services (Pearlman and Uhlmann 1991). In contrast, physicians considered physical and psychological health to be the major contributors to patient quality of life.

In their recommendations about the use of life-sustaining treatment, physicians also appeared to be influenced by their assessments of the patient's quality of life to a greater degree than patients themselves (Uhlmann, Pearlman, and Cain 1988). When patients and their physicians were asked their preferences about receiving (patients) or providing (physicians) cardiopulmonary resuscitation (CPR) under hypothetical conditions of impaired quality of life, the physicians were more inclined than the patients to withhold CPR. Moreover, physicians' preferences for withholding CPR were significantly correlated with their assessments of quality of life under the hypothetical conditions.

Current and Future Applications of Quality of Life in Medical Decision Making

Quality of life has three important roles in medical decision making with older patients. In the first role, quality of life is viewed in the traditional way: the goal of medicine is to enhance quality of life. Unfortunately, oftentimes the benefits of geriatric medicine do not clearly outweigh the burdens of the treatment. This is particularly true for high-technology treatments that blur the distinction between living and dying. In this context, patient-centered quality of life is the major determinant of a benefit (in contrast to a physiological effect such as the maintainance of kidney function within normal parameters). The informed patient is the most appropriate guide in determining whether the benefits of treatment outweigh the burdens. In cases of patient mental incapacitation, the surrogate decision maker can either restate the patient's preferences, offer a judgment of the patient's values, or offer an opinion about what appears to be this or any other patient's best interests. These latter two judgments reflect patient-centered quality of life.

A second role for the quality-of-life concept lies in a determination of medical futility. As mentioned earlier, a judgment of qualitative medical futility finds that a specific treatment is not worthwhile because the treatment outcome is so compromised that it would be considered unacceptable. In a recent article, examples of this condition included persistent vegetative state, as well as abbreviated life confined to an intensive-care unit and dependent on artificial means to sustain life (Schneiderman et al. 1990). Although many would agree with these two examples, the second case presented earlier demonstrates the possibility for abuse. Given this possibility, it is imperative that a professional judgment of qualitative futility (when quality of life appears to fall below a minimum threshold and justifies nontreatment) be communicated to the patient or the surrogate decision maker (if the patient is mentally incapacitated). After all, the judgment of an unacceptable quality of life is subjective and is best left to the patient. If the patient (or surrogate decision maker) disagrees with the professional judgment, it is appropriate to defer initially to the preferences of the patient (or surrogate), review and discuss assumptions and expectations and, if disagreements continue, ask for clarification and advice from an ethics committee or consultant.

The third major application of quality-of-life considerations in caring for geriatric patients takes place in advance care planning. When physicians and their patients communicate about the potential appropriateness of life-sustaining treatments, it is important to remember that the usefulness of advance directives occurs when the patient is no longer able to communicate his or her preferences. These circumstances may occur if the patient becomes comatose, develops a severe stroke with the inability to communicate, develops severe dementia, or experiences delirium in the face of an acute illness. This latter event may occur either in the setting of the patient's current state of health or more likely, when the patient becomes terminally ill. Thus, for the purposes of advance directives, these other states of health, which also reflect health-related quality of life, should be discussed when talking about the potential benefits, burdens, and overall desirability of life-sustaining treatment. Empirical data support the relevance of discussing different conditions. Patients have different preferences for life-sustaining treatment depending on their baseline state of health (Everhart and Pearlman 1990; Uhlmann et al. 1988). Furthermore, even though patients may change their advance care plans and preferences, this possibility does not undermine the importance of eliciting their preferences; it merely reinforces the need to engage in these dialogues whenever the patient experiences a significant change in his or her health or social circumstances.

Another aspect of advance care planning is sufficient disclosure of treatments to allow patients to make authentic, informed decisions. Two important components of this information are the potential side effects of treatment and untoward outcomes, both of which have bearing on a patient's quality of life.

Advance care planning that merely focuses on specific life-sustaining treatments and their likelihood of success however, may require constant updates of information and the patient's understanding of the underlying condition if meaningful discussions are to take place. It might be preferable to discuss states of health and social circumstances that are considered worse than death. The underlying assumption in discussing "states worse than death" in advance care planning is that a person would want treatment if his or her quality of life was better than death, and conversely, would not want treatment or would want the discontinuation of treatment if the quality of life was worse than death. Recent data support the belief that people consider certain common conditions to be worse than death (Pearlman et al. 1993), including coma, dementia, severe pain, a bedridden state, inability to care for oneself, being a significant burden on family, and hopelessness. Discussions between physicians and patients about these or other conditions might contribute to the advance care planning process. If nothing else, these discussions may inform decisions after partially successful life-sustaining treatment results in any of the aforementioned conditions. This information would then help direct the future use of life-sustaining treatment.

Conclusions and Caveats

Quality of life is a central goal of medical care. However, health care providers and patients may be discussing different issues even when they use the same words. The potential for misunderstanding and significant sequelae are heightened when life-sustaining treatments for older patients result in only marginal apparent benefits, while the burdens seem great to the health care provider. To prevent misunderstanding and inappropriate inferences about the patient's quality of life, the health care provider needs to understand what is beneficial from the patient's perspective and align treatment that offers the greatest likelihood of achieving the identified quality of life. These considerations are relevant in obtaining informed consent, in identifying the patient's attitudes about the physician's judgments of qualitative medical futility, and in discussing advance care plans.

Quality of life has intrinsic relevance to the delivery of health care, and that being so, the education of health care providers must address quality-of-life issues. In general, it seems most appropriate for students and trainees to explore the concept with patients in an open-ended manner. It would be helpful to specify a time frame in these discussions and to tailor the discussions either to the informed consent process for a proposed treatment or to advance care planning. It has been noted in the sociology literature that individuals have an easier time thinking about issues that detract from quality of life than about improvements in the quality of life. Similarly, it is easier for patients to identify those conditions that they envision as completely unacceptable—in other words, worse than death. As for concern that patients' attitudes might change, this possibility only reinforces the need to repeat such discussions at timely intervals. Consistent values only serve to support the authenticity of the preferences. If a health care provider has only one opportunity to discuss advance care plans and unacceptable quality of life, the single discussion is better than no communication whatsoever.

Quality of life is a fertile area for further investigation. Research is needed to study interventions that can help potential surrogate decision makers and health care providers to understand patient quality of life and patient preferences regarding life-sustaining treatment. Another area for investigation is the degree to which patients understand "states worse than death" and the degree of internal consistency between this construct and treatment preferences under different states of health or quality of life. Finally, in this era of heightened cost awareness and limited budgets for health care, it would be worthwhile to investigate whether subjective assessments of patient quality of life can be incorporated to some degree into cost-benefit analyses.

Future Educational Considerations

12

The Role of Patient Education in Doctor-Patient Relationships

Marie R. Haug

In conventional social science theory, as embodied in the sociology of the professions, the client or patient is expected to accept a professional's right to control any interaction between them, including the right to give directions in the form of recommendations and advice that will be followed. The authority of the professional in the encounter is taken for granted. It flows from the practitioner's esoteric knowledge and dedication to service, and is institutionalized in legislation and administrative rules that forbid lay performance of many professional activities. In the health care field, Parson's (1951, 1975) concept of the sick role epitomizes this theoretical perspective.

During the 1970s a number of researchers in the United States began to consider that negotiation, rather than an asymmetrical power relationship, would be a more realistic appraisal of what happens when patients and practitioners interact. Some of this work was cast in terms of "deprofessionalization" (Haug 1975, 1976). Others explicitly studied patients' bargaining techniques (Hayes-Bautista 1976; Lazare et al. 1978), while Pratt (1978) outlined in detail the nature of a new consumer-consultant relationship to replace the old doctor-patient concept and argued for its utility in improving health care. Some physicians themselves were willing to have patients challenge their authority and took a more egalitarian stance. Waitzkin and Stoeckle (1976) and Pellegrino (1977) were among those who advocated the demystification of medical expertise and the end of physician paternalism, while Slack (1977) called for "patient power."

Since then the change in doctor-patient relationships has become even more widely documented. Shorter (1985) finds the "post-modern" patient unwilling to accept physician authority, a view echoed by Stoeckle (1987), who pointed out that "patients seeking medical aid are less accepting of professional dominance, since subordinate roles are less acceptable, not only in the relation, but everywhere else in society" (Stoeckle 1987:97). This view has recently been reasserted by Todd (1989) in a study of relationships between physicians and female patients. As she puts it, "Doctors, who were thought to know all, are being questioned. . . . Women, the major consumers of health care in this country, have been in the vanguard of these criticisms. . . . Blind trust in modern medicine has waned" (Todd 1989:2).

   Reasons for the decline in physicians' authority over patients include several factors: the public's unwillingness to accept authority in general, media evidence of physician fallibility, and rising educational levels, which give people more confidence in the validity of their own views. Perhaps the most dramatic evidence of the general decline of authority has been the events in Eastern Europe, where a direct challenge of government authority brought about unprecedented structural changes. In the United States, the anti–Vietnam War movement is another such example, among many that could be cited.

   In a climate where questioning authority has become legitimate as a symbol of the right to autonomy, it is not surprising that patients should refuse blind obedience to physicians. The role of rising public educational levels in these developments is critical, as noted in a recent review of the deprofessionalization hypothesis (Haug 1988). "Despite the continued discovery of new techniques and medical breakthroughs the media have popularized a great deal of the increasing fund of medical knowledge, and made it accessible to a public whose rising educational level permits many people to grasp it, at least in its main outlines" (Haug 1988:50). Moreover, how-to books, slick hospital-sponsored magazines (in my community, there are at least three—from Mt. Sinai, Saint Lukes, and University hospitals), magazines like the 2.5-million-circulation *Prevention*, and special newsletters such as the *Harvard Health Letter* provide information on medical and treatment matters that empowers patients to assert their autonomy by asking informed questions and giving knowledgeable opinions when interacting with a physician.

   At the same time, media reports of successful malpractice suits reveal that physicians can make mistakes, and stories about alcoholic or drug-dependent doctors destroy their ideal image. A recent article, "How Bad Are the Bad Docs?" (Carey 1990), in a popular magazine, and the book *Medicine on Trial* (Inlander, Levin, and Weiner 1988) give multiple examples of physician error. The public is beginning to understand that medicine is not an exact science; instead, as Fox (1957) noted years ago, it contains a large element of uncertainty on the part of both the individual practitioner and the discipline itself. Indeed, more recently Bursztajn and his colleagues (1981) argued convincingly that all medical decision making contains a large element of chance, because of the uncertainty inherent in the discipline.

Empirical studies of these issues first appeared in 1979. In the first survey of public attitudes, about 60% of a midwestern sample ($N = 640$) and over a quarter of a national sample ($N = 1509$) expressed willingness to challenge a physician's authority, and nearly half in each sample reported that they had in fact raised questions about a physician's recommendations during a medical encounter (Haug and Lavin 1979,1983). The relationship between educational level and attitude was monotonic; those with some college education were the most willing to challenge a physician (Haug and Lavin 1983:92). The effect of education on actual reported behavior in confronting and disagreeing with a doctor was equivocal, however, which will be discussed later.

Among the many issues generated by these observations is whether the same types of authority-based doctor-patient relationships, the same trends toward a more egalitarian form of interaction, and the same effects of education characterize countries and cultures other than those of Western industrialized or capitalist form. Some limited data, gathered informally from available informants over a decade ago and largely impressionistic, are available from Great Britain, the former Soviet Union, Cuba, and the Republic of China. The first two are Western industrialized nations, one capitalist and one (at that time) not capitalist. The second two might be considered developing countries, and neither has a capitalist economy. Additional data based on interviews and random samples have recently become available from a survey of older persons in Japan, an Eastern industrialized nation, in connection with studies of self-care. Moreover, in the United States two research projects on self-treatment also investigated attitudes toward physicians, one providing data to compare with the results from Japan and the other yielding information on Hispanics, blacks, and persons of Eastern European origin.

Early Findings

The early work in Britain and in what was then the USSR confirmed the impressions developed in the United States: physicians' traditional authority in interaction with patients was being eroded, and rising levels of patients' formal education affected their relationships with the physician. Those with more schooling were more likely to challenge a physician's authority, an activity resented by many practitioners and indeed considered neurotic or troublesome behavior by many in both societies. A British general practitioner was annoyed because university-educated professionals in a regional think tank raised questions about his recommendations; he considered them difficult patients. As one Soviet physician put it, "The ... educated ... give not only the symptoms but also the diagnosis, it is easier for the doctor if the patient does not try to tell the doctor what to do" (Haug 1976). Significantly, physicians in Britain and the former USSR firmly opposed letting patients see their own records, which might be interpreted as a need to withhold information in order to preserve physician power (Waitzkin and Stoeckle 1976). Consistent with the role of education, in Britain and the former USSR the elderly, who were apt to have lower schooling, were identified as least likely to question medical authority, although their increased health concerns were undoubtedly a contributing factor. These trends seemed to hold regardless of differences in societal structure and ideology. Notably, the classless ideology of the former Soviet Union—in contrast to the hierarchical class structure accepted in Great Britain—apparently had little effect on practitioners' preference for an asymmetrical doctor-patient interaction, and on patients' willingness to question the appropriateness of such asymmetry.

Whether similar trends in doctor-patient relationships exist in two developing countries that also espouse an egalitarian ideology was explored informally by this author in Cuba and China, with the results unpublished. The data from Cuba suggest that acceptance of physician authority in therapeutic encounters is variable, again depending on patient education. Some informants felt that, because universal health care is a new development, the younger, educated "intelligentsia" understand the reasons for treatment more thoroughly than older persons with less schooling, are more conscious of the benefits of care for themselves and their families, and are thus more willing to accept medical advice. For example, one specialist in internal medicine in Havana claimed that the educated more readily understand and accept the need for treatment in the presence of asymptomatic hypertension, whereas those with less schooling think that if there are no symptoms, there is no reason to take medicine. On the other hand, a social scientist noted that the educated also were more apt to question physicians because they were aware of new developments in medicine, and thus would ask for the latest in diagnostic or treatment techniques.

There are many differences between China and Cuba that override, in the medical context, the fact that both are developing countries. Unlike Cuba, China experienced an attack on professionalism in connection with the Cultural Revolution in the late 1960s and early 1970s. At that time, the medical schools were closed down for about three years, and when they reopened with a revised curriculum, entrance examinations were abolished and students were selected on the basis of ideology and election by their factory or farm workmates.

Although medical school examinations have since been reinstated and curricula updated, the legacy of a cohort of physicians perceived as less well-trained remains. Knowledgeable patients, those with more education, try to avoid younger doctors, whose expertise is not trusted. They manipulate the clinic system so that they can be treated by the older practitioners, or at least by those who graduated before 1965. Furthermore, there was anecdotal evidence that blue-collar workers, likely to have fewer years of schooling, had little respect for doctors, were discourteous to them, and on occasion got into a fist fight with a practitioner who failed to meet their treatment demands.

In addition, China has a long tradition of indigenous medicine, including not only acupuncture but also herbal and other folk remedies, dating back many centuries. It persists today, coexisting with Western medicine, which emphasizes scientifically validated practices and modern technology. Older persons and country folk with less education tend to have more confidence in Chinese medicine, while younger, educated people are likely to prefer Western. However, some of the latter as patients are perceived to be apt to challenge physicians' authority, ask more questions, and demand more answers.

Education in China appears to have a somewhat contradictory effect, similar to that noted in Cuba. In contrast to those with little schooling, educated patients were seen as more likely to understand the rationale for a recommended course of treatment, and accordingly, to be willing to follow advice defined as based on scientific knowledge. On the other hand, such patients were said to ask more questions and make more demands on the physicians.

Cultural Variations

In short, challenge to physician authority is not unique to the United States and is appearing in various forms in other societies as well. Moreover, while increased knowledge, as indexed by education, emerged in all four countries as undermining the authority of the doctor to some extent, the complexities of different historical experiences and cultural beliefs produced variance in its effects, both between the two developing countries and between them and the more industrialized societies.

In the developing countries, education was reported to foster understanding of the rationale for diagnosis and treatment, thus encouraging acceptance of a physician's expertise, and also to provide the basis for refusal to accept without question the practitioner's authority. In the industrialized world sectors, on the other hand, informants consistently reported that the more highly educated are inclined to be

Figure 12.1. Relationship between Educational Level and Challenge of Physician Authority in Underdeveloped and Developed Countries

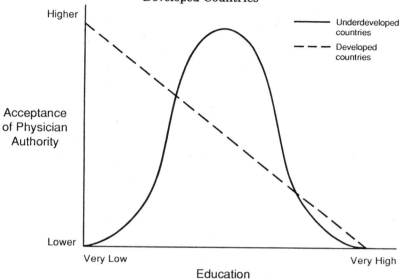

skeptical, to reject physician authority, and to take on a consumer stance. Wilensky (1964) once noted that it was difficult to predict the effect of schooling on patients' response to professional claims. These findings suggest a hypothesis: education's impact depends largely on the developmental stage of a society, with attendant variations in cultural beliefs. Its association with acceptance of physician authority may be curvilinear in developing countries, where the benefits and advantages of scientific medicine are new and often dramatic in improving the nation's health (fig.12.1). People with more schooling, often the younger, whose cultural beliefs are less bound by superstition and fear of the unfamiliar, can comprehend the reasons for diagnosis and treatment, respect the physician's expert knowledge, and be little inclined to argue with it. However, as schooling increases, its effects go beyond this initial stage and produce a more discriminating, less trusting attitude. In industrialized, "modernized" societies, the relationship between schooling and challenge of physician authority is more linear. Those with somewhat higher educational levels are now familiar with the uncertainties and errors of medicine. They have learned that advanced technology and startling scientific breakthroughs cannot always guarantee appropriate care. Last year's wonder drug may this year be withdrawn from the market because of lately discovered disastrous side effects. For those whose cultural beliefs have reached this

Table 12.1. Challenges to Physician Authority by Level of Patient Education

Educational level	Attitudinal (Willingness to challenge physician authority) % of patients very willing to challenge ($N = 640$)	Actual (Behavioral challenge) % of patients who made challenges ($N = 640$)
Less than high school	11	45
Completed high school	19	35
Some college to graduate	32	49

stage of sophistication, challenges to physician authority, intelligent noncompliance, and taking on the role of the consumer may be viewed as the healthiest form of interaction with a doctor.

Recent Research Findings

The formulation of these hypotheses about the interaction between stage of development and education in affecting doctor-patient relationships sparked a new look at the 1979 data from a midwestern survey sample (Haug and Lavin 1979, 1983). Unlike the linear relationship between education and attitudes toward challenging physician authority, the association between education and the reported behavior of actually making such challenges was curvilinear (table 12.1). Persons with the least or the most schooling were more likely to have translated their attitudes into action than those with 'middle-level years of school. This anomaly was dismissed at the time as a nonsignificant result, but it is intriguing as a possible indication that education need not be linearly related to rejection of medical authority even in a developed nation. Those with moderate education might not have had sufficient confidence in their views to translate them into action, just as those in less developed countries with only limited learning are not yet ready to question a physician's authority.

The previously mentioned recent quantitative studies in Japan and the United States offer an opportunity to assess the effect of education on doctor-patient relationships cross-culturally in a less impressionistic and more systematic way than was the case for the studies in Britain, the Soviet Union, Cuba, and China. Because both Japan and the United States are developed countries, it is not possible to test the curvilinear relationship between educational level and acceptance of physician power as modified by stage of development, but it is noteworthy that cultural variations do exist, both within and between countries, thus offering some support to the hypothesis that the relationship between education of patients and the nature of medical encounters is complex. The three studies reported here were each based on random samples of older persons, 900 in Japan, and 728 and 316, respectively in the United States (Haug et al. 1991; Coulton et al. 1990).

Measures of attitudes toward physician authority differed somewhat in the various studies, although all were based on a set of items originally developed in 1979 (Haug and Lavin 1979, 1983). Although items have been grouped in various ways, and with different titles, all measures assessed patients' rights to autonomy in relationships with physicians. An additional variable, claimed experience of medical error, also was included in these projects in Japan and the United States.

Divisions of education levels into lower and higher also varied across countries, depending on their characteristics. In Japan and in one United States sample, the extremes were those with fewer than 8 years of schooling and those with 14 or more years. In another U.S. sample, the break had to be less-than-high-school education versus high-school-or-better education because of the levels reported by the sample.

Cultural variations in the first United States study ($N = 728$) were first analyzed in terms of blacks and whites. Since this 1985 study investigated health behaviors of persons aged 45 and older in a midwestern state (Haug, Wykle, and Namazi 1989), many of the blacks might have emigrated north during World War II, and accordingly might have had a background of southern rural health beliefs, although these data are not available in our secondary analysis. For comparison with a study of health behaviors of older persons in Japan, data for racial groups in the United States were combined. Japan's culture differs from that of the United States in many ways, including, as in China, a belief by some in Eastern herbal medicine and traditional practitioners, in some aspects congruent to views in developing countries. In the second United States study ($N = 316$), health behaviors were evaluated and compared for three groups: Hispanics, blacks, and whites aged 60 and older, all having the chronic disease arthritis. Most elderly Hispanics in the midwestern city that was the locale for the study had emigrated from underdeveloped countries in Central America and from Puerto Rico, and their beliefs in many respects might be considered similar to those of persons living in early stages of industrialization.

Table 12.2. Types of Authority Challenge by Race and Education (USA)

	Years of education		
	% with less than 8 years	% with 14 or more years	Total N
A. Those with high desire for medical information:			
Blacks (N = 16)	13	50	163
Whites (N = 104)	5	39	534
B. Those with high belief in patient right to autonomy:			
Blacks (N = 91)	14	19	163
Whites (N = 281)	5	31	535
C. Those with claimed experience of medical error:			
Blacks (N = 66)	9	24	163
Whites (N = 250)	7	36	536

Cross-cultural Comparisons

Based on quantitative survey results from random samples, comparisons are made here, first within the United States and second between the United States and Japan. In the first United States study, with 725 cases, the effect of educational level on older persons' attitudes to physicians was compared for black and white respondents. Although in both groups those who had more years of education were more apt to express a high desire for medical information, the educated blacks were more likely than the educated whites to do so, perhaps still feeling ill equipped educationally to deal with the knowledgeable physician (table 12.2A). On the other hand, although those with higher education were again more likely to believe in the right to patient autonomy in doctor-patient relations, these views were expressed by only a minority, with relatively more whites likely to do so (table 12.2B).

While information may provide ammunition for questioning a physician's recommendations, not all who desire information are ready to challenge authority. A willingness to pit one's own judgment against that of a physician was implied by respondents who claimed experiences of physician error in diagnosis or treatment. While it is unlikely that doctors make more clinical mistakes when treating the better educated, in both racial groups those who believed they had suffered such events had more education. This suggests that those with more schooling had the confidence to judge medical performance (table 12.2C).

Table 12.3. Types of Authority Challenge by Education, USA and Japan

	Years of education		
	% with less than 8 years	% with 14 or more years	Total N
A. Those with high faith in doctors:			
USA (N = 72)	42	26	703
Japan (N = 98)	40	33	871
B. Those with high belief in health self-reliance:			
USA (N = 45)	11	22	700
Japan (N = 64)	22	28	807
C. Those with claimed experience of medical error:			
USA (N = 76)	7	34	726
Japan (N = 40)	14	16	867

The U.S. data for both racial groups combined were compared with results of the survey of 900 persons aged 45 or older in Japan. Here the items were grouped into two identical scales for intercountry comparison: faith in doctors and self-reliance in health. On the first scale, the direction of effect was the same. Those with more years of schooling were less likely to express high faith in physicians' care and thus were more prepared to question medical authority (table 12.3A). On self-reliance in health, in both countries those with more education were more willing to rely on their own judgment in health decisions (table 12.3B). It appears that cultural differences had little impact on attitudes to physicians' authority in these two highly developed countries. Apparently, stage of development overran differences in cultural background. As for claimed experience of medical error, a similar pattern emerged, although far fewer of the Japanese subjects than those in the United States reported such events, and there was much less effect of education in Japan than in the United States (Table 12.3C). This might be an example of a cultural variation, namely less willingness in Japan, where courtesy is a national value, to criticize physicians or second-guess their conclusions, rather than an indication of the excellence of Japanese medicine in diagnosis and treatment.

In the second U.S. sample, in which the subjects were aged 60 or older and had arthritis, comparisons were made among blacks, whites of second-generation Eastern European origin, and Hispanics, with approximately 100 in each ethnic group. Unlike the larger U.S. sample, these persons had a diagnosed illness. The educational level of the elderly Hispanics was very low, with only 6% having achieved even a

Table 12.4. Elements of Authority Challenge by Ethnicity and Education,
U.S. Residents with Arthritis

	% of total group	% with high school education or more	Total N
A. Those with low faith in doctors:			
Hispanics ($N = 10$)	10	17	100
East Europeans ($N = 37$)	33	41	111
Blacks ($N = 20$)	19	25	105
B. Those with highest belief in health self-reliance:			
Hispanics ($N = 7$)	7	0	100
East Europeans ($N = 24$)	22	30	111
Blacks ($N = 21$)	20	31	105

high school level. In this analysis, comparisons were reported between total group results and results for those with the higher schooling (table 12.4A). With respect to low faith in doctors among those with a high school education, the Hispanics had the fewest with this view, followed by blacks, while the Eastern European group was the most apt to be skeptical.

Since low faith in medical care is consistent with high self-reliance in health, it is not surprising that the results for the self-reliance indicator are similar (table 12.4B). However, none of the few Hispanics at the high school level expressed self-reliance in health matters, compared to about a third of the similarly educated from each of the other two ethnic groups. Even a moderate amount of schooling, in this cultural context, did not justify depending on one's self rather than on doctors when symptomatic.

Discussion

What can one conclude from these various findings? First, it is likely that challenge to physician authority is a pervasive phenomenon, not limited to the United States or even to industrialized countries in general. Moreover, these results, although mixed, are generally congruent with respect to the effect of education among persons in industrialized countries, whether comparing races or ethnic groups in the United States, or comparing national findings for the United States and Japan. Higher education tends to relate to less acceptance of physician power. However, differences emerged that are not inconsistent with the notion that the relationship may vary not only by cultural background, but perhaps also by stage of development. The most relevant findings for this latter point appear in the study of elderly with arthritis. In this sample, the Hispanics might be considered similar to persons in countries in early stages of development. Certainly they had the lowest levels of education. These older persons with little schooling were likely to have emigrated from relatively underdeveloped countries in Central America. They were less likely to have low faith in doctors and were missing among those with high self-reliance in health. In short, they fit the description of the early effects of some degree of education in a developing country, namely increased recognition of the values of science-based professional care, but without sophistication enough to see the flaws in professional claims.

The fact that these data are in part impressionistic and only in part the output of systematic surveys should not obscure their potential theoretical relevance. A doctor-patient relationship has been a power relationship, in which power is exercised not by overt coercion or threat of violence, but by authority grounded in tradition, legitimated by law and regulation, and justified by the mysteries of science. The asymmetry of this relationship is being called into question, sometimes individually by knowledgeable patients, as occurs in many countries, and sometimes by physicians themselves, as is most noticeable in the United States. Even older persons, who are more likely to accept physician power, give evidence of this trend. Moreover, the outlines of that asymmetry can be modified by cultural differences, perhaps by stages of development in the country of origin, and certainly by level of patient sophistication.

The Parsonian model of the sick role is again shown to be bounded in its applicability, this time not by type of illness but by its difficulty in generalizing across cultures and economic systems. In all societies, the concept of professional power over clients is eroded to the extent that clients become more sophisticated about the inadequacies and limitations of professional expertise. As sociologists like Freidson (1961), Johnson (1972), and Starr (1982) have pointed out, the times require reconceptualization of these relationships. The explorations in this paper bear witness to the relevance of their views, not only in Western societies, but also throughout the rest of the world.

Patient power, on the other hand, has its negative side. As Shorter (1985) has noted, loss of faith in doctors has destroyed the placebo effect of trust, responsible for more than one supposed "cure." Moreover, if patients are allowed to win when demanding their own preferred treatment, the result could easily be overuse of unnecessary technological fixes that happen to be popular at the moment (Reiser and Anbar 1984). Stewart and Roter (1989:21) present a model of the doctor-patient relationship that posits high patient control along with low physician control as leading to this kind of negative consumerism, in

Table 12.5. Types of Doctor-Patient Relationship

| Patient control | Physician control | |
	Low	High
Low	Default	Paternalism
High	Consumerist	Mutuality

Source: Stewart, M., and Roter, D., eds. (1989), *Communication with Medical Patients* (Newbury Park, Calif.: Sage), p. 21.

which physicians give in to patients' unreasonable demands (table 12.5). Their ideal form of interaction is "mutuality," in which both parties in the encounter have high control and presumably engage in negotiations to achieve a jointly satisfactory therapeutic outcome.

A final word is in order about two additional trends. First, while the authority of physicians over patients is on the decline, their own autonomy also is in jeopardy, not only in terms of payment limitations—as in the potential application of DRGs (which base hospital payments on type of diagnosis) to private practice Medicare cases—but also in the increasing trend to bureaucratically organized group practices and to more rigorous oversight of physicians' actions by state and regional review groups. Physicians are embattled on more than one front. Being a doctor is not so easy any more. The second factor is the impact of technology on medical practice; no one has yet assessed its potential. On the one hand, it permits even more esoteric medical procedures for diagnosis and treatment. Conversely, technology offers the opportunity for greater patient power. In the future, computerwise patients might have access to stored medical knowledge, including decision trees for determining one's own diagnosis and selecting one's preferred treatment regimen. Computer developments are such that "self-care" at more sophisticated levels than dealing with everyday ailments is theoretically possible, making physician intervention obsolete in many cases. That may not occur in my lifetime or yours, but who knows what the year 2050 will bring?

13

Teaching Communication Skills to Medical Students and House Officers: An Integrated Approach

Richard M. Frankel and Howard B. Beckman

The idea that communication between doctor and patient is an important dimension of medical practice has been a focus of scholarly attention since ancient times (Reiser 1980). Never has it been more important than in the 1990s, the final decade of a century that has witnessed unprecedented advances in the eradication of disease and improvements in both the quality and duration of life. Ironically, at the same time that such sweeping scientific successes have occurred, doctors and the medical profession in general have become the object of increasing dissatisfaction and criticism. Hardly a week goes by without a major news story about the spiraling costs of health care, the malpractice crisis, or ethical issues at the beginning and/or end of life (Gibbs 1989).

The current "crisis" in American medicine also is reflected in the less publicized fact that fewer college graduates are applying to medical schools than at any other time in recent memory. As well, many practicing physicians have chosen to leave medicine rather than face skyrocketing insurance rates and the increasing demands of patients for more autonomy in deciding among alternative courses of treatment (Kassberg 1990). Even more distressing in some ways are reports by significant numbers of young physicians that they experienced physical, sexual, or emotional abuse during their training (Silver and Glicken 1990; Sheehan et al. 1990).

What ties together many elements of the public and professional crisis in medicine is the issue of poor communication—between doctor and patient, citizen and scientist, and teacher and student. In this chapter, we describe three dimensions of doctor-patient communication—historical, research, and educational—with the goal of providing an integrated view of the prospects and problems we face in preparing physicians to practice in the twenty-first century. As well, we will provide recommendations for teaching communication skills to medical students, residents, and practicing physicians.

Doctor-Patient Communication in its Historical Context

As early as the classical age of Greek medicine, it was recognized that different approaches to communication had relative advantages and disadvantages. In a passage that has astonishing relevance for modern medical practice, Plato (cited in Hamilton and Cairns 1961) describes two sets of communication practices that distinguished the care of slaves from that of free men. "Slaves, to speak generally, are treated by slaves who pay them a hurried visit. . . . A physician of this kind never gives a servant any account of his complaint, nor asks him for any; he gives him some empirical injunction with an air of finished knowledge, in the brusque fashion of a dictator, and then is off in hot haste to the next ailing servant." By contrast "The free practitioner, who for the most part attends free men, treats their diseases by going into things thoroughly from the beginning in a scientific way, and takes the patient and his family into confidence. . . . He does not give prescriptions until he has won the patient's support, and when he has done so, he steadily aims at producing complete restoration of health by persuading the sufferer into compliance."

What we find compelling in this statement is that the communication practices that characterized the relationship of physicians to free men in ancient Greece, namely "going into things thoroughly from the beginning," "taking the patient and family into confidence," and "restoring health by persuading the sufferer into compliance," so closely approximate contemporary research findings that relate physician-patient agreement (Starfield et al. 1981), patient-centeredness (Stewart, Brown and Westin 1989), and patient participation (Greenfield, Kaplan, and Ware 1987) to satisfaction and improved outcomes. The parallel contrast also holds. Patients today, like Greek slaves whose autonomy and means of expression were severely limited by a physician-centered, physician-dominated communication style, are described as less satisfied and more likely to bring suit in the face of an undesired outcome (Valente et al. 1988).

In addition to locating deep historical continuities in medical practice, a historical framework is useful in teaching and learning about change and in clarifying conflicting values. One contemporary example is the communication of diagnostic and prognostic information to patients. Reiser (1980), in a seminal paper on this topic, notes that the prevailing view in medicine for the past 2,000 years has been to withhold information because communicating it was assumed to be harmful and not in the best interests of the patient. He cites authorities from Hippocrates, who cautioned physicians to conceal "most things from the patient . . . turning his attention away from what is being done to him," to Thomas Percival, whose views were adopted at the founding meeting of the American Medical Association in 1847 and who counseled that "The life of a sick person can be shortened not only by the acts, but also by the words and manner of a physician."

The assumption that withholding information was correct was tested at the beginning of the twentieth century when Richard Cabot, an American physician in Boston, began telling patients the true nature of their conditions. Contrary to his own expectations, patients were actually grateful for the information and did not seem to get worse as a consequence of knowing. In the six decades that followed Cabot's discovery, attitudes toward disclosure remained virtually unchanged. For example, Oken (1961), in a study of physicians' communication practices after diagnosing cancer, found that almost 90% withheld the diagnosis from the patient. A mere 20 years later, however, a similar study conducted by Novack, et al. (1979), based on the same questions used by Oken, revealed a complete reversal in attitudes, with 98% of the physicians studied affirming the value of being frank with patients who have cancer.

The importance of incorporating a historical perspective in teaching about truth telling, for example, is that it allows trainees to locate their experiences and values in the broader context and traditions of medical practice. In our own experience as teachers, we have found that students and residents are often incredulous to learn that the value they place on telling patients the truth—far from being timeless—is in fact part of an ongoing change that gained momentum less than a generation ago. Such insight often is helpful in reframing conflicts in values, especially between younger and older, more traditional physicians.

From Anecdote to Outcome: Recent Developments in Doctor-Patient Communication Research

While the value of communication has been recognized for millennia, serious systematic inquiry into the subject is of relatively recent origin. Students of the medical interview such as Stoeckle and Billings (1987) mark the beginning of contemporary research on doctor-patient communication in the late 1930s. It was during that period that William F. Murphy and Felix Deutch began recording encounters of psychiatric residents with their patients. Before recordings of actual interviews were available, research on communication was limited to anecdotal experience and case reports, neither of which contained accounts of the actual dialogue that transpired between physician and patient (Deutch and Murphy 1954). The development of audio and video technology made possible moment-by-moment descriptions of the language and dynamics of the interview. From these detailed descriptions, new techniques of supervision and feedback emerged.

In addition to the contributions of technology to research, World War II provided an opportunity for new collaborations among medical specialties and the development of new approaches to disabling emotional conditions such as "shell shock" and "battle fatigue." In general terms, advancing technology and wartime experience led early researchers to focus intensively and descriptively on the doctor-patient relationship and its importance as a social relationship.

In the modern era, research on doctor-patient communication has grown apace, in both scope and sophistication. Currently, some 7,500 articles on doctor-patient communication are listed in the *Index Medicus* and the Social Science Citation Index combined. Inui and Carter (1985, 1988) have recently reviewed the spectrum of research designs used to investigate doctor-patient communication. In addition to increased methodological sophistication, they also note that the field is maturing scientifically, as evidenced by the movement of research methodologies over the past 30 years from developmental-descriptive to subexperimental-etiologic and, most recently, to interventional. A review of the history of progress in research methods will summarize what is currently known about doctor-patient communication and its impact on the process and outcomes of health care, and will also serve as a prologue to our discussion of teaching techniques.

Beginning in the mid-1960s with the analysis of individual visits using direct observation, two-way mirrors, and later audio and video tapes, investigators first began to recognize that verbal and nonverbal behaviors affect the *process* of communication. Because of the focus on process, patient satisfaction quickly became the predominant outcome measure studied. In the late 1960s and early 1970s, Barbara Korsch and her colleagues (Korsch, Gozzi, and Francis 1968; Francis, Korsch, and Morris 1969; Freeman et al. 1971) began to categorize and quantify patient and physician behaviors and to correlate their presence or absence with patient satisfaction. In their studies, conducted in pediatric settings, variables such as meeting patients' expectations and provider warmth were positively correlated with patient satisfaction. Since Korsch's ground-breaking work, many studies have been conducted to further identify variables positively and negatively correlated with patient satisfaction.

The major accomplishment of this exploratory period was the development of increasingly sophisticated and reliable methodologies for categorizing the actions of patient and provider during clinical encounters. Coding schemes, such as the ones developed by Bales (1950) and modified by Roter (1985) and Stiles (1979), permitted enumeration of the types of utterances by participants, their frequency of occurrence, sequence analysis of the discourse, and categorization of both utterances and paralinguistic behaviors. The result was a burst of nonspecific, subexperimental studies, which Inui and Carter (1988) describe as "dredging" for associations between doctor-patient behaviors and outcomes such as satisfaction and compliance. Rather than propose hypotheses, researchers counted an exhaustive number of behaviors, displayed by either patients or provider, and correlated them with desired outcomes, typically satisfaction, intention to comply, or compliance itself. During this period, prospective testing of positively correlated behaviors was not carried out, leading many biomedically oriented researchers to discount the conclusions and recommendations.

Even with the amount of data being generated, a major limitation of work during this period became apparent. Research was conducted in the absence of a unifying conceptual framework to house the burgeoning data. The result was a growing body of information that demanded attention, but was difficult to incorporate into a successful practice model.

The identification of a growing number of provider and patient characteristics associated with satisfaction and compliance, however, paved the way for the next change in the field. Investigators in the late 1970s began to test the specific associations they believed best correlated with outcomes of interest. These types of studies are exemplified by the work of Wasserman et al. (1984), who correlated provider encouragement and empathy, but not reassurance, with patient satisfaction. Using a similar design, Starfield et al. (1979) found a positive association between patient-physician agreement on problems regarding follow-up and subsequent problem resolution.

These subexperimental studies were valuable because they were data driven and permitted the exploration of a particular process in more detail. For example, Wasserman and his colleagues subclassified supportive statements made by pediatricians or clinical nurse specialists into categories of reassurance, empathy, and encouragement. Using this classification scheme, Wasserman et al. were able to relate various types of reassurance with outcome data demonstrating positive or negative effects. For instance, while the pediatricians in Wasserman's study used reassurance most frequently, it bore the weakest association to reductions in maternal concern. By contrast, empathy and encouragement, which were used less frequently, were most highly associated with a reduction in concerns. The findings from

Wasserman's study allowed educators and practitioners to begin to examine such important issues as where, and under what conditions, behaviors such as empathy could be most effectively employed.

Subexperimental studies, although more specific, were still limited by the lack of a conceptual framework that could tie seemingly isolated findings together to significantly improve actual consultations between physicians and patients. From the middle 1980s to the present, researchers have continued, with increasing sophistication, to establish linkages between specific elements of communication in the medical encounter and both short- and longer-term medical care outcomes. Much of this research is informed conceptually by the work of Engel (1977) and others, who have criticized a purely biomedical approach to patient care as failing to recognize the systemic and reciprocal influence of psychosocial factors on the disease process. Investigation of the psychosocial factors, their relationship to the pathophysiology of disease, and their influence on health care outcomes has set the stage for the use of very sophisticated research methodologies to intervene and test hypotheses in a true experimental fashion.

What is already known using these methods may be summarized as follows:

(1) The quality of clinical communication is related to positive health outcomes. In a series of studies using randomized control trials, Kaplan, Greenfield, and Ware (1989) have demonstrated both functional and clinical benefits from a 20-minute coaching intervention designed to teach patients to be more assertive during the medical encounter. For hypertension, diabetes, and peptic ulcer disease, patients in the respective experimental groups had significantly lower blood pressures, blood sugars, and better functional outcomes, such as fewer days missed from work, when compared with patients who received no such communication skills training. A study of the resolution of chronic headache symptoms by the Headache Study Group of the University of Western Ontario (1986) found that the single most powerful predictor of positive outcome was the patients' perception that the physician had listened to all their concerns.

(2) Agreement between physician and patient on the nature of the problem and the proposed solution is related to improving or resolving the problem. Several authors, including Stewart, McWhinney, and Buck (1979); Starfield et al. (1981); and Bass et al. (1986), have noted a strong positive association between doctor-patient discussion of the nature and seriousness of the clinical problem and its resolution.

(3) Explaining patient concerns, even when they cannot be resolved, results in a significant reduction of anxiety. Echoing our earlier discussion of the costs and benefits of delivering bad diagnostic or prognostic news to patients, a number of authors, most recently Mac-

Leod (1991), have demonstrated that patients show a reduction in anxiety when told the truth about their condition. In MacLeod's study the subjects were women with advanced breast cancer.

(4) Greater participation by the patient in the encounter improves satisfaction and compliance. A study by Roter (1977) demonstrated a strong positive association between patients who were more actively involved in asking questions during the encounter and both satisfaction and compliance with medical orders.

(5) The benefits of patient-centered interviewing can be achieved without unduly prolonging visits. A recent study by Stewart, Brown, and Westin (1989) compared biomedically oriented and patient-centered interviewing styles. The authors found that physicians skilled in patient-centered interviewing took an average of only one minute longer than physicians following the narrowly focused biomedical approach. Significantly, the authors also found that for physicians who had not mastered the skills of patient-centered interviewing, the time costs were much more significant. They concluded that physicians learning patient-centered interviewing techniques may need to be supported and encouraged to view the process in developmental terms, with attendant costs and benefits at each stage.

We believe that, if any communication skills program is to be successful, it is important for students and residents to be familiar with basic research strategies that have been employed in the study of doctor-patient communication. In addition, it is important for trainees to recognize the direction in which the field is developing. In this way, it is possible to relate pedagogy to practice in concrete and definable ways. It is also important that trainees be aware of the most important findings of the field today. In the same way that journal articles are used to convey the most recent advances in diagnosis and treatment, the literature on doctor-patient communication can be used to provide guidance and insight, especially about behaviors and techniques of interviewing that influence the process and outcomes of care.

Can Caring Be Taught as a Clinical Communication Skill?

In 1983 the American Board of Internal Medicine (ABIM) published a position paper, "Evaluation of Humanistic Qualities in the Internist" (ABIM 1983). The Board identified three qualities it believed essential to good medical practice and suggested that in the future such skills be demonstrated in a formal way as a condition for licensure. The qualities are: *integrity,* the personal commitment to be honest and trustworthy in evaluating and demonstrating one's own skills and abilities; *respect,* the personal commitment to honor others' choices and rights in their medical care; and *compassion,* an appreciation that suffering and illness engender special needs for comfort and help, without evoking excessive emotional involvement that could undermine professional responsibility.

Publication of this paper was ground-breaking in at least two respects. First, although it was the work of an ad hoc committee that could act only to inform and advise, the very recognition of humanistic qualities as an important dimension of doctoring was significant. Second, the committee recommended some educational strategies for training internal medicine residents including: direct observation and feedback, Balint type physician support groups, discussions of values and feelings, and faculty modeling of key humanistic qualities.

As significant and compelling as the Board's statement was, it did not address several key areas. For example, the qualities of integrity, respect, and compassion, while given global definition, were not identified in terms of specific skills or behaviors that could be tracked across one or several encounters. As well, the educational strategies recommended, while intuitively appealing, were largely untested and unproved.

Since 1983, there have been significant conceptual and practical advances in teaching and evaluating clinical communication skills that lend additional weight to the Board's recommendations. A marker of growing maturity in this area is a recently published consensus statement on doctor-patient communication (Simpson et al. 1991). This statement followed by five years the first international conference on doctor-patient communication and the publication of an edited volume summarizing the state of the field (Stewart and Roter 1989). The consensus statement reviews the current state of knowledge about doctor-patient communication as it relates to both health care outcomes and educational strategies and also identifies the most important unanswered questions and priorities for future research.

With respect to education and training, the consensus statement identifies five characteristics of successful programs: a defined curriculum (Lipkin, Quill, and Napadano 1984); observable criteria for skills training (Maguire 1990); opportunities for observation, practice, and feedback using videotape, audiotape, role playing, and standardized patients (Cohen-Cole 1991); coordinated teaching approaches at all levels of training (Engler et al. 1981); and close attention to trainees' emotional needs via Balint and other support group activities (Quill and Williamson 1984).

The conclusions of the consensus panel are confirmed by our own experience in designing and teaching a course in interviewing for second-year medical students and also in attempting to change resident behavior in the area of humanistic skills. We will briefly review our efforts and findings in each of these areas. From 1985 to 1990, while we were both on the faculty of Wayne State University, we designed and offered a course in basic clinical interviewing skills to year 2 medical students. The course was part of the introduction to physical diagnosis. Our basic goal was to help year 2 students become more comfortable with the dual responsibilities of a physician: eliciting clinical information while establishing a supportive relationship. The course consisted of two introductory lectures to the entire second-year class ($N = 256$), followed by faculty-facilitated small group practice sessions for which the students were divided into groups of six. During these sessions, each student was videotaped for up to five minutes interviewing a professional actor or actress who played one of six patient roles. Each of the tapes was reviewed for approximately 20 minutes per student.

The underlying purposes of our approach were to (1) establish a nonjudgmental, supportive learning environment; (2) emphasize the relevance of the students' existing repertoire of interpersonal skills; and (3) employ a learner-centered "educational alliance" to promote adoption of a patient-centered "therapeutic alliance" for delivering care. The objectives for the course were that, upon completion, students would be able to perform the following tasks: (1) unambiguously greet patients; (2) put patients at ease and, in an open-ended way, solicit their reasons for seeking care; (3) encourage the patient to enumerate a complete list of problems by using silence, continuers, and acknowledgment statements; (4) identify and sensitively explore seven traditional dimensions of a symptom—description, location, onset, severity, precipitators, alleviators, and associated symptoms—and to elicit the patient's attribution of the problem(s); and (5) utilize basic emotion-handling skills such as empathic listening to create a therapeutic alliance.

Small group discussions began with an introduction of learning goals and an explanation of the videotaping process. In addition, there was an attempt to put the students at ease by stressing the nonevaluative nature of the sessions. After soliciting for additional questions and concerns, the faculty preceptor asked for a volunteer to do the first interview. The student interviewer left the group and walked onto a set designed to look like an office in an outpatient clinic. While the student was conducting his or her interview, the rest of the group watched on a remote television monitor. After completing the interview, the student returned to the group for discussion and replay of the videotape. The student was asked to briefly summarize the interview from his or her perspective, focusing particularly on aspects of the interaction that were difficult or rewarding. The student's summary served as a baseline for identifying learning needs and developing a focus for discussion. Before reviewing the tape, the faculty elicited additional feedback from the group on strengths and problem areas in the interview.

The videotape review itself focused on specific aspects of the student's interaction as it related to his or her learning needs and the goals of the course. Stop action and multiple replay of critical communication junctures were used to heighten appreciation of the influence of interviewer's behavior—much of it subtle and nonverbal—on the direction, flow, and completeness of information obtained. Opportunities for open-ended group discussion and the development of alternative strategies for achieving course goals were encouraged. Each replay concluded with a review by the student of the specific skills and strategies that he or she took away from the learning experience.

During the five years that the course was offered, it was enthusiastically received and positively evaluated by the students. Students identified as strengths of the course its small group format, the safety of the learning environment created by the faculty, and the opportunity to practice and discuss specific skills and techniques. Weaknesses of the course that were identified were the lack of follow-up sessions or training, student frustration about having limited clinical exposure and knowledge, and—initially—the large group size. As a result of student feedback, the group size was reduced from eight to six students per session. Another index of success of the course was attendance at the small group sessions, which consistently ran in the 97-98% range for the year 2 class involved.

In the last year that we taught the course, we made an attempt to evaluate a specific area of teaching: the students' success in eliciting patient attribution. To test the effect of our teaching in this area, a standardized patient problem in which attribution played a key role was randomly placed as either the first encounter or the last encounter to be taped and discussed in the small group sessions. Nine of 21 students whose encounters with this patient were taped first elicited attribution. By contrast, when the same scenario was presented last, 17 of 22 students successfully elicited the patient's views. Chi square analysis was highly significant ($P < 0.01$), suggesting a 99% likelihood that improvement in the skill of eliciting attribution was a product of the small group discussion. This type of finding is consistent with those of researchers like Maguire, Fairburn, and Fletcher (1986), who have demonstrated both the short- and long-term benefits of video feedback and in communication skills training. It also confirms the importance of using specifically defined skills as a basis for evaluation.

In the context of residency training, we have attempted to develop and measure changes in humanistic skills in first-year trainees (Beckman, Frankel et al. 1990). The goal of this study was to evaluate an intervention designed to help resident trainees incorporate skills that promote humane patient care. To test this approach, we evaluated residents in nine skill areas derived from the ABIM categories of integrity and respect. We chose a type of medical encounter that is frequently problematic for interns, namely, transition visits from patients who are already established in a clinic but who have been reassigned to the interns as new patients. The skills studied included (1) informing the patient that his or her medical record had been reviewed prior to the visit; (2) introducing oneself as a provider new to the practice; (3) recognizing the patient as having been previously followed in the practice by acknowledging the agenda from previous visits; (4) describing the objectives of the visit; (5) meeting the patient; (6) identifying current problems; (7) collecting relevant history; (8) explaining the need for an extended visit if one was necessary; and (9) soliciting the patient's time constraints for an extended visit.

Prior to the intervention, interns were videotaped during transition visits. The intervention consisted of a one-hour lecture on communication skills, using video vignettes and role playing to illustrate and target each behavior. Following the intervention, interns were again videotaped during transition visits. The videotapes were then coded for the presence or absence of the target behaviors.

The preintervention group performed a mean of 1.38 skills, while the postintervention group performed a mean of 3.56 skills. Overall, there was a consistent increase in the performance of all skills in the postintervention group. When clustered together, the increase in skills performed by this group reached statistical significance (P = 0.03).

From this study we reached several conclusions. First, it was possible, by means of viewing problematic encounters involving first-year trainees, to identify a set of concrete, definable skills that were associated with two of the three qualities of humane care identified by the ABIM in 1983. Exposing the trainees to videotaped examples of the target behaviors and giving them opportunities to practice resulted in better performance when compared with historical controls. While the magnitude of change among the skills was variable, the trend toward improvement in all skill areas for the experimental group suggested that additional training and reinforcement might lead to further improvement.

On the basis of our findings, we concluded that it is possible to identify and change interactional skills associated with humane care, a topic left unaddressed by ABIM in its position paper. In contrast with global assessments, such as "poor empathy skills," which may leave a trainee feeling as though he or she has a character fault, we suggested the use of concrete, observable actions as the basis for feedback. In retrospect, it appears that our approach to humanistic skills is quite similar to that of others, such as Maguire (1990), Lipkin (1987), and Cohen-Cole (1991), who have reported success in teaching more generalized clinical communication skills.

Conclusions

We began this chapter by noting that there is both a public and professional crisis in American medicine today. Given the current state of doctor-patient communication studies, we believe there is reason to be cautiously optimistic about the skills, attitudes, and values of future physicians regarding the doctor-patient relationship and its importance to the health care process and its outcomes. Historically, we are at a point where the motivation to disclose and the desire to know the truth about diagnosis and prognosis complement one another. This represents an enormous change in values and attitudes and holds the potential for physicians and patients to develop true partnerships and shared responsibility for life-and-death decisions. Similarly, with respect to research on doctor-patient communication, we have developed enormously sophisticated techniques for relating specific elements of communication to both biomedical and functional outcomes of care. Increased methodological and theoretical sophistication is rapidly moving us toward a comprehensive and integrated theory of what matters in the doctor-patient relationship, and how to use it to best advantage. Finally, there is growing consensus among both scholars and educators about the most effective ways to teach clinical communication skills to trainees and young clinicians.

In our own experience, we have found the use of history, research, and innovative educational techniques to be most effective in teaching and modeling communication skills at all levels of training. We believe that traditional medical education has fundamentally failed to address the current crisis. Our hypothesis, and the educational experiment that will test it, assumes that students and residents who are respected, nurtured, and empowered in their educational process will become physicians who will bring those same skills, and the attendant positive outcomes, to the practice of medicine in the twenty-first century.

Concluding Commentary

14

Toward a Social Medicine

James E. Lewis and J. Claude Bennett

The papers in this book on the physician-patient relationship give the reader a wide array of viewpoints presented by scholars from several social science disciplines and medicine. These scholars are committed to furthering our understanding of the complex relationship at the heart of clinical medicine—the interaction of an individual patient with an individual physician. Their questions, their approaches to answering them, and the way they interpret their data are shaped by the philosophies that underlie their disciplines, training, and subsequent experience as investigators and teachers. Thus, in this volume, we have at least twelve approaches to investigating, understanding, reacting to, and making suggestions for improving the interaction between physician and patient in light of widely differing expectations for such encounters.

Focusing on the encounter, this intimate event, provides a starting point, perhaps the best starting point, for melding a "social medicine" out of this array of academic disciplines. The melding process will be neither quick nor easy. One of the essentials, besides learning one's own discipline, is developing a thorough working knowledge of the intricacies of the structure and organization of health care: how it is financed, what and how physicians and other health professionals are taught, how they are socialized into their profession, and, perhaps most important, how rapidly everything in the "health industry" changes.

Social change may be one of the most important factors giving rise to concern about physician-patient communication. We shall discuss in depth how changes in what physicians are technically able to do alters, over time, the balance between the art and the science of medicine. When technical ability and biological knowledge are limited, the physician has little to offer but "art," that is, the caring and concern that nourish hope that disease will be overcome and health restored.

What we all want is that such caring and concern not be overlooked or lost as technical ability and biological knowledge advance.

Reading these papers a year after hearing them presented and discussed at a symposium, "Patient Care Relationships and Ethics" (Clair and Wilson 1990), makes even the assigned title of this commentary the basis for a series of questions:

(1) Rather than "concluding," it is clear that the discussion is in its opening stages: What do physicians view themselves as able to give the patient and how does that compare with what the patient, the patient's family, and society expect? Are the latter three expectations congruent? Moreover, how do the measures and interpretations of those expectations, and the varying degrees to which physicians meet them, vary among social scientists and physicians and between social and medical disciplines?

(2) What is "social medicine" and how can it help make the everyday practice of medicine more humane, more sensitive and responsive to the patient's psychosocial concerns and needs and more appreciative of the possible relationships between the patient's socioeconomic milieu and the medical problems he or she presents to the physician?

(3) In a more complex vein, is it appropriate and realistic to cast the physician as the primary representation of the health care system in any country? Jeffrey Clair's reference (chap. 1) caused us to read Kafka's (1971) "A Country Doctor." In the story, an overworked, exhausted physician is called out at night during a snowstorm to the cottage of a patient whose infected wound will prove to be beyond the physician's ability to help. The physician's own horses are exhausted and his groom has found another, but unruly, team. The doctor's groom refuses to accompany him, preferring to stay behind, intent on a physical relationship with the doctor's housekeeper. Although the story was written in the winter of 1916-17, many contemporary physicians may well see the blizzard, the overpowering horses, the recalcitrant groom, the patient beyond professional help, and the housemaid whom the doctor is unable to protect as transcultural anticipation of circumstances in the late twentieth century: storms of paperwork; forces of competition, cost control, and technological advance; hospital, practice, and third-party payer administrative bureaucracies; patients whom all of a century's advances in medical science cannot help; and physicians' families and loved ones sacrificed to the "god" of healing others. They will have special appreciation for the physician, who, having been stripped of most of his clothes at the patient's cottage, rides off disheveled and nearly naked astride one of the steeds. How much more out of control could a physician be? The concept of physician power and control described by social scientists and other observers may be just an illusion. While it may not be intended by the physician,

the illusion may be sought and held by patients as a part of their desire for restoration to a prior healthy state, or to an otherwise acceptable quality of life. Or it may be projected by observers, perhaps reflecting their own experiences as patients.

(4) From the standpoint of the processes of medical education, the past year has seen an unparalleled succession of high-level national conferences.[1] These have been driven by fundamental questions: What do physicians need to know? How, in four short years, is that body of information to be integrated into their being, along with the sense of responsibility for constantly replenishing and renewing it? And how can the profession and society assure themselves that these mortals, their sons and daughters, have committed themselves to meeting the standards and the expectations of the profession, including that of effective communication with patients?

What do we think should be the aim of social medicine? Why do we think that aim is worthy of wide study? How do these authors' excellent and representative views of patient-physician communication, as an element of social medicine, contribute to our understanding of what might be and what can be? The ideas put forth here should propel further interdisciplinary work toward a social medicine.

Balancing the Art and Science of Medicine

Jeffrey Clair's description (chap. 1) of Sir Luke Fildes's 1891 painting *The Doctor* reveals that there is little beyond "art," in the sense of his physical presence, visible concern, and caring, that the physician can offer the apparently deathly ill child, the stoic father, and the sobbing, prayerful mother. The setting is a workingman's cottage, not a hospital, which in the 1890s was still a place where people went only to die. Medical science is represented by an obviously medicinal liquid in a clear glass bottle with a cork stopper. A cup with a fiddle-handled pewter spoon (coffee for the doctor?), an orange crockery mixing bowl holding a larger spoon, and a large pitcher are the sum total of the (possibly) medical tools shown. Not even a doctor's black bag is visible; perhaps the child is beyond help.

This painting, in all its somber hues and shadows, with the light focused on the physician and the child-patient, epitomizes the disparity between art and science that characterized medicine until the discovery of sulfonamides in the late 1930s and penicillin in the early 1940s and their widespread battlefield use in World War II. In the twilight of the twentieth century, with medical miracles at every hand, it is often difficult to realize that the "century of medical progress" since *The Doctor* was painted has in fact been a bare half century of greater than geometric rates of growth in medical knowledge, medical technology, and, in spite of our failing to serve everyone, of access not just to caring hands but in many cases to curing ones as well.

It has been suggested that the child in *The Doctor* is dying of diphtheria. Hardly anyone in industrialized societies has died of diphtheria in three or four decades; infants are vaccinated against it soon after birth. The World Health Organization believes that goal is achievable worldwide before the year 2000 for diphtheria as well as for polio, whooping cough, and most of the other diseases of childhood. There is reason to hope that, like smallpox, these diseases can be eradicated. To be sure, we now have AIDS and its ravages of babies, children, and adults; substance abuse; and, in the United States at least, an epidemic of homicides. Medical science is almost powerless against these diseases; curing them seems to be an almost meaningless idea. The only workable approach is prevention, which implies changes in human behavior.

In figure 14.1 we have represented the changing imbalances between the art and science of medicine over the past century or century and a half. We say "imbalances" because the art and the science have never been equal. For millennia, as Charlotte Borst (chap. 4) points out, the healer's art was great caring, empathy, humane concern, and occasionally an empirically derived cure, near-cure, or alleviation (perhaps coincidental or spontaneous) of symptoms. The basis for a medical science, which grew slowly, was laid by the discoveries that the body consisted of interconnected organs, that blood circulated, that microorganisms could cause disease, and that in its healthy, properly fed, exercised, and cared-for state the body was wonderfully self-regulating.

For centuries, diagnostic acumen was largely guesswork enhanced by experience that improved only slightly with each major technological advance: the stethoscope (1816), the thermometer (1868), roentgenography or X-rays (1895), the sphygmomanometer (1895), and clinical laboratory studies of blood (ca. 1918) and urine (ca. 1930). While, as Hughes Evans points out in chapter 5, adoption of those devices often was slow, meeting resistance from the medical profession, the accumulation of this intellectual and technical base provided a firm foundation for the discovery of antimicrobial agents—a scant 50 years ago. But in the last half century the science of medicine has loomed so large that the art—despite the lives saved and the quality-of-life improvements for so many—has, in both appearance and reality, diminished. Hence, there has followed a public and professional outcry for caring as well as curing, and that concern has been recognized in recently expanded professional requirements for certification—for example, those of the American Board of Internal Medicine (1991).

Figure 14.1. Shifting Cultures of Medicine

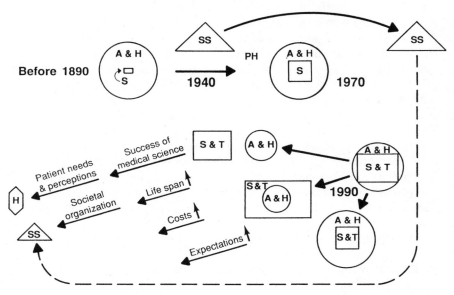

Note: Size of geometric figures represents proportional relationships.

A & H - Art and humanistic aspects of medicine
S - Scientific aspects of medicine
T - Technical aspects of medicine
S & T - Scientific and technological aspects of medicine
PH - Public health
SS - Social sciences
H - Humanities

Figure 14.1 shows the changing relationships between the art and science of medicine over the past century. The starting point in figure 14.1 was arbitrarily set in 1890, which, as it happens, is the year before Fildes's painting. The imbalances between the art and humanities (A&H) and the science (S) of medicine are shown by the sizes of the circles and rectangles; the major contributions of pharmaceutical and public health (PH) advances occurred at midcentury, causing science to grow larger relative to art and humanity. About this same period, the social sciences (SS) began their parallel course of growth and relatively modest interaction with medicine.

By 1990 medical science and technology (S&T) and art and humanities are close to being in balance, but only in an aggregate that does not exist in reality. In some situations, some medical specialties experience a separation of them, in others science and technology far outweigh the art and humanities, and in the third case, the current state of science and technology leaves us still with only the physician's art and humanity as weapons against certain diseases—AIDS being a prominent example. But if we focus on the success of medical science, we have, along with a longer life span (and greater quality of life), much greater medical and health care costs and vastly increased expectations of what physicians can do and, to some degree, how they should go about it.

Medicine must learn and benefit from a more humane, socially sensitive approach to patients' needs and perceptions. The social sciences can contribute greatly to that understanding, yet they also bear a major responsibility for helping all of us understand how societal organization influences physicians, patients, their interactions, and their relative satisfaction or dissatisfaction.

Our aim for a more "social" medicine is the establishment and maintenance of a balance between the art and the science of medicine. Our aim for the discipline of "social medicine" is to help all of us understand how to accomplish that goal.

Patient-Physician Communication: Variations on a Theme

Allman, Yoels, and Clair (chap. 2) contrast what the physician and the patient expect from their interaction. It is worth repeating in summary form:

Physician's Agenda: Make a diagnosis after defining diagnostic possibilities, based on chief complaint, history of present illness, past medical history, family history, review of systems, and complete physical examination; develop an evaluation and management plan; develop a relationship with the patient.

Patient's Agenda: Learn explanation for the cause of illness; seek therapy and cure; be kept informed by the doctor; participate in decision making when desired; maintain autonomy as much as possible; gain health education; get help with life stresses, depression, or social isolation.

Allman, Yoels, and Clair note (chap. 2) that "the traditional clinical method does not insure that the physician will pay attention to these [the patient's] issues." Most medical educators agree that some improvement in communication is needed on the physician's side, especially if it will help elicit more useful information from the patient, help the patient feel that the physician has listened to him or her, help the patient understand what the physician has said, and increase the patient's compliance with a prescribed therapeutic regimen. At the same time, we must recognize that time for training is both limited and jammed full and that, once in practice, time is the physician's only item of exchange.

The realities of medical education must be taken into account. It is widely accepted among medical educators that the student needs to memorize less and instead to learn more about how to organize and critically analyze information. But there are some basics that to a physician have to be as much second nature as knowing one's own name. In emergency situations, critically ill patients cannot wait for the physician to look up facts and organize them. There has to be an immediate reflex response that is right for that problem at that time. Granted, the art of medicine has been overwhelmed by the science of medicine in the past few decades. But how much of the art should be devoted to ills of societal etiology, and what should we teach medical students to do about such ills beyond what is taught to all other students to enhance their sense of social responsibility and humanity?

The encounter transcripts provided by Howard Waitzkin, Theron Britt, and Constance Williams (chap. 8) are both illuminating and cause for concern, for they put critical points in concrete terms. The videotapes presented at the symposium by Frankel and Beckman should be seen by all physicians and medical educators. Time will not blot out the image of a young adult female patient holding closed her open-throated blouse as a male obstetrician-gynecologist a few years older than she off-handedly asks intimate details about her sexual activity without knowing, in fact, whether she is sexually active with her boyfriend.

Reforming medical curricula is a continuing challenge. In recent decades, there have been serious efforts to shorten the curriculum to more quickly provide the additional physicians that society said it wanted, and possibly to reduce the costs of medical education. There have been major revisions designed to bring about a more orderly, that is, logical, presentation of curriculum content and to introduce advances in modern biology earlier. There have been efforts to involve medical students with patients at the beginning of their medical school careers rather than waiting, usually until the clerkship and acting intern years. Few schools believe that communication skills can (or need) be taught; most believe those skills come through observation of others during the training years. Although major reform efforts are under way, there is immense inertia in the medical education system, and true reform will be slow.

The financial realities of medical practice cannot be ignored. Dissatisfied patients go to other physicians either directly or by enrolling in other health care plans. If their dissatisfaction is great enough, they complain to their family and friends, who also may choose another physician or health plan, and if they have been medically injured, they may sue for malpractice. In a well-run health maintenance organization, where in effect the organization has a bargain with the patient (or his employer) that it can keep the patient satisfied and healthy for less than the amount of the annual subscription, the future costs of current dissatisfaction are high, perhaps unaffordable. And that is true whether the disjunction between the patient's expectations and the physician's offerings leads to merely greater utilization, to inappropriate malpractice litigation, or to disenrollment, all of which cost the organization time and money beyond the amount budgeted for the average subscriber.

For the physician in traditional practice, the penalties of patient dissatisfaction, excluding increased utilization costs, are the same, but there is no real mechanism of payment for keeping patients well, for spending more time than is required to deal with a patient's current problem (chief complaint), or for social and counseling services. This is not to suggest that the physician does not see the need for a longer visit or for supportive services; rather, there is simply no mechanism to pay for the time that the physician and his or her staff might spend on them. And, fundamentally, time is all the physician has to exchange for money or bartered goods. If that time is not rewarding, both professionally and economically, the physician is not going to be satisfied with his or her career choice. Anecdotally, in the past year we have encountered the following examples of physicians' frustrations:

(1) An excellent internist with whom we worked left practice after eight years for a residency in a surgical subspecialty, largely because the economics of practice would not permit him the time with patients that he and they thought appropriate.

(2) We have heard of middle-class suburban patients who demand of their physicians, whose offices are adjacent to what is known in the trade as a "green pastures" hospital, whatever new drugs or diagnostics or therapeutic maneuvers are reported in the weekly *New England Journal of Medicine*. Their physicians' rejections of their demands may help contain overall health costs but are unlikely to improve the patients' perception of physicians' communication skills.

(3) A highly regarded senior internist in a medium-sized community is abandoning his practice because he cannot meet either his or his patients' expectations and operate an economically viable practice.

(4) We have heard that one surgeon, as a matter of practice, does not talk to patients or their families after surgery.

Thus, the disjunction between what the physician intends to offer and what the patient expects from an encounter has many roots.

Toward a Social Medicine

Reading these papers fires the imagination and the desire for future studies. Jeffrey Clair in chapter 1 raises the question of "whether doctor-patient communication really matters." The extended, and not merely glib, response is: "Matters how, to what end, and to whom?" At one level, we want to know: Did the patient's medical situation objectively improve as a result of the encounter? At the subjective level: Do patients feel that their medical situation has improved? At still another: Are patients satisfied with their encounters with physicians? And yet another: Has the patient's ability to cope with life stresses increased? In other words, there are many possibilities for study. How can we justify medical intervention if the patient still feels sick afterward?

There are also questions, apparently unstudied as yet, as to differences among medical specialties with respect to communicating with patients. Are problems in communication associated more with one specialty than another? Where does the physician's (or the patient's) personality enter the equation? What more do we need to know about family involvement with older and younger patients and also with those who are terminally ill but do not want their families to know? Studies are needed of the roles of nonphysician health professionals in the patient-physician communication process.

Observational and impressionistic studies can provide valuable insights and assist in generating hypotheses. Explicit, controlled trials and other carefully designed experiments are needed to strengthen arguments for changing education programs, payer practices, and physician behavior. Fundamental to such studies is some philosophical agreement on what is desirable in a physician-patient encounter. The gulf between the patient's and the physician's agendas described by Allman, Yoels and Clair (chap. 2) is too wide to be accidental, and it cannot be bridged until there is wide agreement on the expected outcomes of the event for each party. Until such agreement is reached, medical educators will continue to teach physicians what they now believe to be important, and patients and patient advocates will continue to wonder why their expectations are not being met.

Attributing the failures of agreement to power imbalances, as reported in William Cockerham's review (chap. 3) of early medical sociological thinking, may deserve critical reconsideration. People who wait in lines at supermarkets and auto dealership service departments and who describe properly used legal language as "mumbojumbo" often feel powerless, just as they do when they tackle their annual income tax report. Are there studies or theories that indicate these power imbalances also are deliberate? Cockerham correctly observes that physician autonomy is declining particularly relative to communicating with patients of higher socioeconomic status.[2] Patients are better educated; many have a great and growing interest in health and biomedical science; and social class separations between professional and other occupational groups are less distinct and less accepted or sought than was the case a few decades ago.

On the other hand, the general public often is not aware that even in the 1950s and 1960s it was common for a small-town or suburban banker to look askance at a new physician's credit-worthiness, deny a loan, and, in so doing, inadvertently plant some of the seeds of the rural health "crisis" of the past two decades. Or that in the 1920s and 1930s, as physicians moved their offices from their homes to "medical arts" buildings to gain "prestige," newspaper advertisements urged them to buy an appropriate, i.e., sound, solid, but not ostentatious, "doctor's car" for the commute (Knox, Bohland, and Shumsky 1984). As Hughes Evans points out (chap. 5), a century ago physicians were warned that being seen doing manual labor would diminish their respectability. Referring again to *The Doctor,* note this quote from the era when it was painted, made by a physician lecturing to his students (Treuherz 1987:89): "What do we not owe to Mr. Fildes for showing to the world the typical doctor, as we would all like to be shown—an honest man and a gentleman, doing his best to relieve suffering? A library of books written in our honor would not do what this picture has done and will do for the medical profession in making the hearts of our fellow-men warm to us with confidence and affection." The question is put: When did physicians reach the peak of their supposed power and autonomy, what were the roots of their power and autonomy, and was the supposed power and autonomy real or an unfounded assumption that led to an unchallenged theory?

William Cockerham (chap. 3) also forces the recognition that simultaneous with the desires and efforts of medical educators to reduce the imbalances between the art and the science of medicine, educated patients of higher socioeconomic status desire to modify the "art" through increased participation in decision making relative to their own medical needs. As Cockerham points out, this desire is variable, depending on whether the illness is acute or chronic. In a recent patient-oriented news article, Peter M. Schur (1992:11), who specializes in chronic diseases such as rheumatoid arthritis and systemic lupus erythematosus, states another view: "When the patient thinks he or she knows more about a particular subject but really doesn't, dialogue is well-nigh impossible and irreconcilable conflict can easily result."

Robert Ohsfeldt's discussion of economics and agency relationships (chap. 6) describes two alternatives for physicians' behavior in the context of acting as agents for patients: The physician should either make the choice the patient would make given the information available to the physician, or act in the best interests of society to attain a just allocation of resources. Physicians in training are not taught to follow either alternative, and while some of us may consider that wrong, most do not. First and foremost, physicians (in the United States at least) are taught the sanctity of human life, which is to be preserved at virtually any cost. As recent events demonstrate, no state allows a physician to act overtly to end a patient's life, even if that is what the patient might choose.

Allocation of resources can be "just" only if there is an agreed-upon goal, presumably established nationally, against which resource allocation alternatives can be evaluated. As the current debate over national health programs illustrates, there is no agreed-upon and accepted national health goal at present and the Oregon experience demonstrates how difficult it is to find a societally acceptable resource allocation scheme even in a relatively small and homogeneous population.[3] The debate is worthwhile, however, because it begins with the question of whether an explicit resource allocation scheme is acceptable to the American people.

When people talk about withholding care or achieving the most effective and efficient outcomes of care, the discussion is made difficult by the ethical issues involved. Perhaps thinking about the differential contributions of medical art and medical science would advance the discussion. For example, in figure 14.2 we suggest a decreasing applicability and appropriateness of medical science and an increasing need for the art of medicine as the patient's age advances. We have hypothesized a curvilinear relationship among these variables but leave it to others to define, assess, and specify the exact relationship, if indeed, one exists.

The thirteen papers in this book are linked by the theme of patient-physician communication. Their differences are great enough that they have been organized into four sections. Yet their focus is that core event in health care—the encounter between a physician and a patient. Much remains to be learned, and more scholarship is needed, but these papers throw much light on many paths both worthy and in need of exploration.

There is a great need for those who would undertake social medicine as a field of scholarly endeavor to develop an early and deep understanding of the structure and organization of the health care system. How do the parts fit? How did they get that way? What are the flows of authority and responsibility, power, and money? How do things look from the inside as well as from the outside? What do colleagues in other fields say? What is the historical background of contemporary issues? What are the political science, the economic, the geographic, the psychosocial, and the socioeconomic views that can help illuminate some of the most complex issues in what might be the

Figure 14.2. The Relationship of Medical Art, Medical Science, and Patient Age

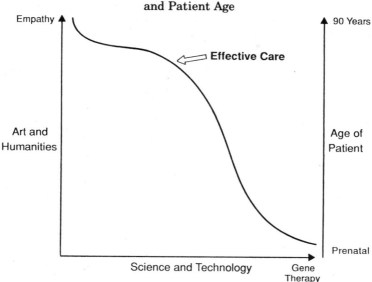

most complex system humanity ever created? There are many insightful responses to these questions within this book.

Social medicine should provide the opportunity for members of these related, but still separately focused, fields of study to come much closer together, to spend time in each others' libraries, to experience each others' seminars and conferences, so as to improve their ability to understand and explicate the intricacies of this marvelously complex system, at the heart of which is nothing more, and nothing less, than one patient and one physician talking together.

Notes

1. American Board of Internal Medicine, summer retreat, August 1991; proceedings published by ABIM. Association of Professors of Medicine/Association of American Medical Colleges, Retreat on Internal Medicine Curriculum Reform, Lansdowne Conference Center, Virginia, Sept. 19-21, 1991; meeting proceedings in *Annals of Internal Medicine* (June 15, 1992), *Supplement on Internal Medicine Curriculum Reform,* 116, No. 12: 1041-1116. Association of Professors of Medicine/Association of Program Directors in Internal Medicine, Teaching in Internal Medicine, Chicago, October 1991.

2. In the past decade, physician autonomy has been greatly limited by third-party payers, who decide whether, how much, and in what setting they will pay for a patient care service that the physician believes necessary and appropriate.

3. The health literature includes many articles about Oregon's attempt to balance public health care expenditures with presumed benefits to society. Four articles in *Health Affairs* 10, no. 2 (Summer 1992) introduce the subject and the problem: D.M. Fox, and H.M. Leichter, "Rationing Care in Oregon: The New Accountability," pp. 7-27; L.D. Brown, "The National Politics of Oregon's Rationing Plan," pp. 28-51; D. Callahan, "Ethics and Priority Setting in Oregon," pp. 78-87; and A. Etzioni, "Health Care Rationing: A Critical Evaluation," pp. 88-95.

References

Abbott, Andrew. 1988. *The System of Professions*. Chicago: University of Chicago Press.

Ackerknecht, E.H. 1948. "Anticontagionism between 1821 and 1867." *Bulletin of the History of Medicine* 22:569.

Ackerman, T. 1988. "Moral Dilemmas Involving Duties to Patients and Family." *Clinical Report on Aging* 2:3-4.

Adamson, T.; Tschann, J.; Gullion, D.; and Oppenberg, A. 1989. "Physician Communication Skills and Malpractice Claims: A Complex Relationship." *Western Journal of Medicine* 150:356-60.

Aiken, L., and Mechanic, D., eds. 1986. *Applications of Social Science to Clinical Medicine and Health Policy*. New Brunswick, N.J.: Rutgers University Press.

Allen, J., and Allen, M. 1979. "Discovering and Accepting Hearing Impairment: Initial Reactions of Parents." *Volta Review* 81:279-85.

American Board of Internal Medicine. 1983. "Evaluation of Humanistic Qualities in the Internist." *Annals of Internal Medicine* 99:720-24.

American Board of Internal Medicine. 1991. *Guide to the Awareness and Evaluation of Humanistic Qualities in the Internist: 1991-1995*. Philadelphia: ABIM.

American Medical Association. 1991a. *Issues Related to Graduate Education: AMA House of Delegates and Council on Medical Education*. Chicago: AMA.

American Medical Association. 1991b. *Socioeconomic Characteristics of Medical Practice 1990/91*. Chicago: AMA.

Amundsen, D.W. 1977. "The Duty of the Physician in Classical Legal Theory and Practice." *Journal of the History of Medicine and Allied Sciences* 32:202.

———. 1978. "The Physician's Obligation to Prolong Life: A Medical Duty Without Classical Roots." *Hastings Center Report* 8:23-30.

———. 1979. "Medicine and Surgery as Art or Craft: The Role of Schematic Literature in the Separation of Medicine and Surgery in the Late Middle Ages." *Transactions and Studies of the College of Physicians* 51:43-57.

———. 1981. "Casuistry and Professional Obligations: The Regulation of Physicians by the Court of Conscience in the Late Middle Ages." *Transactions and Studies of the College of Physicians* 5:93-94.

———— . 1982. "Medicine and Faith in Early Christianity." *Bulletin of the History of Medicine* 56:326-50.

Anderson, R.; House, D.; and Ormiston, M. 1981. "A Theory of Physician Behavior with Supplier-Induced Demand." *Southern Economic Journal* 47:124-33.

Annandale, Ellen C. 1989. "The Malpractice Crisis and the Doctor-Patient Relationship." *Sociology of Health and Illness* 11:1-23.

Applegate, W.B. 1986. "Physician Management of Patients With Adverse Outcomes." *Archives of Internal Medicine* 146:2249-52.

Arnott, R., and Stiglitz, J. 1991. "Moral Hazard and Non-market Institutions: Dysfunctional Crowding Out or Peer Monitoring." *American Economic Review* 81:179-90.

Auster, R., and Oaxaca, R. 1981. "The Identification of Supplier-Induced Demand in the Health Care Sector." *Journal of Human Resources* 16: 327-42.

Baader, G. 1985. "Early Medieval Latin Adaptations of Byzantine Medicine in Western Europe." Pp. 251-59 in *Symposium on Byzantine Medicine,* edited by J. Scarborough. Washington, D.C: Dumbarton Oaks Research Library and Collection.

Bales R. 1950. *Interaction Process Analysis.* Cambridge: Addison Wesley.

Ballester, L.G. 1981. "Galen as a Medical Practitioner: Problems in Diagnosis." Pp. 13-46 in *Galen: Problems and Prospects,* edited by Vivian Nutton. London: Welcome Institute for the History of Medicine.

Bangs, J.K. 1924. "A Man and His Car." *Hospital Social Service* 10:95.

Barsky, A.J. 1981. "Hidden Reasons Some Patients Visit Doctors." *Annals of Internal Medicine* 94:492-98.

Bartlett, E.E. 1990. "Improving Patient Communications for Malpractice Prevention." *Medical Encounter* 7:5-6.

Bass, M.; Buck, C.; Turner, L.; Dickie, G.; Pratt, G.; and Robinson, H. 1986. "The Physician's Actions and the Outcome of Illness in Family Practice." *Journal of Family Practice* 23(1):43-47.

Baxter, C. 1986. "Intellectual Disability: Parental Perceptions and Stigma as Stress." Doctoral diss., Monash University, Victoria, Australia.

Bayles, Michael D. 1981. "Physicians as Body Mechanics." Pp. 665-75 in *Concepts of Health and Disease: Interdisciplinary Perspectives,* edited by Arthur L. Caplan, H. Tristram Englehardt, Jr., and James J. McCartney. London: Addison-Wesley.

Beckman, H.B., and Frankel, R.M. 1984. "The Effect of Physician Behavior on the Collection of Data." *Annals of Internal Medicine* 101:692-96.

Beckman, H.B; Frankel, R.M; Kihm, J.; Kulesza, G.; and Geheb, M. 1990. "Measurement and Improvement of Humanistic Skills in First Year Trainees." *Journal of General Internal Medicine* 5:42-45.

Beckman, H.B.; Kaplan, S.H.; and Frankel, R.M. 1989. "Outcome-Based Research on Doctor-Patient Communication: A Review." Pp. 223-27 in *Communicating with Medical Patients,* edited by Moira Stewart and Debra Roter. Newbury Park, Calif. Sage.

Begley, C.E. 1987. "Prospective Payment and Medical Ethics." *Journal of Medicine and Philosophy* 12:107-22.

Beland, F., and Maheux, B. (1990). "Medical Care for the Elderly: Attitudes of Medical Caregivers." *Journal of Aging and Health* 2:194-214.

Bellet, P., and Maloney, M. 1991. "The Importance of Empathy as an Interviewing Skill in Medicine." *Journal of the American Medical Association* 266:1831-32.

Belli, M.M. 1989. *Belli: For Your Malpractice Defense.* Oradell, N.J.: Medical Economic Books.

Berg, J.M.; Gilderdale, S.; and Way, J. 1969. "On Telling Parents of the Diagnosis of Mongolism." *British Journal of Psychiatry* 115:1195-96.

Berry, C.; Held, P.J.; Kehrer, B.; et al. 1980. "Canadian Physicians' Supply Response to Universal Health Insurance." Pp. 56-70 in *Physicians and Financial Incentives,* edited by J.R. Gabel, et al. Washington, D.C.: U.S. Government Printing Office.

Bertakis, K.D.; Roter, D.; and Putman, S.M. 1991. "The Relationship of Physician Medical Interview Style to Patient Satisfaction." *Journal of Family Practice* 32:175-81.

Biegel, D.; Sales, E.; and Schulz, R. 1991. *Family Caregiving in Chronic Illness.* Newbury Park, Calif.: Sage.

Blascovich, J. 1982. "Social Psychology in Family Medicine." Pp. 279-300 in *Applied Social Psychology Annual,* edited by L. Bickman. Newbury Park, Calif.: Sage.

Blendon, R.J. 1989. "Three Systems: A Comparative Survey." *Health Management Quarterly* 11:2-10.

Blomqvist, Ake. 1991. "The Doctor as Double Agent: Information Asymmetry, Health Insurance, and Medical Care." *Journal of Health Economics* 10(4):411-32.

Bloom, S. 1989. "The Medical School as a Social Organization: The Sources of Resistance to Change." *Medical Education* 23:228-41.

―――. 1990. "Episodes in the Institutionalization of Medical Sociology: A Personal View." *Journal of Health and Social Behavior* 31(1):1-10.

Booth, W.A. 1849-50. "Quinine: The Importance of Understanding, and a Theory Relating to, its Modus Operandi." *New Orleans Medical News and Hospital Gazette* 6:251.

Boreham, P., and Gibson, D. 1978. "The Informative Process in Private Medical Consultation: A Preliminary Investigation." *Social Science and Medicine* 12:409-15.

Borell, Merriley. 1985. "The Kymograph and the Origins of the Graphic Method." *Electric Quarterly* 7 (Summer): 2-3.

―――. 1986. "Extending the Senses: The Graphic Method." *Medical Heritage* 2:114-21.

―――. 1987. "Instrumentation and the Rise of Modern Physiology." *Science and Technology Studies* 5 (2):53-62.

Borell, Merriley; Coon, Deborah J.; Evans, Hughes; and Hornstein, Gail A. 1988. "Selective Importation of the 'Exact Method': Experimental Physiology and Psychology in the United States, 1860-1910." Pp 189-96 in *Program, Papers, and Abstracts,* joint conference, 11-15 July 1988, British Society for the History of Science, Manchester, England; and the History of Science Society, Madison, Wisconsin.

Bosk, C.L. 1979. *Forgive and Remember: Managing Medical Failure*. Chicago: University of Chicago Press.

Boulton, M.; Tuckett, David; Olson, Coral; and Williams, Anthony. 1986. "Social Class and the General Practice Consultation." *Sociology of Health and Illness* 8:325-50.

Brandt, Allan M. 1985. Pp. 40 and 152 in *No Magic Bullet: A Social History of Venereal Disease in the United States since 1880*. New York and Oxford: Oxford University Press.

Brecher, Ruth, and Brecher, Edward. 1969. *The Rays: A History of Radiology in the United States and Canada*. Baltimore: Williams and Wilkens.

Breunlin, D.C.; Mann, B.J.; Richtsmeier, A.; Lillian, Z.; Richman, J.S.; and Bernotas, T. 1990. "Pediatricians' Perceptions of Their Behavioral and Developmental Training." *Journal of Developmental and Behavioral Pediatrics* 11:165-69.

Brim, Charles J. 1930. "The Story of Blood Pressure." *Medical Life* 37:72.

Brock, D.W., and Wartman, S.A. 1990. "When Competent Patients Make Irrational Choices." *New England Journal of Medicine* 322:1595-99.

Brockliss, L.W.B. 1978. "Medical Teaching at the University of Paris." *Annals of Science* 35:239-46.

Brody, D.S. 1980. "The Patient's Role in Clinical Decision-Making." *Annals of Internal Medicine* 93:718-22.

Brody, J. 1989. "Toward Quantifying the Health of the Elderly." *American Journal of Public Health* 79 (6):685-86.

Brook, R.E., and Williams, K.N. 1978. "Malpractice and the Quality of Care." *Annals of Internal Medicine* 88:836-38.

Brooten, K.E., and Chapman, S. 1987. *Malpractice: A Guide to Avoidance and Treatment*. New York: Harcourt Brace Jovanovich.

Broussais, F.J.V. 1831. P. 20 in *On Irritation and Insanity, a Work wherein the Relations of the Physical with the Moral Conditions of Man, are Established on the Basis of Physiological Medicine*. trans. Cooper. Columbia, S.C.

Brown, N.K., and Thompson, D.J. 1979. "Nontreatment of Fever in Extended Care Facilities." *New England Journal of Medicine* 300:1245-50.

Buller, M.K., and Buller, D.B. 1987. "Physicians' Communication Style and Patient Satisfaction." *Journal of Health and Social Behavior* 28:375-88.

Bullough, V. 1959. "Training of the Non-University-Educated Medical Practitioners in the Later Middle Ages." *Journal of the History of Medicine and Allied Health Sciences* 14:447.

———. 1966. *The Development of Medicine as a Profession: The Contribution of the Medieval University to Modern Medicine*. Basel: Karger.

Bunker, J., and Brown, B. 1974. "The Interview Instruments: The Physician-Patient as an Informed Consumer of Surgical Services." *New England Journal of Medicine* 290:1051-55.

Burke, P. 1991. "Identity Processes and Social Stress." *American Sociological Review* 56:836-49.

Bursztajn, H.; Hamm, R.M.; Feinbloom, R.I.; and Brodsky, A. 1981. *Medical Choices, Medical Chances*. New York: Delacorte Press/Seymour Lawrence.

Bylebel, J. 1978. "William Harvey, a Conventional Medical Revolutionary." *Journal of the American Medical Association* 239:1295-98.

Campbell, A.; Converse, P.E.; and Rodgers, W.L. 1976. *The Quality of American Life: Perceptions, Evaluations and Satisfactions.* New York: Russell Sage Foundation.

Carey, B. 1990. "How Bad Are the Bad Docs?" *Health* 4:82.

Carr, J. 1970. "Mongolism—Telling the Parents." *Developmental Medicine and Child Neurology* 12:213.

Carter, W.; Inui, T.; Kukull, W.; and Haigh, V. 1982. "Outcome-Based Doctor-Patient Interaction Analysis." *Medical Care* 20:550-56.

Cassell, Eric J. 1986. "The Changing Concept of the Ideal Physician." *Daedalus* 15:185-208.

Cathell, Daniel W. 1900. P.93 in *Book on the Physician Himself and Things that Concern his Reputation and Success,* 10th ed. Philadelphia: F.A. Davis.

Charles, S.C.; Wilbert, J.R.; and Franke, K.J. 1985. "Sued and Nonsued Physicians' Self-Reported Reactions to Malpractice Litigation." *American Journal of Psychiatry* 142:437-40.

Charles, S.C.; Wilbert, J.R.; and Kennedy, E.C. 1984. "Physicians' Self-Reports of Reactions to Malpractice Litigation." *American Journal of Psychiatry* 141:563-65.

Charmaz, K. 1983. "The Grounded Theory Method: An Explication and Interpretation." Pp. 109-26 in *Contemporary Field Research,* edited by R. Emerson. Boston: Little, Brown.

Chassin, M.R., Kosecoff, J.; Park, R.E.; et al. 1987. "Does Inappropriate Use Explain Geographic Variation in the Use of Health Services?" *Journal of the American Medical Association* 258:2533-37.

Clair, J. 1990a. "Regressive Intervention: The Discourse of Medicine during Terminal Encounters." *Advances in Medical Sociology Research Annual* 1:57-97.

——— . 1990b. "Old Age Health Problems and Long Term Care Policy." Pp. 24-48 in *The Legacy of Longevity: Health, Illness, and Long Term Care in Later Life,* edited by S. Stahl. Newbury Park, Calif.: Sage.

——— . 1991. *Old Age Communication Problems During Medical Encounters.* Washington, D.C.: AARP Andrus Foundation.

Clair, J., and K. Wilson. 1990. *Patient Care Relationships and Ethics: Advancing the Use of Social Theory and Methodology in Behavioral and Biomedical Research.* Washington, D.C.: American Sociological Association/ National Science Foundation.

Clark, E.; Fritz, J.; and Rieker, P., eds. 1990. *Clinical Sociological Perspectives on Illness and Loss: The Linkage of Theory and Practice.* Philadelphia: Charles Press.

Cleary, P., and McNeil, B. 1988. "Patient Satisfaction as an Indicator of Quality Care." *Inquiry* 25:25-36.

Cockerham, William C. 1992. *Medical Sociology.* 5th ed. Englewood Cliffs, N.J.: Prentice-Hall.

Cockerham, William C.; Kunz, Gerhard; and Lueschen, Guenther. 1988. "Social Stratification and Health Lifestyles in Two Systems of Health Care

Delivery: A Comparison of the United States and West Germany." *Journal of Health and Social Behavior* 29:113-26.

Cockerham, William C.; Lueschen, Guenther; Kunz, Gerhard; and Spaeth, Joe L. 1986. "Social Stratification and Self-Management of Health." *Journal of Health and Social Behavior* 27:1-14.

Cohen-Cole, S., and Wills, T. 1985. "Stress, Social Support, and the Buffering Hypothesis." *Psychological Bulletin* 98:310-57.

Cohen-Cole, S. 1991. *The Medical Interview: The Three Function Approach*. St. Louis: Mosby.

Colombotos, J. 1988. "Continuities in the Sociology of Medical Education: An Introduction." *Journal of Health and Social Behavior* 29 (4):271-78.

Combs, A.W., and Avila, D.L. 1985. *Helping Relationships: Basic Concepts for the Helping Professions*. 3rd ed. Boston: Allyn & Bacon.

Comstock, L.; Hooper, E.; Goodwin, J.M.; and Goodwin, J.S. 1982. "Physician Behaviors that Correlate with Patient Satisfaction." *Journal of Medical Education* 57:105-12.

Conrad, Peter. 1988. "Health and Fitness at Work." *Social Science and Medicine* 26:545-50.

————. 1990. "Report of the Medical Sociology Section." *Footnotes* 18 (2):15.

Consumer Reports. 1986. "The Manufactured Crisis: Liability Insurance Companies Have Created a Crisis and Dumped It on You." August, 5444-49.

Cook, Henry. W. 1903a. "Blood Pressure Determinations in General Practice." *Journal of the American Medical Association* 40:1200-1202.

————. 1903b. "The Clinical Value of Blood-Pressure Determinations as a Guide to Stimulation in Sick Children." *Johns Hopkins Hospital Bulletin* 14:37.

————. 1903c. "The Accurate Estimation of Pulse Tension." *Old Dominion Journal of Medicine and Science* 2:106.

Cook, M.; Coe, R.; and Hanson, K. 1990. "Physician-Elderly Patient Communication: Processes and Outcomes of Medical Encounters." Pp. 291-309 in *The Legacy of Longevity: Health, Illness, and Long Term Care in Later Life*, edited by S. Stahl. Newbury Park, Calif.: Sage.

Coulton, C.J.; Milligan, S.; Chow, J.; and Haug, M. 1990. "Ethnicity, Self Care and Use of Medical Care Among the Elderly with Joint Symptoms." *Arthritis Care and Research* 3 (1):19-28.

Crane, D. 1975. *The Sanctity of Social Life: Physicians' Treatment of Critically Ill Patients*. New York: Russell Sage Foundation.

Cranefield, Paul. 1957. "The Organic Physics of 1847 and the Biophysics of Today." *Journal of the History of Medicine and Allied Sciences* 12:407-23.

————. 1966. "The Philosophical and Cultural Interests of the Biophysics Movement of 1847." *Journal of the History of Medicine and Allied Sciences* 21:1-7.

Crawford, Robert. 1984. "A Cultural Account of Health: Control, Release, and the Social Body." Pp. 60-103 in *Issues in the Political Economy of Health Care*, edited by J. Mckinley. New York: Tavistock.

Cromwell, J., and Mitchell, J. 1986. "Physician-Induced Demand for Surgery." *Journal of Health Economics* 5:293-313.

Cross, A.W., and Churchill, L.R. 1982. "Ethical and Cultural Dimensions of Informed Consent: A Case Study and Analysis." *Annals of Internal Medicine* 96:110-13.

Cunningham, C.C.; Morgan, P.A.; and McGucken, R.B. 1984. "Down's Syndrome: Is Dissatisfaction with Disclosure of Diagnosis Inevitable?" *Developmental Medicine and Child Neurology* 26:33-39.

Curran, W.J. 1981. "Retaliatory Actions in Malpractice: Doctors Against Lawyers and Patients." *New England Journal of Medicine* 304:211-12.

Cushing, Harvey. 1903. "On Routine Determinations of Arterial Tension in Operating Room and Clinic." *Boston Medical and Surgical Journal* 148: 250-54.

Danzon, P.M. 1985. *Medical Malpractice: Theory, Evidence and Public Policy.* Cambridge: Harvard University Press.

————. 1987. "Overview of the Liability System." Pp.1-22 in *Medical Practice,* edited by Duncan Yaggy and Patricia Hodgson. Durham, N.C.: Duke University Press.

D'Arcy, E. 1968. "Congenital Defects: Mothers' Reaction to First Information." *British Medical Journal* 3:796-98.

Darling, R.B. 1979. *Families against Society: A Study of Reactions to Children with Birth Defects.* Newbury Park, Calif.:Sage.

————. 1983. "Parent-Professional Interactions: The Roots of Misunderstanding." Pp. 95-121 in *The Family with a Handicapped Child: Understanding and Treatment,* edited by N. Seligman. New York: Grune & Stratton.

————. 1989. "Using the Social System Perspective in Early Intervention: The Value of a Sociological Approach." *Journal of Early Intervention* 13:24-35.

Davies, A.R.; Ware, J.E., Jr.; and Brook, R.H. 1986. "Consumer Acceptance of Prepaid and Fee-for-Service Medical Care: Result from a Randomized Controlled Trial." *Health Services Research* 21:429-52.

Davis, Audrey B. 1981. *Medicine and Its Technology: An Introduction to the History of Medical Instrumentation.* Westport, Conn., and London: Greenwood Press.

Davis, F. 1960. "Uncertainty in Medical Prognosis, Clinical and Functional." *American Journal of Sociology* 66:41-47.

Demaitre, L. 1976. "Nature and the Art of Medicine in the Later Middle Ages." *Mediaevalia* 2:23-47.

Department of Health, Education and Welfare (Health and Human Services). 1973. *Medical Malpractice: Report of the Secretary's Commission.* Washington, D.C.: U.S. Government Printing Office.

Deutch, F., and Murphy, W. 1954. *The Clinical Interview.* Vol.1, *Diagnosis: A Method of Teaching Associative Exploration.* New York: International University Press.

DeVries, M.; Berg, R.; and Lipkin, M. 1982. *The Use and Abuse of Medicine.* New York: Praeger.

Dewey, J. [1929] 1960. *Quest for Certainty: A Study in the Relation of Knowledge and Action.* New York: Capricorn Books.

Doherty, E.G., and Haven, C.O. 1977. "Medical Malpractice and Negligence." *Journal of the American Medical Association* 238:1656-58.

Doherty, W., and Baird, M. 1987. *Family-centered Medical Care: A Clinical Casebook*. New York: Guilford Press.

Douglas, M. 1966. *Purity and Danger: An Analysis of Concepts of Pollution and Taboo*. London: Penguin.

Dranove, D. 1988. "Demand Inducement and the Physician/Patient Relationship." *Economic Inquiry* 26:281-98.

Dreher, B.B. 1987. *Communication Skills for Working with Elders*. New York: Springer.

Edelstein, L. 1937. "Greek Medicine in Its Relation to Religion and Magic." *Bulletin of the History of Medicine* 5:201-46.

——— . 1967. *Ancient Medicine: Selected Papers of Ludwig Edelstein*. Edited by O. Temkin and C. Temkin. Baltimore: Johns Hopkins University Press.

Edwards, K.S. 1985. "Defensive Medicine: Health Care with a Pricetag." *Ohio State Medical Journal* 81:38-42.

Eisenberg, J.M. 1979. "Sociologic Influences on Decision-Making by Clinicians." *Annals of Internal Medicine* 90:957-64.

——— . 1986. *Doctors' Decisions and the Cost of Medical Care*. Ann Arbor, Mich.: Health Administration Press.

Eisenberg, L. 1977. "Disease and Illness: Distinctions between Professional and Popular Ideas of Sickness." *Culture, Medicine and Psychiatry* 1:9-23.

——— . 1988. "Science in Medicine: Too Much or Too Little and Too Limited in Scope?" *American Journal of Medicine* 84:483-91.

Eisenberg, L., and Kleinman, A. 1981. *The Relevance of Social Science for Medicine*. Boston: D. Reidel.

Ellis, R.P., and McGuire, T.G. 1990. "Optimal Payment Systems for Health Services." *Journal of Health Economics* 9:375-96.

Elston, J.; Koch, G.; and Weissert, W. 1991. "Regression-adjusted Small Area Estimates of Functional Dependency in the Noninstitutionalized American Population Age 65 and Over." *American Journal of Public Health* 81:335-43.

Ende, J.; Kazis, L.; Ash, A.; and Moskowitz, M.A. 1989. "Measuring Patients' Desire for Autonomy." *Journal of General Internal Medicine* 4:23-30.

Engel, G. 1977. "The Need for a New Medical Model: A Challenge for Biomedicine." *Science* 196:535-44.

——— . 1980. "The Clinical Application of the Biopsychosocial Model." *American Journal of Psychiatry* 137:534-44.

——— . 1988. "How Much Longer Must Medicine's Science Be Bound by a 17th Century World View?" Pp. 113-36 in *The Task of Medicine: Dialogue at Wickenburg*. Menlo Park, Calif.: Henry J. Kaiser Family Foundation.

Engler, C.; Saltzman, G.; Walker, M.; and Wolf, F. 1981. "Medical Student Acquisition and Retention of Communication and Interviewing Skills." *Journal of Medical Education* 56:572-79.

Ensel, W., and Lin, N. 1991. "The Life Stress Paradigm and Psychological Distress." *Journal of Health and Social Behavior* 32:321-41.

Epstein, A.M.; Begg, C.B.; and McNeil, B.J. 1986. "The Use of Ambulatory Testing in Prepaid and Fee-for-Service Group Practices." *New England Journal of Medicine* 314:1089-94.

Epstein, R.A. 1992. "Why is Health Care Special?" *University of Kansas Law Review* 40:307-24.

Erlanger, Joseph. 1904. "A New Instrument for Determining the Minimum and Maximum Blood Pressures in Man." *Johns Hopkins Hospital Reports* 12:56.

Ermann, D. 1988. "Hospital Utilization Review: Past Experience and Future Directions." *Journal of Health Politics, Policy and Law* 12:683-704.

Estes, J.W. 1991. "Quantitative Observations of Fever and its Treatment before the Advent of Short Clinical Thermometers." *Medical History* 35: 189-216.

Evans, Hughes H. Forthcoming. "Losing Touch: The Controversy over the Introduction of Blood Pressure Instruments into Medicine." *Technology & Culture.*

Evans, R. 1974. "Supplier-Induced Demand: Some Empirical Evidence and Implications." Pp. 161-73 in *The Economics of Health and Medical Care,* edited by N. Pearlman. New York: Wiley.

Evans-Pritchard, E.E. 1937. *Witchcraft, Oracles and Magic Among the Azande.* Oxford: Clarendon.

Everhart, M.A., and Pearlman, R.A. 1990. "Stability of Patient Preferences Regarding Life Sustaining Treatments." *Chest* 97:159-64.

Feldstein, M.S. 1970. "The Rising Price of Physician Services." *Review of Economics and Statistics* 52:121-33.

Fink, A.; Siu, A.; Brook, R.; Park, R.; and Solomon, D. 1987. "Assuring the Quality of Health Care for Older Persons: An Expert Panel's Priorities." *Journal of the American Medical Association* 258 (14):1905-8.

Fleckenstein, Karen. 1984a. "The Early ECG in Medical Practice." *Medical Instrumentation* 18:191-92.

―――. 1984b. "The Mosso Plethysmograph in Nineteenth-Century Physiology." *Medical Instrumentation* 18:330-31.

Flint, Austin. 1866. "Remarks on the Use of the Thermometer in Diagnosis and Prognosis." *New York Medical Journal* 4:6-82.

Folstein, M.; Folstein, S.; and McHugh, P. 1975. " 'Mini-mental State': A Practical Method for Grading the Cognitive State of Patients for the Clinician." *Journal of Psychiatric Research* 12:189-98.

Forrer, G.R. 1959. "The Mother of a Defective Child." *Psychoanalytic Quarterly* 28:59-63.

Fox, R.C. 1957. "Training for Uncertainty." Pp. 207-41 in *The Student Physician,* edited by R.K. Merton et al. Cambridge: Harvard University Press. Reprinted (1988) as pp. 19-50 in *Essays in Medical Sociology.* New Brunswick, N.J.: Transaction Books.

―――. 1976. "Medical Evolution." Pp. 773-87 in *Explorations in General Theory in Social Science: Essays in Honor of Talcott Parsons,* edited by Jan J. Loubser, Rainer C. Baum, Andrew Effrat, and Victor Meyer Lidz. New York: Free Press.

―――. 1985. "Reflections and Opportunities in the Sociology of Medicine." *Journal of Health and Social Behavior* 26 (1):6-14.

―――. 1989. *The Sociology of Medicine: A Participant Observer's View.* Englewood Cliffs, N.J.: Prentice.

————. 1990. "Training in Caring Competence: The Perennial Problem in North American Medical Education." Pp. 199-216 in *Educating Competent and Humane Physicians,* edited by H. Hendrie and C. Lloyd. Bloomington: Indiana University Press.

Francis, V.; Korsch, B.M.; Morris, M.J. 1969. "Gaps in Doctor-Patient Communication: Patients' Response to Medical Advice." *New England Journal of Medicine* 280:535-40.

Frank, Robert G., Jr. 1988. "The Telltale Heart: Physiological Instruments, Graphic Methods, and Clinical Hopes, 1854-1914." Pp. 211-90 in *The Investigative Enterprise: Experimental Physiology in Nineteenth-Century Medicine,* edited by William Coleman and Frederic L. Holmes. Berkeley and Los Angeles: University of California Press.

Frankel, R., and Beckman, H. 1989. "Evaluating the Patient's Primary Problem(s)." Pp. 86-98 in *Communicating with Medical Patients,* edited by M. Stewart and D. Roter. Newbury Park, Calif: Sage.

Frech, H.E. 1991. *Regulating Doctors' Fees: Competition, Benefits, and Control under Medicare.* Washington, D.C.: American Enterprise Institute.

Freeman, B.; Negrett, V.; Davis, M.; and Korsch, B. 1971. "Gaps in Doctor-Patient Communication: Doctor-Patient Interaction Analysis." *Pediatric Research* 5:298.

Freeman, H., and Levine, S. 1989. "The Present Status of Medical Sociology." Pp. 1-13 in *Handbook of Medical Sociology.* 4th Ed. Edited by H. Freeman and S. Levine. Englewood Cliffs, N.J.: Prentice-Hall.

Freidin, R.B.; Goldman, L.; Cecil, R.R. 1980. "Patient-Physician Concordance in Problem Identification in the Primary Care Setting." *Annals of Internal Medicine* 93:490-93.

Freidson, E. 1961. *Patients' Views of Medical Practice.* New York: Russell Sage Foundation.

————. 1970a. *Profession of Medicine.* New York: Dodd, Mead.

————. 1970b. *Professional Dominance.* Chicago: Aldine.

————. 1986. "The Medical Profession in Transition." Pp. 63-79 in *Applications of Social Science to Clinical Medicine and Health Policy,* edited by L. Aiken and D. Mechanic. New Jersey: Rutgers University Press.

————. 1989. *Medical Work in America: Essays on Health Care.* New Haven, Conn.: Yale University Press.

Fretwell, M. 1990. "Comprehensive Functional Assessment (CFA) in Everyday Practice." Pp. 218-23 in *Principles of Geriatric Medicine and Gerontology,* edited by W. Hazzard, R. Andres, and E. Bierman. New York: McGraw-Hill Information Services.

Fries, J. 1990. "Medical Perspectives upon Successful Aging." Pp. 35-49 in *Successful Aging: Perspectives from the Behavioral Sciences,* edited by P. Baltes and M. Baltes. Cambridge: Cambridge University Press.

Fritz, J. 1991. "The Contribution of Clinical Sociology in Health Care Settings." *Sociological Practice* 9:15-29.

Fuchs, V. 1978. "The Supply of Surgeons and the Demand for Operations." *Journal of Human Resources* 13:35-56.

Gallagher, Eugene B. 1988. "Modernization and Medical Care." *Sociological Perspectives* 31:59-87.

Gargiulo, R.M. 1985. *Working with Parents of Exceptional Children: A Guide for Professionals.* Boston: Houghton Mifflin.

Garnick, D.W.; Luft, H.S.; Gardner, L.B.; et al. 1990. "Services and Charges by PPO Physicians for PPO and Indemnity Patients." *Medical Care* 28: 894-906.

Gaynor, M., and Kleindorfer, P.R. 1987. "Misperceptions, Equilibrium and Optimal Incentives with Many Agents." Pp. 389-414 in *Agency Theory, Information, and Incentives,* edited by G. Bamberg and K. Spremann. Berlin: Springer-Verlag.

Gaynor, M., and Pauly, M.V. 1990. "Compensation and Productive Efficiency in Partnerships: Evidence from Medical Group Practice." *Journal of Political Economy* 98:544-73.

Geddes, L.A. 1976. "Perspectives in Physiological Monitoring." *Medical Instrumentation* 10:91-97.

Gerrity, M.S.; Earp, J.A.L.; DeVellis, R.; and Light, D. 1992. "Uncertainty and Professional Work: Perceptions of Physicians in Clinical Practice." *American Journal of Sociology* 97:1022-51.

Geyman, J.P. 1985. "Malpractice Liability Risk and the Physician-Patient Relationship." *Journal of Family Practice* 20:231-32.

Gibbs, N. 1989. "Doctors and Patients: Image vs. Reality." *Time,* July 31, 48-53.

Giddens, A. 1990. *The Consequences of Modernity.* Stanford, Calif.: Stanford University Press.

————. 1991. *Modernity and Self-Identity.* Cambridge, Eng.: Polity Press.

Glaser, B. 1978. *Theoretical Sensitivity: Advances in the Methodology of Grounded Theory.* Mill Valley, Calif.: Sociology Press.

Glaser, B., and Strauss, A. 1967. *Toward a Grounded Theory.* Chicago: Aldine.

Glasscock, S.; O'Brien, S.; Friman, P.C.; Christophersen, E.R.; and MacLean, W.E. 1989. "Residency Training in Behavioral Pediatrics (Commentary)." *Journal of Developmental and Behavioral Pediatrics* 10:262-63.

Glassner, Barry. 1988. *Bodies.* New York: G.P. Putnam.

Glover, J.J., and Povar, G.J. 1991. "The Ethics of Cost-Conscious Physician Reimbursement." Pp. 13-24 in *Paying the Doctor: Health Policy and Physician Reimbursement,* edited by J.D. Moreno. New York: Auburn House.

Goffman, E. 1963. *Notes on the Management of Spoiled Identity.* Englewood Cliffs, N.J.: Prentice-Hall.

Gourevitch, D. 1969. "Suicide among the Sick in Classical Antiquity." *Bulletin of the History of Medicine* 43:501-18.

Gray, B.H., and Field, M.J. 1989. *Controlling Costs and Changing Patient Care: The Role of Utilization Management.* Washington, D.C.: National Academy Press for the Institute of Medicine.

Green, J.A. 1988. "Minimizing Malpractice Risks by Role Clarification." *Annals of Internal Medicine* 109:234-41.

Greene, M.G.; Adelman, R.; Charon, R.; and Friedmann, E. 1989. "Concordance between Physicians and Their Older and Younger Patients in the Primary Care Medical Encounter." *Gerontologist* 29:808-13.

Greene, M.G.; Adelman, R.; Charon, R.; and Hoffman, S. 1986. "Ageism in the Medical Encounter: An Exploratory Study of the Doctor-Patient Relationship." *Language and Communication* 6:113-24.

Greene, M.G.; Hoffman, S.; Charon, R.; and Adelman, R. 1987. "Psychosocial Concerns in the Medical Encounter: A Comparison of the Interactions of Doctors with Their Old and Young Patients." *Gerontologist* 27:164-68.

Griffith, R.L. 1985. "Malpractice Avoidance Techniques." *Texas Medicine* 81: 50-51.

Grigg, E.R.N. 1965. *The Trail of the Invisible Light: From X-Strahlen to Radiobiology.* Springfield, Ill.: Charles C. Thomas. Gutheil, T.G.; Bursztajn, H.; and Brodsky, A. 1984. "Malpractice Prevention through the Sharing of Uncertainty." *New England Journal of Medicine* 311:49-51.

Gutheil, T.; Bursztajn, H; and Brodsky, H. 1984. "Malpractice Prevention through the Sharing of Uncertainty." *New England Journal of Medicine* 311:49-51

Haber, Samuel. 1964. *Efficiency and Uplift.* Chicago: University of Chicago Press.

Hahn, R., and Kleinman, A. 1983. "Biomedical Practice and Anthropological Theory: Frameworks and Directions." *Annual Review of Anthropology* 12:305-33.

Haley, W.; Clair, J.; and Saulsberry, K. 1992. "Family Caregiver Satisfaction with Medical Care of Their Demented Relatives." *Gerontologist* 32:219-26.

Hall, J.A.; Roter, D.L.; and Katz, N.R. 1988. "Meta-analysis of Correlates of Provider Behavior in Medical Encounters." *Medical Care* 26:657-75.

Hall, M.A., and Anderson, G.F. 1992. "Health Insurers' Assessment of Medical Necessity." *University of Pennsylvania Law Review* (in press).

Halpern, S.A. 1992. "Dynamics of Professional Control: Internal Coalitions and Cross-professional Boundaries." *American Journal of Sociology* 97: 994-1021.

Hamarneh, S. 1971. "The Physician and the Health Professions in Medieval Islam." *Bulletin of the N.Y. Academy of Medicine* 47:1088-1110.

Hamilton, E., and Cairns, H., eds. 1961. *The Collected Dialogues of Plato.* New York: Bollingen Foundation.

Harrison, Louis B.; Worth, Melvin H., Jr.; and Carlucci, Michael A. 1985. "The Development of the Principles of Medical Malpractice in the United States." *Perspectives in Biology and Medicine* 29:41-72.

Harvey, L.K., and Shubat, S.C. 1989. *Physician Opinion on Health Care Issues.* Chicago: American Medical Association.

Haug, M.R. 1975. "The Deprofessionalization of Everyone." *Sociological Focus* 8:197-213.

——— . 1976. "The Erosion of Professional Authority: A Cross-cultural Inquiry in the Case of the Physician." *Milbank Quarterly* 54:83-106.

——— . 1988. "A Re-examination of the Hypothesis of Physician Deprofessionalization." *Milbank Quarterly* 66:48-56.

Haug, M.R.; Akiyama, H.; Tryban, G.; Sonoda, K.; and Wykle, M. 1991. "Self Care: Japan and the U.S. Compared." *Social Science and Medicine* 33 (9):1011-22.

Haug, M.R., and Lavin, B. 1979. "Public Challenge of Physician Authority." *Medical Care* 17:844-58.

——— . 1981. "Practitioner or Patient—Who's in Charge?" *Journal of Health and Social Behavior* 22:212-29.

——— . 1983. *Consumerism in Medicine*. Newbury Park, Calif.: Sage.

Haug, M.R., and Ory, M.G. 1987. "Issues in Elderly Patient-Provider Interactions." *Research on Aging* 9:3-44.

Haug, M.R.; Wykle, M.L.; and Namazi, K.H. 1989. "Self-Care among Older Adults." *Social Science and Medicine* 29:171-83.

Hay, J., and Leahy, M. 1982. "Physician-Induced Demand: An Empirical Analysis of the Consumer Information Gap." *Journal of Health Economics* 1:231-43.

Hayes-Bautista, D.S. 1976. "Modifying the Treatment: Patient Compliance, Patient Control and Medical Care." *Social Science and Medicine* 10: 233-38.

Headache Study Group of the University of Western Ontario. 1986. "Predictors of Outcome in Headache Patients Presenting to Family Physicians—A One Year Prospective Study." *Headache Journal* 26:285-94.

Headen, A.E. 1990. "Wage, Returns to Ownership, and Fee Responses to Physician Supply." *Review of Economics and Statistics* 2472:30-37.

Heitzmann, C. 1879. "The Aid which Medical Diagnosis Receives from Recent Discoveries in Microscopy." *Archives of Medicine (New York)* 1:65-66.

Hellman, S. 1991. "The Intellectual Quarantine of American Medicine." *Academic Medicine* 66 (5):245-48.

Helman, C. 1978. " 'Feed a Cold, Starve a Fever'—Folk Models of Infection in an English Suburban Community and Their Relation to Medical Treatment." *Culture, Medicine and Psychiatry* 2:107-37.

Hemenway, D.; Killen, A.; Cashman, S. B.; et al. 1990. "Physicians' Responses to Financial Incentives: Evidence from a For-Profit Ambulatory Care Center." *New England Journal of Medicine* 322:1059-63.

Hershey, Nathan. 1982. "The Defensive Practice of Medicine." In Law and Ethics in Health Care, edited by John McKinlay. Cambridge: MIT Press.

Hickson, G.B.; Altemeier, W.A.; and Perrin, J.M. 1987. "Physician Reimbursement by Salary of Fee-for-Service: Effect on Physician Practice Behavior in a Randomized Prospective Study." *Pediatrics* 80:344-50.

Hillman, A.L. 1987. "Financial Incentives for Physicians in HMOs: Is There a Conflict of Interest?" *New England Journal of Medicine* 317: 1743-48.

——— . 1990. "HMOs, Financial Incentives, and Physicians' Judgements." *Annals of Internal Medicine* 112:891-93.

——— . 1991. "Managing the Physician: Rules versus Incentives." *Health Affairs* 10:138-46.

Hillman, A.L.; Pauly, M.V.; and Kerstein, J.J. 1989. "How Do Financial Incentives Affect Physicians' Clinical Decisions and the Financial Performance of HMOs." *New England Journal of Medicine* 321:86-92.

Hillman, B.J.; Joseph, C.A.; Mabry, M.R.; et al. 1990. "Frequency and Costs of Diagnostic Imaging in Office Practice—A Comparison of Self-Referring and Radiologist-Referring Physicians." *New England Journal of Medicine* 323:1604-8.

Hinkle, L.; Redmont, R.; Plummer, N.; and Wolf, H. 1960. "An Examination of the Relation between Symptoms, Disability, and Serious Illness in Two

Homogeneous Groups of Men and Women." *American Journal of Public Health* 50:1327-36.

Hippocrates. 1886. "On Airs, Places, and Waters." P. 156 in *The Genuine Works of Hippocrates,* vol. 1. Translated and edited by Francis Adams, with a preliminary discourse and annotations. New York: William Wood.

Hirsch, P.J.; Stuart, A.H.; and Reedman, L. 1987. "25 Ways to Avoid Malpractice Suits." *New Jersey Medicine* 84:857-58.

Howard, J.; Davis, F.; Pope, C.; and Ruzek, S. 1977. "Humanizing Health Care: The Implications of Technology, Centralization, and Self-Care." *Medical Care* 15 (5):11-26.

Howell, Joel D. 1986. "Early Use of X-ray Machines and Electrocardiographs at the Pennsylvania Hospital." *Journal of the American Medical Association* 255:2320-23.

———. 1987. "Machines' Meanings: British and American Uses of Technology, 1880-1930." Ph.D. diss., University of Pennsylvania.

———. 1988. Pp. 86-87 in *Technology and American Medical Practice, 1880-1930: An Anthology of Sources.* New York and London: Garland Publishing.

———. 1991. "An Elective Course in Medical History." *Academic Medicine* 66:668-69.

Howell, J.; Lurie, N.; and Wooliscroft, J. 1987. "Some Thoughts to be Delivered to House Officers on the First Day of Clinic." *Journal of the American Medical Association* 258 (4):502-3.

Hoy, E.W.; Curtis, R.E.; and Rice, T. 1991. "Change and Growth in Managed Care." *Health Affairs* 10:18-36.

Huddle, Thomas. 1991. "Review of Educating Competent and Humane Physicians." Edited by H. Hendrie and C. Lloyd. *Journal of General Internal Medicine* 7:129-30.

Hughes, J. 1991. *"The Doctor-Patient Relationship: Does It Really Matter?"* Proceedings of American Sociological Association Annual Meetings, Cincinnati, Ohio.

Hunt, G., and Sobal, J. 1990. "Teaching Medical Sociology in Medical Schools." *Teaching Sociology* 18 (3):319-28.

Iglehart, J.K. 1989. "Physician Ownership of Health Care Facilities." *New England Journal of Medicine* 321:198-204.

———. 1990. "Congress Moves to Regulate Self-Referral and Physicians' Ownership of Clinical Laboratories." *New England Journal of Medicine* 322:1682-87.

———. 1991. "The Struggle over Physician-Payment Reform." *New England Journal of Medicine* 325:823-28.

Illich, Ivan. 1976. *Medical Nemesis: The Expropriation of Health.* Toronto, New York, and London: Bantam Books.

Imershein, Allen W.; Rond, Phillip C. III; and Mathis, Mary P. 1992. "Restructuring Patterns of Elite Dominance and the Formation of State Policy in Health Care." *American Journal of Sociology* 97:970-93.

Inlander, C.B.; Levin, L.S.; and Weiner, E. 1988. *Medicine on Trial.* New York: Prentice Hall.

Inui, T., and Carter, W. 1985. "Problems and Prospects for Health Services Research on Provider-Patient Communication." *Medical Care* 23:521-38.

Inui, T., and Carter, W. 1988. "Design Issues in Research on Doctor-Patient Communication." In *Communicating with Medical Patients,* edited by M. Stewart and R. Roter. Newbury Park, Calif: Sage.

Irvin, M.A.; Kennell, J.H.; and Klaus, M.H. 1982. "Caring for the Parents of an Infant with a Congenital Malformation." Pp. 227-58 in *Parent-Infant Bonding,* 2nd ed. Edited by M.H. Klaus and J.H. Kennell. St. Louis, Mo.: Mosby.

Jakobson, R. 1985. *Verbal Art, Verbal Sign, Verbal Time.* Minneapolis: University of Minnesota Press.

James, W. [1909] 1970. "A Pluralistic Universe" in *Essays in Radical Empiricism and Pluralistic Universe.* Gloucester: Peter Press.

Jameson, F. 1981. *The Political Unconscious: Narrative as a Socially Symbolic Act.* Ithaca, N.Y.: Cornell University Press.

Jamieson, D.W., and Zann, M.P. 1989. "Need for Structure in Attitude Formation and Expression." Pp. 383-406 in *Attitude Structure and Function,* edited by Anthony R. Pratkanis, Steven J. Breckler, and Anthony G. Greenwald. Hillsdale, N.J.: Lawrence Erlbaum.

Janeway, Theodore C. 1901. "Some Observations on the Estimation of Blood Pressure in Man, with Especial Reference to the Value of the Results Obtained with the Newer Sphygmomanometers." *New York University Bulletin of the Medical Sciences* 1:XXXX.

———. 1904. *The Clinical Study of Blood-Pressure: A Guide to the Use of the Sphygmomanometer in Medical, Surgical, and Obstetrical Practice, with a Summary of the Experimental and Clinical Facts Relating to the Blood-Pressure in Health and Disease.* New York: D. Appleton.

Jensen, G.A., and Morrisey, M.A. 1990. "Group Health Insurance: An Hedonic Approach." *Review of Economics and Statistics* 72:38-44.

Jensen, G.A.; Morrisey, M.A.; and Marcus, J. 1987. "Cost Sharing and the Changing Patterns of Employer-sponsored Health Insurance." *Milbank Quarterly* 65:521-50.

Johnson, E.A. 1991. "Ethical Considerations for Business Relationships of Hospitals and Physicians." *Health Care Management Review* 16:7-13.

Johnson, T.J. 1972. *Professions and Power.* London: Macmillan.

Joint Commission on Accreditation of Health Care Organizations. 1992. *Accreditation Manual for Hospitals.* Oakbrook Terrace, Ill.

Jonsen, A.R.; Siegler, M.; and Winslade, W.J. 1982. *Clinical Ethics.* New York: Macmillan.

Kafka, F. 1971. "A Country Doctor." Pp. 220-25 in *Franz Kafka: The Complete Stories,* edited by Nahum N. Glatzer. New York: Shocken Books.

Kaplan, S.H.; Greenfield, S.; and Ware, J.E., Jr. 1989. "Impact of the Doctor-Patient Relationship on the Outcomes of Chronic Disease." Pp. 228-45 in *Communicating with Medical Patients,* edited by Moira Stewart and Debra Rotter. Newbury Park, Calif.: Sage.

Kaplan, S.H.; Greenfield, S.; Ware, J.E., Jr. 1989. "Assessing the Effects of Physician-Patient Interactions on the Outcomes of Chronic Disease." *Medical Care* 27:S110-S127.

Kassberg, M. 1990. "The Perfect Ob/Gyn." *OBG Management.* April, pp. 29-35.

Kasteler, J.; Kane, R.; Olsen, D.; and Thetford, C. 1976. "Issues Underlying the

Prevalence of 'Doctor-Shopping' Behavior." *Journal of Health and Social Behavior* 17:328.

Katz, S.; Branch, L.; Branson, M.; Papsidero, J.; Beck, J.; and Greer, D. 1983. "Active Life Expectancy." *New England Journal of Medicine* 309: 1218-24.

Keele, Kenneth D. 1963. *The Evolution of Clinical Methods in Medicine.* Springfield, Ill: Charles C. Thomas.

Kelly, J.; St. Lawrence, J.; Smith, S.; et al. 1987. "Stigmatization of AIDS Patients by Physicians." *American Journal of Public Health* 77:789.

Kemper, P., and Murtaugh, C. 1991. "Lifetime Use of Nursing Home Care." *New England Journal of Medicine* 324:595-600.

Kenkel, D. 1990. "Consumer Information and the Demand for Medical Care." *Review of Economics and Statistics* 72:587-95.

Kessler, D. 1991. "Communicating with Patients about Their Medications." *New England Journal of Medicine* 325:1650-52.

Khandker, R.K., and Manning, W.G. 1991. "The Impact of Utilization Review on Costs and Utilization." Pp. 47-62 in *Health Economics Worldwide,* edited by P. Zweifel and H.E. Frech. Boston: Kluwer Academic.

Kimball, C. 1982. *Biopsychosocial Approach to the Patient.* Baltimore: Williams and Wilkins.

King, L.S. 1963. Pp. 91-95 in *The Growth of Medical Thought.* Chicago: University of Chicago Press.

———. 1982. *Medical Thinking: A Historical Preface.* Princeton, N.J.: Princeton University Press.

Kleinman, A. 1980. *Patients and Healers in the Context of Culture.* Berkeley and Los Angeles: University of California Press.

———. 1986. *Social Origins of Distress and Disease.* New Haven: Yale University Press.

———. 1988. *The Illness Narratives.* New York: Basic Books.

Kleinman, Arthur; Eisenberg, Leon; and Good, Byron. 1978. "Culture, Illness, and Care: Clinical Lessons from Anthropologic and Cross-Cultural Research." *Annals of Internal Medicine* 88:251-58.

Knox, P.; Bohland, James; and Shumsky, Larry. 1984. "Urban Development and the Geography of Personal Services: The Example of Medical Care in the United States." Pp. 164-70 in *Public Provision and Urban Development,* edited by A. Kinby, P. Knox, and S. Pinch. London: Croom Helm.

Korsch, B.; Gozzi, E.; and Francis, V. 1968. "Gaps in Doctor-Patient Communication: I. Doctor-Patient Interaction and Patient Satisfaction." *Pediatrics* 42:855-71.

Kotarba, Joseph A., and Bentley, Pamela. 1988. "Workplace Wellness Participation and the Becoming of Self." *Social Science and Medicine* 26:551-58.

Kübler-Ross, Elizabeth. 1969. *On Death and Dying.* New York: MacMillan.

LaBelle, R.; Hurley, J.; and Rice, T. 1989. *Financial Incentives and Medical Practice: Evidence from Ontario on the Effect of Changes in Physician Fees on Medical Care Utilization.* Background paper no.89-3, Physician Payment Review Commission, Washington, D.C.

Lachs, M.S.; Sindelar, J.L.; and Horwitz, R.I. 1990. "The Forgiveness of Coinsurance: Charity or Cheating?" *New England Journal of Medicine* 322:1599-1602.

Lacombé, Michael. 1991. "The Bag Lady." *American Journal of Medicine* 90:622-27.

Laénnec, R.T.H. 1827. *A Treatise on the Diseases of the Chest, and on Mediate Auscultation.* 2nd ed. Translated by John Forbes. London: T. & G. Underwood.

Langwell, K.M., and Werner, J.L. 1981. "Professional Liability Environment and Physicians' Responses." *Medical Care* 19:233-42. La Puma, John, and Schiedermayer, David L. 1989. "Outpatient Clinical Ethics." *Journal of General Internal Medicine* 4:413-20.

La Puma, John, and David Schiedermayer. 1989. "Outpatient Clinical Ethics." *Journal of General Internal Medicine* 4:413-20.

Laqueur, T. 1987. "Orgasm, Generation, and the Politics of Reproductive Biology." Pp. 1-41 in *The Making of the Modern Body: Sexuality and Society in the Nineteenth Century,* edited by Catherine Gallagher and Thomas Laqueur. Berkeley and Los Angeles: University of California Press.

Larson, C. 1990. "Applied/Practical Sociological Theory: Problems and Issues." *Sociological Practice Review* 1 (1):8-18.

Last, J. 1963. "The Iceberg: Completing the Clinical Picture in General Practice." *Lancet* 2:28-31.

Lavery, J.P. 1988. "The Physician's Reaction to a Malpractice Suit." *Obstetrics and Gynaecology* 71:138-41.

Lawrence, Christopher. 1978. "Physiological Apparatus in the Wellcome Museum. 1. The Marey Sphygmograph." *Medical History* 22:196-200.

———. 1979. "Physiological Apparatus in the Wellcome Museum. 2. The Dudgeon Sphygmograph and Its Descendants." *Medical History* 23:96-101.

———. 1979a. "Physiological Apparatus in the Wellcome Museum. 3. Early Sphygmomanometers." *Medical History* 23:474-78.

———. 1985a. "Incommunicable Knowledge: Science, Technology and the Clinical Art in Britain, 1850-1914." *Journal of Contemporary History* 20:503-20.

———. 1985b. "Modern and Ancients: The 'New Cardiology' in Britain, 1880-1930." In *The Emergence of Modern Cardiology,* supplement 5 to *Medical History,* edited by W.F. Bynum, C. Lawrence, and V. Nutton. London: Wellcome Institute.

Lawrence, V.A., and Clark, G.M. 1987. "Cancer and Resuscitation. Does the Diagnosis Affect the Decision?" *Archives of Internal Medicine* 147:1637-40.

Lazare, A.; Eisenthal, S.; Frank, A.; and Stoeckle, J.D. 1978. "Studies on a Negotiated Approach to Patienthood." Pp. 119-39 in *The Doctor Patient Relationship in the Changing Health Scene,* edited by Eugene Gallagher. Washington, D.C.: Department of Health, Education and Welfare (NIH).

Lazarus, E. 1988. "Theoretical Considerations for the Study of the Doctor-Patient Relationships: Implications of a Perinatal Study." *Medical Anthropology Quarterly* 2:34-58.

Leavitt, J.W. 1986. Pp.171-95 in *Brought to Bed: Childbearing in America, 1750-1950.* New York: Oxford University Press.

Lee, A. 1979. "The Services of Clinical Sociology." *American Behavioral Scientist* 22 (1):487-511.

Lemert, C. 1991. "The End of Ideology, Really." *Sociological Theory* 9: 131-46.

Levenstein, J.H.; Brown, J.B.; Weston, W.W.; Stewart, M.; McCracken, E.C.; and McWhinney, I. 1989. "Patient-Centered Clinical Interviewing." Pp. 107-20 in *Communicating with Medical Patients,* edited by M. Stewart and D. Roter. Newbury Park, Calif.: Sage.

Levine, S. 1987. "The Changing Terrains in Medical Sociology: Emergent Concern with Quality of Life." *Journal of Health and Social Behavior* 28:1-6.

Lewis, Sinclair 1925. *Arrowsmith.* New York: Harcourt Brace.

Lieberson, S. 1992. "Einstein, Renoir, and Greeley: Some Thoughts about Evidence in Sociology." *American Sociological Review* 57:1-15.

Light, D. 1989. "Social Control and the American Health Care System." Pp. 456-74 in *Handbook of Medical Sociology,* 4th ed., edited by H. Freeman and S. Levine. Englewood Cliffs, N.J.: Prentice Hall.

———. "Introduction: Stengthening Ties between Specialties and the Discipline." *Americal Journal of Sociology* 97:909-18.

Light, D., and Levine, S. 1988. "The Changing Character of the Medical Profession: A Theoretical Overview." *Milbank Quarterly* 66:10-32.

Link, Bruce. 1983. "Reward System of Psychotherapy: Implications for Inequities in Service Delivery." *Journal of Health and Social Behavior* 24: 61-69.

Lipkin, M., Jr. 1987. "The Medical Interview and Related Skills." Pp. 287-306 in *The Office Practice of Medicine,* edited by W.T. Branch. Philadelphia: W.B. Saunders.

Lipkin, M.; Quill, T.; and Napodano, R. 1984. "The Medical Interview: A Core Curriculum for Residencies in Internal Medicine." *Annals of Internal Medicine* 100 (2):277-84.

Lloyd, G.E.R. 1983. "Treatment of Women in the Hippocratic Corpus." Pp. 109-10 in *Science, Folklore, and Ideology.* Cambridge: Cambridge University Press.

Lonergan, E., ed. 1991. *Extending Life, Enhancing Life: A National Research Agenda on Aging.* Washington, D.C.: National Academy Press.

Longrigg, J. 1981. "Superlative Achievement and Comparative Neglect: Alexandrian Medical Science and Modern Historical Research." *History of Science* 19:155-200.

Ludmerer, K. 1985. *Learning to Heal: The Development of American Medical Education.* New York: Basic Books.

Ludwig, E.G., and Gibson, G. 1969. "Self Perception of Sickness and the Seeking of Medical Care." *Journal of Health and Social Behavior* 10:125-33.

Lukács, G. 1971a. *History and Class Consciousness.* Cambridge: MIT Press.

———. 1971b. *The Theory of the Novel.* Cambridge: MIT Press.

McCarthy, E.G.; Finkel, M.L.; and Ruchlin, H.S. 1981. *Second Opinion Elective Surgery.* Boston: Auburn House.

McCue, J.D. 1982. "The Effects of Stress on Physicians and Their Medical Practice." *New England Journal of Medicine* 306:458-63.

McDowell, T.N. 1989. "Physician Self-Referral Arrangements: Legitimate Business or Unethical 'Entrepreneuralism'?" *American Journal of Law and Medicine* 15:61-109.

McGoldrick, M., and Gerson, R. 1985. "Constructing Genograms." Pp.9-38 in *Genograms in Family Assessment.* New York: W.W. Norton.

McGuire, T.G., and Pauly, M.V. 1991. "Physician Responses to Fee Changes with Multiple Payers." *Journal of Health Economics* 10 (4):385-410.

McHugh, D. 1968. *Defining the Situation: The Organization of Meaning in Social Interaction.* Indianapolis: Bobbs-Merrill.

McKay, M., and Hensey, O. 1990. "From the Other Side: Parents' Views of Their Early Contacts with Health Professionals." *Child Care, Health and Development* 16:373-81.

McKinlay, J. 1988. "The Changing Character of the Medical Profession: Introduction." *Milbank Quarterly* 66:1-9.

McKinlay, J.; McKinlay, S.; and Beaglehole, R. 1989. "Trends in Death and Disease and the Contribution of Medical Measures." Pp. 14-45 in *Handbook of Medical Sociology,* edited by H. Freeman and Sol Levine. Englewood Cliffs, N.J.: Prentice Hall.

McLeod, R. 1991. "Patients with Advanced Breast Cancer: The Nature and Disclosure of Their Concerns," Ph.D. Diss. University of Manchester.

McWhinney, I. 1989. "The Need for a Transformed Clinical Method." Pp.25-40 in *Communicating with Medical Patients,* edited by M. Stewart and D. Roter. Newbury Park, Calif.: Sage.

Maguire, P. 1990. "Can Communication Skills Be Taught?" *British Journal of Hospital Medicine* 43:215-16.

Maguire, P.; Fairburn, S.; and Fletcher C. 1986. "Consultative Skills of Young Doctors: Benefits of Feedback Training in Interviewing Skills Persist." *British Medical Journal* 292:1573-76.

Maloney, T., and Paul, B. 1991. "The Emerging Science of Patient Care." Pp. 29-43 in *Annual Report of the Commonwealth Fund.* New York, N.Y.

Manning, W.G.; Newhouse, J.P.; Duan, N.; et al. 1987. "Health Insurance and the Demand for Medical Care: Evidence from a Randomized Experiment." *American Economic Review* 77:251-77.

Manton, K., and Stallard, E. 1990. "Changes in Health Functioning and Mortality." Pp. 140-62 in *The Legacy of Longevity: Health, Illness, and Long Term Care in Later Life,* edited by S. Stahl. Newbury Park, Calif.: Sage.

———. 1991. "Cross-Sectional Estimates of Active Life Expectancy for the U.S. Elderly and Oldest-Old Populations." *Journal of Gerontology* 46:S170-82.

Marey, E.J. 1878. *La Méthode graphique dans les Sciences Expérimentales et principalement en physiologie et en médecine.* Paris: G. Mason.

Maulitz, Russell C. 1979. "Physician vs Bacteriologist: The Ideology of Science in Clinical Medicine." Pp. 91-107 in *The Therapeutic Revolution: Essays in the Social History of American Medicine,* edited by Morris J. Vogel and Charles E. Rosenberg. Philadelphia: University of Pennsylvania Press.

Maynard, D. 1991. "Interaction and Asymmetry in Clinical Discourse." *American Journal of Sociology* 97:448-95.

Matthews, J. 1983. "The Communication Process in Clinical Settings." *Social Science and Medicine* 17:1371-78.

Mechanic, D. 1989. "Medical Sociology: Some Tensions among Theory, Method, and Substance." *Journal of Health and Social Behavior* 30 (2):147-60.

———. 1990. "The Role of Sociology in Health Affairs." *Health Affairs* 9: 85-97.

Mechanic, D., and Aiken, L., eds. 1986. "Social Science, Medicine, and Health Policy." Pp. 1-9 in *Applications of Social Science to Clinical Medicine and Health Policy.* New Brunswick, N.J.: Rutgers University Press.

Medical Economics. 1986. March 31, 70-73.

Mendelsohn, Everett. 1964. "The Biological Sciences in the Nineteenth Century: Some Problems and Sources." *History of Science* 3:39-59.

Mercer, J.R. 1965. "Social System Perspective and Clinical Perspective: Frames of Reference for Understanding Career Patterns of Persons Labeled as Mentally Retarded." *Social Problems* 13:18-34.

Meyers, A.R. 1987. " 'Lumping It': The Hidden Denominator of the Medical Malpractice Crisis." *American Journal of Public Health* 77:1544-48.

Mishler, E.G. 1984. *The Discourse of Medicine: Dialectics of Medical Interviews.* Norwood, N.J.: Ablex.

Mishler, E.G.; Clark, J.A.; Ingelfinger, J.; and Simon, M.P. 1989. "The Language of Attentive Patient Care: A Comparison of Two Medical Interviews." *Journal of General Internal Medicine* 4:325-35.

Mitchell, J.M., and Sass, T.R. 1992. "Physician Ownership of Ancillary Services: Referral for Profit or Quality Assurance?" Paper presented at the annual meeting of the American Economic Association, New Orleans, Louisiana.

Mitchell, Weir S. 1891. "The Early History of Instrumental Precision in Medicine." *Transactions of the College of American Physicians and Surgeons* 2:164.

Montgomery, C. 1987. "MDs: Treat Your Patients and Their Naivete." *Michigan Medicine* 86:447-48.

Morantz-Sanchez, Markell, R. 1985. *Sympathy and Science: Women Physicians in American Medicine.* New York: Oxford University Press.

Murray, J.P.; Greenfield, S.; Kaplan, S.H.; and Yano, E.M. 1992. "Ambulatory Testing for Capitation and Fee-for-Service Patients in the Same Practice Setting." *Medical Care* 30 (March): 252-61.

Nagi, S.A. 1976. "An Epidemiology of Disability among Adults in the United States." *Milbank Quarterly* 54:439-68.

Nalebuff, B., and Stiglitz, J. 1983. "Prizes and Incentives: Toward a General Theory of Compensation and Competition." *Bell Journal of Economics* 14:21-43.

Nelkin, D., and Tancredi, Laurence. 1989. *Dangerous Diagnostics: The Social Power of Biological Information.* New York: Basic Books.

Nicolson, E.P. 1898. "Medical Progress." Pp.99-109 in *Transactions of Medical Association of State of Alabama.*

Nicolson, M. 1989. "Medicine and Racial Politics: Changing Images of the New Zealand Maori in the Nineteenth Century." Pp.66-104 in *Imperial Medicine and Indigenous Societies,* edited by D. Arnold.Delhi: Oxford University Press.

Niklas, D. 1982. "Methodological Controversies between Social and Medical Sciences." *Social Science and Medicine* 16:659-65.

Northouse, P.G., and Northouse, L.L. 1985. *Health Communication.* Englewood Cliffs, N.J.: Prentice Hall.

Novack, D.H. 1987. "Therapeutic Aspects of the Clinical Encounter." *Journal of General Internal Medicine* 2:346-55.

Novack, D.H.; Detering, B.; Arnold, R.; et al. 1989. "Physicians' Attitudes toward Using Deception to Resolve Difficult Ethical Problems." *Journal of the American Medical Association* 261:2980-85.

Novack, D.H.; Plummer, R.; Smith, R.L.; Ochitillh, H.; Morrow G.R.; and Bennett, J.M. 1979. "Changes in Physicians' Attitudes toward Telling the Cancer Patient." *Journal of the American Medical Association* 241:897-900.

Nursey, A.D.; Rhode, J.R.; and Farmer, R.D.T. 1990. "A Study of Doctors' and Patients' Attitudes to People with Mental Handicaps." *Journal of Mental Deficiency Research* 34:143-55.

Nutton, V. 1985a. "From Galen to Alexander, Aspects of Medicine and Medical Practice in Late Antiquity." Pp. 1-14 in *Symposium on Byzantine Medicine,* edited by J. Scarborough. Washington, D.C.: Dumbarton Oaks Research Library and Collection.

———. 1985b. "Murders and Miracles: Lay Attitudes towards Medicine in Classical Antiquity." P. 48 in *Patients and Practitioners,* edited by Roy Porter. Cambridge: Cambridge University Press.

Nyman, J.A.; Feldman, R.; Shapiro, J.; et al. 1990. "Changing Physician Behavior: Does Medical Review of Part B Medicare Claims Make a Difference?" *Inquiry* 27:127-37.

Ohio Medicine. 1990. "Common Practice Errors Identified as Factors in Malpractice Lawsuits." *Ohio Medicine* 86:541-42.

Oken D. 1961. "What to Tell Cancer Patients: A Study of Medical Attitudes." *Journal of the American Medical Association* 175:1120-28.

Olshansky, S. 1962. "Chronic Sorrow: A Response to Having a Mentally Defective Child." *Social Casework* 43:190-93.

Omnibus Budget Reconciliation Act of 1990. Public Law No. 101-508 4206, 4751 (codified in scattered sections of 42 U.S.C., 1395cc, 1396a; West Supplement 1991).

Pagel, W. 1958. *Paracelsus: An Introduction to Philosophical Medicine in the Era of the Renaissance.* Basel: S. Karger.

———. 1974. "Paracelsus." *Dictionary of Scientific Biography* 10:304-13.

Pappas, G. 1990. "Some Implications for the Study of Doctor-Patient Interaction: Power, Structure, and Agency in the Works of Howard Waitzkin and Arthur Kleinman." *Social Science and Medicine* 30:199-204.

Parsons, T. 1951. *The Social System.* New York: Free Press.

———. 1975. "The Sick Role and the Role of the Physician Reconsidered." *Milbank Quarterly* 53:257-78.

Pauly, M.V. 1980. *Doctors and Their Workshops.* Chicago: University of Chicago Press.

———. 1986. "Taxation, Health Insurance, and Market Failure in the Medical Economy." *Journal of Economic Literature* 25:629-75.

Pauly, M.V.; Hillman, A.L.; and Kerstein, J. 1990. "Managing Physician Incentives in Managed Care: The Role of For-Profit Ownership." *Medical Care* 28:1013-24.

Peabody, F.W. 1927. "The Care of the Patient." *Journal of the American Medical Association* 88:877-82.

Pearlman, R.A.; Cain, K.; Patrick, D.; Starks, H.; Appelbaum-Maizel, M.; Jecker, N.S.; and Uhlmann, R. 1993. "Insights into Treatment Preferences: States Worse than Death." *Journal of Clinical Ethics.* April.

Pearlman, R.A.; Inui, T.S.; and Carter, W.B. 1982. "Variability in Physician Bioethical Decision-Making: A Case Study of Euthanasia." *Annals of Internal Medicine* 97:420-25.

Pearlman, R.A., and Jonsen, A.R. 1985. "The Use of Quality of Life: A Consideration in Medical Decision-Making." *Journal of the American Geriatrics Society* 33:344-52.

Pearlman, R.A., and Speer, J.B. 1983. "Quality of Life Considerations in Geriatric Care." *Journal of the American Geriatrics Society* 31:113-20.

Pearlman, R.A., and Uhlmann, R.F. 1988. "Quality of Life in Chronic Diseases: Perceptions of Elderly Patients." *Journal of Gerontology* 43:M25-30.

——— . 1991. "Quality of Life in Elderly Chronically Ill Outpatients." *Journal of Gerontology* 46:M31-38.

Pellegrino, E.D. 1977. "Medicine and Human Values." *Yale Alumni Magazine and Journal* 41:10-11.

Phelps, C.E. 1986. "Physician-Induced Demand—Can We Ever Know Its Extent?" *Journal of Health Economics* 5:355-65.

Pickering, G. 1979. "Therapeutics: Art or Science?" *Journal of the American Medical Association* 242:649-53.

Porter, R. 1985. "Doing Medical History from Below." *Theory and Society* 14:175-98.

Powell, F.D. 1975. Theory of Coping Systems: Changes in Supportive Health Organizations. Cambridge, Mass.: Scherkman.

Powers, J.T., and Rickert, N. 1979. *Physician Perceptions of In-Service Training Needs: A Working Paper.* Evanston, Ill.: American Academy of Pediatrics.

Pratt, L.V. 1978. "Reshaping the Consumer's Posture in Health Care." Pp. 197-214 in *The Doctor-Patient Relationship in the Changing Health Scene,* edited by E.B. Gallagher. Washington, D.C.: Department of Health, Education and Welfare (NIH).

Putman, S.M.; Stiles, W.B.; Jacob, M.C.; James, S.A. 1988. "Teaching the Medical Interview: An Intervention Study." *Journal of General Internal Medicine* 3:38-47.

Quill, T.E., and Williamson, P.R. 1990. "Healthy Approaches to Physician Stress." *Archives of Internal Medicine* 150:1857-61.

Quine, L., and Pahl, J. 1987. "Parental Reaction to Diagnosis of Severe Handicap." *Developmental Medicine & Child Neurology* 29:232-42.

Rabkin, M.T. 1983. "Control of Health Care Costs: Targeting and Coordinating the Economic Incentives." *New England Journal of Medicine* 309:982-84.

Ramsey, J.B., and Wasow, B. 1986. "Supplier-Induced Demand for Physician Services: Theoretical Anomaly or Statistical Artifact?" Pp. 49-77 in *Advances in Econometrics,* vol. 5, edited by G.F. Rhodes. Greenwich, Conn.: JAI Press.

Reeder, Leo G. 1972. "The Patient-Client as Consumer: Some Observations on the Changing Professional-Client Relationship." *Journal of Health and Social Behavior* 13:406-12.

Reiser, S.J. 1978. *Medicine and the Reign of Technology.* Cambridge: Cambridge University Press.

——— . 1979. "The Medical Influence of the Stethoscope." *Scientific American* 240:148-56.

——— . 1980. "Words As Scalpels: Transmitting Evidence in the Clinical Dialogue." *Annals of Internal Medicine* 92:837-42.

Reiser, S.J., and Anbar, M. 1984. *The Machine at the Bedside*. Cambridge: Cambridge University Press.

Relman, A.S. 1988. "Salaried Physicians and Economic Incentives." *New England Journal of Medicine* 319:784.

Rice, T.H. 1983. "The Impact of Changing Medicare Reimbursement Rates on Physician-Induced Demand." *Medical Care* 21:803-15.

Richards, E.P., and Rathbun, K.C. 1983. *Medical Risk Management: Preventive Legal Strategies for Health Care Providers*. Rockville, Md.: Aspen.

Richardson, L. 1991. "Post-modern Social Theory: Representational Practices." *Sociological Theory* 9:173-79.

Richmond, J. 1992. "Re-Dedication, Department of Social Medicine." Harvard University, Cambridge, Mass. Unpublished manuscript.

Risse, G.B. 1979. "Epidemics and Medicine: The Influence of Disease on Medical Thought and Practice." *Bulletin of the History of Medicine* 53: 505-19.

Ritchey, F.J. 1979. "Physicians' Perception of Suit-Prone Patients." *Human Organization* 38:160-68.

———. 1980. "Case Management of Patients Perceived as Suit-Prone." *Social Science and Medicine* 7 (Part F):37-48.

———. 1981. "Medical Rationalization, Cultural Lag, and the Malpractice Crisis." *Human Organization* 40:97-112.

Ritzer, G., and Walczak, D. 1988. "Rationalization and the Deprofessionalization of Physicians." *Social Forces* 67:1-22.

Riva-Rocci, Scipione. 1896. "Un nouvo Sfigmomanometro." *Gazz Meddi Torino* 47:981, 1001.

Rizzo, J.; Marder, W.; and Willke, W. 1990. "Physician Contact with and Attitudes toward HIV-Seropositive Patients." *Medical Care* 28 (3):251-60.

Robert Wood Johnson Foundation Commission on Medical Education. 1991. "Environment for Learning: The Sciences of Medical Practice." A discussion workshop of the interim report presented in Princeton, N.J.

Rodwin, M.A. 1989. "Physicians' Conflicts of Interests: The Limitations of Disclosure." *New England Journal of Medicine* 321:1405-08.

Rosen, George. 1944. *The Specialization of Medicine, with Particular Reference to Ophthalmology*. New York: Froben Press.

———. 1979. "The Evolution of Social Medicine," Pp. 23-50 in *Handbook of Medical Sociology*, 2nd ed., edited by H. Freeman, S. Levine, and L. Reeder. Englewood Cliffs, N.J.: Prentice-Hall.

Rosenberg, C.E. 1962. *The Cholera Years: The United States in 1832, 1849, and 1866*. Chicago: University of Chicago Press.

———. 1979. "The Therapeutic Revolution: Medicine, Meaning, and Social Change in Nineteenth-Century America." Pp. 3-26 in *The Therapeutic Revolution: Essays in the Social History of American Medicine*, edited by Morris J. Vogel and Charles E. Rosenberg. Philadelphia: University of Pennsylvania Press.

Rosenberg, Smith. 1973. "Puberty to Menopause: The Cycle of Feminity in Nineteenth-Century America." *Feminist Studies* 1:58-72.

Rosenkrantz, B.G. 1985. "The Search for Professional Order in 19th-Century American Medicine." Pp. 219-32 in *Sickness and Health in America:*

Readings in the History of Medicine and Public Health. 2nd ed., edited by Ronald L. Numbers and Judith Walzer Leavitt. Madison: University of Wisconsin Press.

Rosenthal, Marilyn M. 1988. *Dealing with Medical Malpractice: The British and Swedish Experience*. Durham N.C.: Duke University Press.

Ross, Catherine E., and Duff, Raymond. 1982. "Returning to the Doctor: The Effect of Client Characteristics, Type of Practice, and Experiences with Care." *Journal of Health and Social Behavior* 23:119-31.

Rost, K.; Carter, W.; and Inui, T. 1989. "Introduction of Information during the Initial Medical Visit: Consequences for Patient Follow-through with Physician Recommendations for Medication." *Social Science & Medicine* 28:315-21.

Rost, K., and Roter, D. 1987. "Predictors of Recall of Medication Regimens and Recommendations for Lifestyle Change in Elderly Patients." *Gerontologist* 27:510-15.

Roter, D. 1977. "Patient Participation in Patient-Provider Interactions: The Effects of Patient Question-asking on the Quality of Interaction, Satisfaction and Compliance." *Health Education Monographs* 5:281-315.

———. 1985. "The Roter Method of Interaction Process Analysis." Unpublished manuscript. Department of Behavioral Sciences and Health Education, Johns Hopkins University, Baltimore, Md.

———. 1989. "Which Facets of Communication Have Strong Effects on Outcome—A Meta-Analysis." Pp. 183-96 in *Communicating with Medical Patients*, edited by Moira Stewart and Debra Rotter. Newbury Park, Calif.: Sage.

Roter, D., and Hall, J.A. 1989. "Studies of Doctor-Patient Interaction." *Annual Review of Public Health* 10:163-80.

Rubel, A.J.; O'Nell, C.W.; and Ardon, R. 1984. *Susto: A Folk Illness*. Berkeley and Los Angeles: University of California Press.

Rubin, B. 1978. "Medical Malpractice Suits Can Be Avoided." *Hospitals* 52: 86-88.

Rublee, D.A., and Rosenfield, R.H. 1987. "Organization Aspects of Physician Joint Ventures." *American Journal of Medicine* 82:518-24.

Rucker, William C. 1971. *A History of the Ophthalmoscope*. Rochester, Minn.: Whiting Printers.

Rueben, D.; Novach, D.; Wachtel, T.; and Wartman, S. 1984. "A Comprehensive Support System for Reducing House Staff Distress." *Psychosomatics* 25:815-20.

Ruggie, Mary. 1992. "The Paradox of Liberal Intervention: Health Policy and the American Welfare State." *American Journal of Sociology* 97: 919-44.

Russell, L.B. 1989. *Medicare's New Payment System: Is It Working?* Washington, D.C.: Brookings Institution Press.

Sappington, D.E.M. 1991. "Incentives in Principal-Agent Relationships." *Journal of Economic Perspectives* 5:45-66.

Savitt, T.L. 1978. *Medicine and Slavery: The Disease and Health of Blacks in Antebellum Virginia*. Urbana: University of Illinois Press.

———. 1989. "Black Health on the Plantation: Masters, Slaves, and Physicians." Pp. 327-55 in *Science and Medicine in the Old South,* edited by R.L. Numbers and T.L. Savitt. Baton Rouge: Louisiana State University Press.

Scambler, G., and Scambler, A. 1984. "The Illness Iceberg and Aspects of Consulting Behavior." Pp 32-53 in *The Experience of Illness,* edited by R. Fitzpatrick, J. Hinton, S. Newman, G. Scambler, and J. Thompson. New York: Tavistock.

Schanze, E. 1987. "Contract, Agency, and the Delegation of Decision Making." Pp. 461-80 in *Agency Theory, Information, and Incentives,* edited by G. Bamberg and K. Spremann. Berlin: Springer-Verlag.

Scheffler, R.M.; Sullivan, S.; and Ko, T.H. 1991. "The Impact of Blue Cross and Blue Shield Plan Utilization Management Programs, 1980-88." *Inquiry.* 28:263-75.

Scheper-Hughes, N. 1990. "Three Propositions for a Critically Applied Medical Anthropology." *Social Science and Medicine* 30 (2):189-97.

Schneiderman, L.J.; Jecker, N.S.; and Jonsen, A.R. 1990. "Medical Futility: Its Meaning and Ethical Implications." *Annals of Internal Medicine* 112: 949-54.

Schroeder, S.A., and Showstack, J.A. 1978. "Financial Incentives to Perform Medical Procedures and Laboratory Tests." *Medical Care* 16:289-98.

Schulz, R.; Visintainer, P.; and Williamson, G. 1990. "Psychiatric and Physical Morbidity Effects of Caregiving." *Journal of Gerontology* 45:181-91.

Schur, P. 1992. "Patient-Doctor Relationships." *Lupus News* 12:11.

Schwalbe, M. 1986. *The Psychosocial Consequences of Natural and Alienated Labor.* Albany: State University of New York Press.

Schwartz, B. 1975. *Queuing and Waiting.* Chicago: University of Chicago Press.

Schwartz, D.H. 1976. "Social Responsibility for Malpractice." *Milbank Quarterly* 54:469-88.

Scotchmer, S. 1990. "Professional Advice and Other Hazards." *Journal of Economic Perspectives* 4:189-95.

Seeman, Melvin, and Seeman, Teresa E. 1983. "Health Behavior and Personal Autonomy: A Longitudinal Study of Sense of Control in Illness." *Journal of Health and Social Behavior* 24:144-60.

Seidman, S. 1991. "The End of Sociological Theory: The Postmodern Hope." *Sociological Theory* 9:131-46.

Seligman, M., and Darling, R.B. 1989. *Ordinary Families, Special Children.* New York: Guilford Press.

Sennett, R., and Cobb, J. 1972. *The Hidden Injuries of Class.* New York: Vintage.

Shaffert, T.; Mitchell, S.; and Schlenker, R. 1980. "Study of Reimbursement and Practice Arrangements of Provider-Based Physicians." Pp. 87-93 in *Physicians and Financial Incentives,* edited by J.R. Gabel et al. Washington, D.C.: U.S. Government Printing Office.

Shalin, D. 1986. "Pragmatism and Symbolic Interactionism." *American Sociological Review* 51:9-29.

Shapiro, Robyn S.; Simpson, D.S.; Lawrence, S.L.; Talsky, A.M.; Sobocinski, K.A.; and Schiedermayer, D.L. 1989. "A Survey of Sued and Nonsued Physicians and Suing Patients." *Archives of Internal Medicine* 149:2190-96.

Sheehan, D.; Harnett, K.; White, K.; Leibowitz, A.; and Baldwin, D. 1990. "A Pilot Study of Medical Student Abuse: Student Perceptions of Mistreatment and Misconduct in Medical School." *Journal of the American Medical Association* 263:533-37.

Shorter, E. 1985. *Bedside Manners: The Troubled History of Doctors and Patients.* New York: Simon and Schuster.

————. 1991. *Doctors and Their Patients: A Social History.* New Brunswick, N.J.: Transaction Publishers.

Shryock, R.H. 1979. *The Development of Modern Medicine: An Interpretation of the Social and Scientific Factors Involved.* Madison: University of Wisconsin Press.

Sigerist, H.E. 1946. *The University at the Crossroads.* New York: Henry Shuman.

————. 1961. *A History of Medicine,* vol. 2. New York: Oxford University Press.

Silliman, R. 1989. "Caring for the Frail Older Patient: The Doctor-Patient-Family Caregiver Relationship." *Journal of General Internal Medicine* 4:237-41.

Silliman, R., and Sternberg, J. 1988. "Family Caregiving: Focus on Patient Functioning and Underlying Causes of Dependency." *Gerontologist* 28:377-82.

Silver, H., and Glicken, A. 1990. "Medical Student Abuse: Incidence, Severity, and Significance." *Journal of the American Medical Association* 263:527-32.

Simons, R.C., and Hughes, C.C., eds. 1985. *The Culture Bound Syndrome: Folk Illnesses of Psychiatric and Anthropologic Interest.* Dordrecht, Holland: Reidel Publishing.

Simpson, M.; Buckman, R.; Stewart, M.; Maguire, P.; Lipkin, M.; Novack, O.; and Till, J. 1991. "Doctor-Patient Communication: The Toronto Consensus Statement." *British Medical Journal* 303:1385-87.

Simpson, R. 1956. "A Modification of the Functional Theory of Social Stratification." *Social Forces* 35:132-37.

Slack, W.V. 1977. "The patient's right to decide." *Lancet* 2(8031)30 (July):240.

Sloan, F.A.; Morrisey, M.A.; and Valvona, J. 1988. "Effects of the Medicare Prospective Payment System on Cost Containment: An Early Assessment." *Milbank Quarterly* 66:191-220.

Smith, R.C., and Hoppe, R.B. 1991. "The Patient's Story: Integrating the Patient- and Physician-Centered Approaches to Interviewing." *Annals of Internal Medicine* 115:470-71.

Somers, Herman M. 1977. "The Malpractice Controversy and the Quality of Patient Care." *Milbank Quarterly* 55:193-232.

Sommers, P.A. 1985. "Malpractice Risk and Patient Relations." *Journal of Family Practice* 20:299-301.

Sonnefeld, S.T.; Waldo, D.R.; Lemieux, J.A.; and McKusick, D.R. 1991. "Projections of National Health Spending through the Year 2000." *Health Care Financing Review* 13:1-27.

Spitzer, Walter O.; Dobson, Annette J.; Hall, Jane; Chesterman, Esther; Levi, John; Shepherd, Richard; Battista, Rinaldo N.; and Catchlove, Barry R. 1981. "Measuring the Quality of Life of Cancer Patients." *Journal of Chronic Disease* 34:858-97.

Spremann, K. 1987. "Agent and Principal." Pp. 3-37 in *Agency Theory, Information, and Incentives,* edited by G. Bamberg and K. Spremann. Berlin: Springer-Verlag.

Stafford, R.S. 1990. "Alternative Strategies for Controlling Rising C-Section Rates." *Journal of the American Medical Association* 263:683-87.

Stano, M. 1987. "A Further Analysis of the Physician Inducement Controversy." *Journal of Health Economics* 6:227-38.

Starfield, B.; Steinwachs, D.; Morris, I.; Bause, G.; Siebert, S.; and Westin, C. 1979. "Patient-Doctor Agreement about Problems Needing Follow-up." *Journal of the American Medical Association* 242:344-46.

Starfield, B.; Wray, C.; Hess, K.; Gross, R.; Birk, P.; and D'Lugoof, B. 1981. "The Influence of Patient-Physician Agreement on Outcome of Care." *American Journal of Public Health* 71:127-32.

Starr, P. 1982. *The Social Transformation of American Medicine.* New York: Basic Books.

Starr, T.J.; Pearlman, R.A.; and Uhlmann, R.F. 1986. "Quality of Life Factors in Resuscitation Decisions." *Journal of General Internal Medicine* 1:373-79.

Stewart, M. 1984. "What Is a Successful Doctor-Patient Interview? A Study of Interactions and Outcomes." *Social Science and Medicine* 19:167-75.

Stewart, M.; Brown, J.; and Westin, W. 1989. "Patient-Centered Interviewing, Part III: Five Provocative Questions." *Canadian Family Physicians* 35:159-61.

Stewart, M., and Roter, D., eds. 1989. *Communication with Medical Patients.* Newbury Park, Calif.: Sage.

Stewart, M.; McWhinney, I.; and Buck, C. 1979. "The Doctor-Patient Relationship and Its Effect on Outcome." *Journal of the Royal Cell of General Practice* 29:77-82.

Stiles, W.B. 1979. "Discourse Analysis on the Doctor-Patient Relationship." *International Journal of Psychiatry in Medicine* 9 (3&4):263-74.

———. 1987. "Evaluating Medical Interview Process Components: Null Correlations with Outcomes May Be Misleading." *Medical Care* 27:212-20.

Stoeckle, J.D. 1987. Introduction, *Encounters between Patients and Doctors,* edited by J.D. Stoeckle. Cambridge: The MIT Press. ———. 1988. "Reflections on Modern Doctoring." *Milbank Quarterly* 66:76-91.

Stoeckle, J.D., and Billings, J.A. 1987. "A History of History-Taking: The Medical Interview." *Journal of General Internal Medicine* 2:119-27.

Strahlman, E. 1990. "The Next Generation." *Journal of the American Medical Association* 264:1157.

Strauss, A.; Fagerhaugh, S.; Suczek, B.; and Wiener, C. 1985. *Social Organization of Medical Work.* Chicago: University of Chicago Press.

Straus, R. 1957. "The Nature and Status of Medical Sociology." *American Sociological Review* 22 (2):200-204.

———. 1979. "Clinical Sociology: An Idea Whose Time Has Come. . . . Again." *Sociological Practice* 3 (1):21-43.

Sudnow, D. 1967. *Passing On*. Englewood Cliffs, N.J.: Prentice-Hall.

Sui, A.L.; Sonnenberg, F.A.; Manning, W.G.; et al. 1986. "Inappropriate Use of Hospitals in a Randomized Trial of Health Insurance Plans." *New England Journal of Medicine* 315:1259-66.

Susser, M.; Watson, W.; and Hooper, K. 1985. *Sociology in Medicine*. New York: Oxford University Press.

Svarstad, B.L., and Lipton, H.L. 1977. "Informing Parents about Mental Retardation: A Study of Professional Communication and Parent Acceptance." *Social Science and Medicine* 11:645-51.

Szasz, T.S., and Hollander, M.H. 1956. "A Contribution to the Philosophy of Medicine: The Basic Models of the Doctor-Patient Relationship." *Archives of Internal Medicine* 97:585-92.

Task Force on Doctor and Patient. 1991. "Ideal Medical Interviewing Curriculum." Faculty Development Course. Rochester, N.Y.: Society of General Internal Medicine.

Taussig, M.T. 1980. "Reification and the Consciousness of the Patient." *Social Science & Medicine* 14B:3-13.

Temkin, O. 1953. "Greek Medicine as Science and Craft." *Isis* 44:213-25.

————. 1973. *Galenism: Rise and Fall of a Medical Philosophy*. Ithaca, N.Y.: Cornell University Press.

————. 1977. *On Galen's Pneumatology: Double Face of Janus and Other Essays in the History of Medicine*. Baltimore: Johns Hopkins University Press.

————. 1985. "Byzantine Medicine." P. 210 in *Symposium on Byzantine Medicine*, edited by J. Scarborough. Washington, D.C.: Dumbarton Oaks Research Library and Collection.

Thomas, Lewis. 1983. *The Youngest Science: Notes of a Medicine Watcher*. New York: Viking Press.

Todd, A.D. 1989. *Intimate Adversaries: Cultural Conflict between Doctors and Women Patients*. Philadelphia: University of Pennsylvania Press.

Traube, L. 1871-78. *Gesammelte Beiträge zur Pathologie und Physiologe*. 3 vols. Berlin: August Hirschwald.

Treuherz, J. 1987. *Hard Times: Social Realism in Victorian Art*. London: Lund Humpries.

Turner, Barry. 1981. "Some Practical Aspects of Qualitative Data Analysis: One Way of Organizing the Cognitive Process Associated with the Generation of Grounded Theory." *Quality and Quantity* 5:225-47.

Turner, Bryan S. 1987. *Medical Power and Social Knowledge*. London: Sage.

Twaddle, A. 1982. "From Medical Sociology to the Sociology of Health." Pp. 323-58 in *Sociology: The State of the Art*, edited by T. Bottomore, S. Nowak, and M. Sokolowska. Newbury Park, Calif.: Sage.

Uhlmann, R.F.; Pearlman, R.A.; and Cain, K.C. 1988. "Ability of Physicians and Spouses to Predict Resuscitation Preferences of Elderly Patients." *Journal of Gerontology* 43:M115-21.

U.S. General Accounting Office. 1986. *Medical Malpractice: No Agreement on the Problems or Solutions*. GAO/HRD-86-50. Washington, D.C: U.S. Government Printing Office.

Uzych, L. 1988. "Physicians and the Dispensing of Drugs for Profit." *New York State Journal of Medicine* 88:119-20.

Valente, C.M.; Antlitz, A.M.; Boyd, M.D.; and Troisi, A.J. 1988. "The Importance of Physician-Patient Communication in Reducing Medical Liability." *Maryland Medical Journal* 37:75-78.

Varian, H. 1990. "Monitoring Agents with Other Agents." *Journal of Institutional and Theoretical Economics* 2:153-74.

Verbrugge, L. 1990. "The Iceberg of Disability." Pp. 55-75 in *The Legacy of Longevity: Health, Illness, and Long Term Care in Later Life,* edited by S. Stahl. Newbury Park, Calif.: Sage.

Vogel, Morris. 1980. *The Invention of the Modern Hospital: Boston, 1879-1930.* Chicago: University of Chicago Press.

Wachter, R.M.; Luce, J.M.; Hearst, N.; and Lo, B. 1990. "Decisions about Resuscitation: Inequities among Patients with Different Diseases but Similar Prognoses." *Annals of Internal Medicine* 111:525-30.

Wadsworth, M.E.J.; Butterfield, W.J.H.; and Blaney, R. 1971. *Health and Sickness: The Choice of Treatment.* London: Tavistock.

Waitzkin, H.B. 1983. *The Second Sickness: Contradictions of Capitalist Health Care.* New York: Free Press.

———. 1984. "Doctor-Patient Communication: Clinical Implications of Social Scientific Research." *Journal of the American Medical Association* 252:2441-46.

———. 1985. "Information Giving in Medical Care." *Journal of Health and Social Behavior* 26:81-101.

———. 1986. "Research on Doctor-Patient Communication: Implications for Practice." *Internist* 27 (7):7-10.

———. 1989a. "A Critical Theory of Medical Discourse: Ideology, Social Control, and the Processing of Social Context in Medical Encounters." *Journal of Health and Social Behavior* 30:220-39.

———. 1989b. "A Critical Theory of Medical Discourse: Ideology, Social Control, and the Processing of Social Context in Medical Encounters." *Journal of Health and Social Behavior* 30:220-39.

———. 1990. "On Studying the Discourse of Medical Encounters: A Critique of Quantitative and Qualitative Methods and a Proposal for Reasonable Compromise." *Medical Care* 28:473-88.

———. 1991. *The Politics of Medical Encounters: How Patients and Doctors Deal with Social Problems.* New Haven: Yale University Press.

Waitzkin, H.B., and Britt, T. 1989a. "A Critical Theory of Medical Discourse: How Patients and Health Professionals Deal with Social Problems." *International Journal of Health Services* 19:577-97.

———. 1989b. "Changing the Structure of Medical Discourse: Implications of Cross-national Comparisons." *Journal of Health and Social Behavior* 30:436-49.

Waitzkin, H.B., and Stoeckle, J. 1976. "Information Control and the Micro-Politics of Health Care: Summary of an Ongoing Research Project." *Social Science and Medicine* 10:263-76.

Waldo, D.R.; Sonnefeld, S.T.; Lemieux, J.A.; and McKusick, D.R. 1991. "Health Spending Through 2030: Three Scenarios." *Health Affairs* 10:231-42.

Walker, J.H. 1971. "Spina Bifida—and the Parents." *Developmental Medicine and Child Neurology* 13:462-76.

Walker, L.R.; Broyles, Robert W.; and Furrow, Barry. 1990. "The Effect of Malpractice Litigation on Patient Access to Specialty Physician Services." *Journal of Legal Medicine* 11:199-223.

Wallace, S. 1990. "Institutionalizing Divergent Approaches in the Sociology of Health and Healing: A Review of Medical Sociology Readers." *Teaching Sociology* 18 (3):377-84.

Wallander, J.L. 1991. "Stressful Events Experienced by Mothers of Children with Chronic Physical Conditions." Research in progress, University of Alabama at Birmingham.

Wallander, J.L., and VanBuskirk, A. 1991. "Stress and Adaptation of Mothers of Children with and without Chronic Physical Conditions: A Matched Comparison." Research in progress, University of Alabama at Birmingham.

Wallander, J.L.; Pitt, L.C.; and Mellins, C.A. 1990. "Child Functional Independence and Maternal Psychosocial Stress as Risk Factors Threatening Adaptation in Mothers of Physically and Sensorially Handicapped Children." *Journal of Consulting and Clinical Psychology* 58:818-24.

———. 1991. "Risk Factors for Maladaptation in Mothers of Physically HandicappedChildren: Disability Status, Functional Care Strain, and Psychosocial Stress." Paper presented at the Florida Conference on Child Health Psychology, Gainesville, Fla.

Wardell, W. 1982. "The State of Medical Sociology: A Review Essay." *Sociological Quarterly* 23:563-71.

Ware, J.E., Jr; Davies, A.R.; Kane, R.L.; et al. 1978. "Effects of Differences in Quality of Care on Patient Satisfaction and Behavioral Intentions: An Experimental Simulation." Paper presented at Research in Medical Education Annual Meeting, New Orleans.

Warner, Harley. 1985. "Science in Medicine." *Osiris* 1:37-58.

———. 1986. *The Therapeutic Perspective: Medical Practice, Knowledge and Identity in America, 1820-1885.* Cambridge: Harvard University Press.

Warner, J.H. 1983. "A Southern Medical Reform: The Meaning of the Antebellum Argument for Southern Medical Education." *Bulletin of the History of Medicine* 57:364-81.

———. 1986. *The Therapeutic Perspective: Medical Practice, Knowledge, and Identity in America, 1820-1885.* Cambridge: Harvard University Press.

———. 1989. "The Idea of Southern Medical Distinctiveness: Medical Knowledge and Practice in the Old South." Pp. 364-81 in *Science and Medicine in the Old South,* edited by R.L. Numbers and T.L. Savitt. Baton Rouge: Louisiana State University Press.

Wasserman, R.; Inui, T.; Barriana, B.; Carter, W.; and Lipincott, B. 1984. "Pediatric Clinicians' Support for Parents Makes a Difference: An Outcome-Based Analysis of Clinician-Patient Interaction." *Pediatrics* 74 (6):1047-53.

Weber, M. 1946. *Max Weber: Essays in Sociology,* edited and translated by Hans Gerth and C. Wright Mills. New York: Oxford University Press.

Weber, M. 1978. *Economy and Society.* 2 vols. Edited by G. Roth and C. Wittich. Berkeley: University of California Press.

Webster, C. 1979a. "William Harvey and the Crisis of Medicine in Jacobean England." Pp. 1-27 in *William Harvey and His Age,* edited by Jerome Bylebel. Baltimore: Johns Hopkins University Press.

———. 1979b. "Alchemical and Paracelsian Medicine." Pp. 301-34 in *Health, Medicine, and Mortality in the Sixteenth Century.* Cambridge: Cambridge University Press.

Weinberger, M.; Greene, J.; and Mamlin, J. 1981. "The Impact of Clinical Encounter Events on Patient and Physician Satisfaction." *Social Science and Medicine* 15E:239-44.

Weisman, Carol S.; Morlock, Laura L.; Teitelbaum, Martha Ann; Klassen, Ann C.; and Celentano, David D. 1989. "Practice Changes in Response to the Malpractice Litigation Climate." *Medical Care* 27:16-24.

Weiss, K. 1985. "The Biology of Aging and the Quality of Life." Pp. 29-49 in Aging 2000: Our Health Care Destiny. vol. 1, *Biomedical Issues,* edited by C. Gaitz, G. Niederehe, and N. Wilson. New York: Springer-Verlag.

Wenger, N.K.; Mattson, M.E.; Furberg, C.D.; and Elinson, J. 1984. *Assessment of Quality of Life in Clinical Trials of Cardiovascular Therapies.* New York: Le Jacq.

Wennberg, J.E.; Barnes, B.A.; and Zubkoff, M. 1980. "An Epidemiologic Perspective on the Problem of Supplier-Induced Demand: The Case of Surgery and Surgical Second Opinions." Pp. 107-20 in *Physicians and Financial Incentives,* edited by J.R. Gabel. Washington, D.C.: U.S. Government Printing Office.

———. 1982. "Professional Uncertainty and the Problem of Supplier-Induced Demand." *Social Science and Medicine* 16:811-24.

———. 1987. "Population Illness Rates Do Not Explain Population Hospitalization Rates." *Medical Care* 25:354-59.

West, C. 1984. *Routine Complications: Troubles with Talk between Doctors and Patients.* Bloomington: Indiana University Press.

Wickizer, T.M. 1990. "The Effect of Utilization Review on Hospital Use and Expenditures: A Review of the Literature and an Update on Recent Findings." *Medical Care Review* 47 (Fall): 327-63.

Wiebe, Robert H. 1967. *The Search for Order.* New York: Hill and Wang.

Wilensky, H. 1964. "The Professionalization of Everyone." *American Journal of Sociology* 70:137-58.

Wilensky, G., and Rossiter, L. 1983. "The Relative Importance of Physician-Induced Demand on the Demand for Medical Care." *Milbank Quarterly* 6:252-77.

Williams, L. 1907-8. "The Practical Value of Blood-Pressure Estimation." *Clinical Journal* 31:197.

Wirth, L. 1931. "Clinical Sociology." *American Journal of Sociology* 37:49-66.

Wolinsky, F. 1988. "The Professional Dominance Perspective Revisited." *Milbank Quarterly* 66:33-47.

Wolraich, M.L. 1980. "Pediatric Practitioners' Knowledge of Developmental Disabilities." *Journal of Developmental and Behavioral Pediatrics* 1:133-36.

—————. 1982. "Communication between Physicians and Parents of Handicapped Children." *Exceptional Children* 48:324-29.

Woodward, R.S., and Warren-Boulton, F. 1984. "Considering the Effects of Financial Incentives and Professional Ethics on 'Appropriate' Medical Care." *Journal of Health Economics* 3:223- 37.

Wunderlich, Carl. 1871. *On the Temperature in Diseases: A Manual of Medical Thermometry.* Translated by W. Bathurst Woodman. London: New Sydenham Society.

Yesavage, J.; Brink, T.; Rose, T.; et al. 1982. "Development and Validation of a Geriatric Depression Screening Scale: A Preliminary Report." *Journal of Psychiatric Research* 17:37-49.

Young, K. 1989. "Disembodiment: The Phenomenology of the Body in Medical Examinations." *Semiotica* 73:43-66.

Zaner, R. 1990. "Medicine and Dialogue." *Journal of Medicine and Philosophy* 303-25.

Zola, I.K. 1972. "Studying the Decision to See a Doctor." *Advances in Psychosomatic Medicine* 8:216-36.

—————. 1983a. "Culture and Symptoms: An Analysis of Patients Presenting Complaints." Pp. 86-108 in *Socio-Medical Inquiries.* Philadelphia: Temple University Press. Originally published in 1966 in *American Sociological Review* 31:615-30.

—————. 1983b. "Structural Constraints in the Doctor-Patient Relationship: The Case of Non-compliance." Pp. 215-26 in *Socio-Medical Inquiries.* Philadelphia: Temple University Press. Originally published in 1981 in *The Relevance of Social Science for Medicine,* edited by Leon Eisenberg and Arthur Kleinman. Dordrecht, Holland: D. Reidel.

—————. 1991. "Bringing Our Bodies and Ourselves Back In: Reflections on a Past, Present, and Future 'Medical Sociology.' " *Journal of Health and Social Behavior* 32 (1):1-16.

Zuckerman, S. 1984. "Medical Malpractice: Claims, Legal Costs, and the Practice of Defensive Medicine." *Health Affairs* 3:128-33.

Contributors

Richard M. Allman, M.D., is associate professor of medicine, director of the Center for Aging, director of the Division of Gerontology and Geriatric Medicine, chief of Geriatric Medicine, Department of Veterans Affairs Medical Center in Birmingham, Alabama, as well as the curriculum development and evaluation coordinator for the Primary Care Training Program at the University of Alabama at Birmingham. He completed his M.D. and internship and residency in internal medicine at West Virginia University and then served as a fellow in general internal medicine at Johns Hopkins University. He serves as an associate editor for the *American Journal of Medicine*. He is currently a co-investigator with Jeffrey Clair in a study of doctor-older patient-caregiver communication. He and Clair also are working on a medical interviewing curriculum for the Primary Care Internal Medicine Program at the University of Alabama at Birmingham.

Howard B. Beckman, M.D., F.A.C.P., is associate professor of medicine in the Department of Internal Medicine at the University of Rochester School of Medicine and Dentistry. He also is chief of medicine at Highland Hospital of Rochester, New York. He received his M.D. from Wayne State University School of Medicine. He has consistently published in major medical journals on teaching medical interviewing. His current interests include physician satisfaction, the use of videotapes in internal medicine, and rethinking the art of the medical interview.

J. Claude Bennett, M.D., is professor and chairman of the Department of Medicine at the University of Alabama, Birmingham School of Medicine. He received his M.D. from Harvard Medical School and took further training in rheumatology and immunology at Massachusetts General Hospital, the National Institutes of Health, and Cal Tech. At UAB he served concurrently as director, Division of Clinical Immunology and Rheumatology; founding director, Multipurpose Arthritis Center; and chairman, Department of Microbiology. During his tenure, these three entities reached the height of national and international recognition, a position which has been maintained by his successors. He holds many honors, including membership in the Institute of Medicine, the American Board of Internal Medicine, the American Society for Clinical Investigation, the Association of American Physicians, and the American College of Rheumatology. He has served in high leadership positions in these and other organizations and currently is president, Association of Professors of Medicine. A current major interest is the reform of internal medicine education.

Charlotte G. Borst, Ph.D., is assistant professor in the Department of History at the University of Alabama at Birmingham. She completed her Ph.D. in the history of science at the University of Wisconsin at Madison. She has numerous publications on women, health, and history and is currently working on a book documenting the change from midwife- to physician-attended childbirth.

Theron Britt, Ph.D., is assistant professor of English at Memphis State University, where he teaches contemporary American literature and critical theory. He received his Ph.D. in English with a critical theory emphasis from the University of California at Irvine. His research applies perspectives from critical theory to the fields of law, mental health, and medicine. He is working on a book, *Lawful Fictions: Schizophrenia, Law and Literature.*

Jeffrey Michael Clair, Ph.D., is assistant professor of sociology and medicine serving in the Department of Sociology, the Division of General and Preventive Medicine, and the Division of Gerontology and Geriatrics at the University of Alabama at Birmingham. He serves as director of the Medical Sociology Program, as well as the director of the Social and Behavioral Sciences/Center for Aging Gerontology Education Program. His current applied experience includes work as the Medical Interviewing Preceptor for the Primary Care Training Program at UAB. He completed an N.I.A. Postdoctoral Research Fellowship in Health and Aging at the Andrus Gerontology Center, University of Southern California, after completing his Ph.D. in Sociology at Louisiana State University, with a National Science Foundation Dissertation Research Award for a study on doctor-patient-family communication. His substantive areas of specialization are medical sociology, social gerontology, social psychology, and triangulated research techniques.

William C. Cockerham, Ph.D., is professor of sociology and medicine at the University of Alabama at Birmingham. He received his Ph.D. from the University of California at Berkeley. He has published in major social science and medical journals and is the solo author of numerous books, including *Medical Sociology* 5th ed. (1992), *Sociology of Mental Disorder,* 3rd ed. (1992), *This Aging Society* (1991), and the forthcoming *The Global Society: A Sociological Analysis* (1993). His current work focuses on the survey of health and illness behavior and the integration of health policy in the European Community (Germany, Netherlands, France, Belgium, and Spain).

John R. Durant, M.D., is vice president for health affairs, director of the Medical Center, and professor of Medicine, Division of Hematology and Oncology, at the University of Alabama at Birmingham. He received his B.A. in Biology from Swarthmore College and his M.D from Temple University. He is a member of the National Cancer Advisory Board, currently serving a six-year term. He has served as an American Cancer Society Fellow. He has been active at the national level of the National Cancer Institute, American Cancer Society, American Board of Internal Medicine, American College of Physicians, Association of American Cancer Institutes, American Society of Clinical Oncology, and the American Association for Cancer Research. He has more than 200 scientific publications and a long-standing interest in social medicine.

H. Hughes Evans, M.D., Ph.D., is assistant professor of medicine and in the Department of History at the University of Alabama at Birmingham. She received her M.D. from the Harvard Medical School and Ph.D in the history of science department from Harvard. Her interests are in the history of medicine and science, and she has been published in the *New England Journal of Medicine, Social Science and Medicine,* and *Technology and Culture.*

Richard M. Frankel, Ph.D., is associate professor of medicine at the University of Rochester School of Medicine and Dentistry and is codirector of the Internal Medicine Residency Program at Highland Hospital in Rochester, New York. After completing his Ph.D. in sociology at the Graduate School and University Center of the City University of New York, he was a postdoctoral fellow in qualitative approaches to mental health research at Boston University. In 1986, he was a Fulbright Senior Research Fellow in sociolinguistics and social medicine at the University of Uppsala in Sweden. He has lectured and published widely on face-to-face communication in a number of contexts, including developmental disabilities and a range of medical encounters.

Eugene B. Gallagher, Ph.D., is professor of medical sociology at the University of Kentucky, holding a primary appointment in the Department of Behavioral Science and a joint appointment in the Department of Sociology. He received his Ph.D. in sociology from Harvard University. He has been active in the work of the Medical Sociology Section of the American Sociological Association. During 1985-89 he served as editor of the *Journal of Health and Social Behavior* of the American Sociological Association. He has held visiting appointments at Bristol University in England, the Fogarty International Center of the National Institutes of Health, King Faisal University in Saudi Arabia, and United Arab Emirates National University. His research interests include psychosocial aspects of end-stage renal disease, community mental health, cross-national comparisons of health care, and the socioeconomics of health care.

Denise F. Hardy, M.A., is a doctoral student in the clinical-medical psychology program at the University of Alabama at Birmingham. She received a masters degree in developmental psychology from the University of Houston in 1990. Her research focuses on coping in children and the generational transmission of competence to children.

Marie R. Haug, Ph.D., is professor emerita of sociology at Case Western Reserve University and director emerita of the University Center on Aging and Health. She received her Ph.D. in sociology from Western Reserve University. She is internationally known as a gerontologist and has pioneered research activities in the area of doctor-patient relationships. She is widely recognized as an expert in research design and methods and has served on the research committees of NIA and NIMH. She is past chair of the Medical Sociology Section of the American Sociological Association and a fellow of the Behavioral and Social Science Section of the Gerontological Society of America. She currently has a merit award from NIA for her study of stress and health among the elderly.

James E. Lewis, Ph.D., is professor and senior executive officer of the Department of Medicine at the University of Alabama School of Medicine. He received his doctorate in geography from the University of Georgia. In addition to teaching and program direction at the University of Virginia and the University of Oklahoma, he worked at the Institute of Medicine on national studies of the organization and financing of academic medical institutions and graduate medical education. He has served as consultant to the National Institute of Arthritis and Musculoskeletal Disease, the Health Care Financing Administration, and many professional, voluntary health, and academic medical organizations. He has served as president of the Lupus Foundation of America and is the immediate past president of Administration of Internal Medicine. His current academic interests are the structure and organization of health care and the management of academic medical organizations.

Robert L. Ohsfeldt, Ph.D., is associate professor in Health Care Organization and Policy, School of Public Health, University of Alabama at Birmingham. He received his Ph.D. in economics from the University of Houston. He recently received a Robert Wood Johnson Foundation Faculty Fellowship in health care finance at Johns Hopkins University. He is widely published on such substantive topics as physicians, the insurance industry, medicare, and public health policy.

Robert A. Pearlman, M.D., M.P.H., is associate professor of medicine and adjunct professor of health services at the University of Washington, Seattle. He is currently serving as a fellow at Harvard University in the Program of Ethics and the Professions. He received his M.D. from Boston University. He has published more than 50 articles in major medical and interdisciplinary journals. He has received funding for his research in quality-of-life considerations in medical decision making for older patients. He has a long-standing interest in physician bioethical decision making and geriatric patient care issues.

Ferris J. Ritchey, Ph.D., is associate professor in the Department of Sociology at the University of Alabama at Birmingham, with secondary appointments in the Department of Health Services Administration and the Center for Health Risk Assessment and Disease Prevention. He received his doctorate from the University of Texas at Austin. He has published in major medical sociology, medicine, public health, clinical pharmacy, and physical therapy journals. He is most recognized for his research on changing role relationships among health professionals, and for his work on the health of homeless persons.

Rebecca A. Silliman, M.D., Ph.D., M.P.H., recently moved from Brown University to accept an appointment as scientist with the Institute for the Improvement of Medical Care and Health at the New England Medical Center in Boston. She received her M.D. and M.P.H. degrees from the University of Washington and her Ph.D. in epidemiology from the University of North Carolina-Chapel Hill. Her clinical observations as geriatrician have served as the cornerstone of research on interactions between frail older patients and their families. More recently, this focus has expanded to include the exploration of these interactions within the context of the medical encounter.

Howard Waitzkin, M.D., Ph.D., currently serves as chief of General Internal Medicine and Primary Care, and professor of medicine and the social sciences, at the University of California at Irvine. He received his M.D. in medicine and Ph.D. in sociology from Harvard University while working with Talcott Parsons and Renne Fox. He has served as a National Science Foundation Fellow, Fulbright Fellow, and Robert Wood Johnson Foundation Fellow, as well as receiving NIH and NIA Service awards (senior fellowships). He is an international expert on doctor-patient communication. He has published in every major medical, sociological, public health, and health sciences journal. His research has received wide press coverage. Yale University Press recently published his *Politics of Medical Encounters: How Patients and Doctors Deal with Social Problems.*

Jan L. Wallander, Ph.D., is associate professor of psychology at the Civitan International Research Center of the University of Alabama at Birmingham. A licensed clinical psychologist, he has previously practiced in the area of developmental disabilities and other childhood disorders and family stress at the Sparks Center for Developmental and Learning Disorders, a university affiliated program at UAB. Currently, he holds a Research Career Development Award from National Institute of Child Health and Human Development. His research program, which investigates stress, coping, and adjustment in children and adolescents with chronic disease or handicapping conditions and in their parents, has produced more than 50 publications. He is president-elect of the Society of Pediatric Psychology and an associate editor of *Journal of Pediatric Psychology.* He has recently coedited *Stress and Coping with Pediatric Conditions* (Guilford Press) and *Family Issues in Pediatric Psychology* (Lawrence Erlbaum Associates).

Constance Williams, M.D., M.P.H., is a fellow in geriatric medicine at the Division on Aging, Harvard Medical School, and a research associate at the Harvard Injury Control Center, School of Public Health. She completed medical school and public health training at the University of California-San Francisco and Berkeley Joint Medical Program and residency training at the University of California at Irvine in primary-care internal medicine. Previously, she worked extensively in advocacy for the rights of nursing home patients. Her current research focuses on injury control strategies for the elderly, concentrating specifically on driving for the medically and mentally impaired.

William C. Yoels, Ph.D., is professor of sociology at the University of Alabama at Birmingham. He also is a research associate at the Birmingham VA Medical Center, serving as a social psychologist on the Interdisciplinary Geriatrics Assessment Unit. He received his Ph.D. from the University of Minnesota. He has coauthored the following books: *Being Urban* (1991); *Sociology and Everyday Life* (1993); and *Experiencing the Life Cycle* (1993). He is currently collecting field observational data while working on a medical interviewing project with the primary-care residents training program.

Author Index

Subject Index

functional independence. *See* activities of daily living; independence; instrumental activities of daily living; quality of life

gastroenterology, 153

gender: Galen's system of, 75; and higher education, 77; historical perspectives on, 75-76; and homosexuality, 80; and medical encounters, 159-61, 199; modern perspectives on, 76; theory of, 75-77

genograms, 166

geriatric assessment units, 160

geriatrics: family-centered medical care, 162-73; increasing interest in, xiii, xiv; social problems affecting patient care, 6. *See also* aging; patients, elderly

Great Britain, 8, 38-39, 200

Greek medicine, 4, 61-64, 212

grief, 122, 170. *See also* bereavement

handicapped children, xiv. *See also* disabled children

health: and aging, 19; control over, 51; deterioration of, 144-58; equilibrium, 62; and experience, 32; judging, 1, 19; as a multidimensional concept, 17-18; outcomes, 19-20, 37, 39-40, 44, 232; and patient satisfaction, 37; physical, 191; and prevention, 16, 50; psychological, 191; Pythagorean ideals of, 62; restoration of, 226; self-reported, 40, 42; sociology of, 17-18; status of, 19, 40; and symptomatic experience, 32. *See also* illness; mental health

health care seeking behavior: and cultural meanings, 42-43; and emergency room visits, 20; and self-treatment, 32, 38. *See also* behavior; illness; patients

health care service utilization, 191

health insurance. *See* insurance

health maintenance organizations (HMOs), 104, 107, 109, 230

heart disease, 54-55, 70, 186

Hippocrates: and Hippocratic corpus, 69; ideal of experience, 70; and physiological and pathological systems, 62-64

historians, medical, 63

history: of biomedicine, 8-9; clinical, 44; role in medical care, 1; of technology, 5

HMOs. *See* health maintenance organizations (HMOs)

holistic medicine, 4; and consequences of humoral physiology, 63; and pathology, 63; and physiology, 63

hospital admissions, 110

housing, 140

humanistic mandates, 1, 2, 14, 19, 27, 46, 218

humanities, 1, 15, 141, 228

humoral physiology, 62-64

hygiene, 62

hypertension, 40, 187

identity, of physician, 5. *See also* stereotypes

ideology: Aristotelian, 64; biological, 76-77; definition of, 141; individualism, 6, 153; in medical education, 201; in medical encounters, 141-42; political, 201; stoicism, 6, 153, 157-58; therapeutic, 62

illness: acute, 163; as an experienced social construction, 15; biomedical, 168; cause of, 32-33; in children, 7; chronic, 7, 163, 174; consulting a physician about, 32; and correlates of health, 16; cure of, 32-33; definition of, xi-xii; disabling, 32, 174-85; vs. disease, xi-xii, 15, 33-34, 41; experience of, 13; folk, 42; and formal context, 13; Galenic doctrines of, 67; and health-related behaviors, 15; and help seeking, 16; as a human experience, 14; identification of, 16; and informal context, 13; information about, 33; and interpersonal relationships, 13; judging, 1, 19; and language, 13; and pathophysiological processes, 15; perceived likelihood of, 101; personal aspects of, 93; physical aspects of, 25; self-diagnosis in, 101; and selfhood, xii; self-limiting, ix; and social class, 15; social psychological factors in, 15, 25; societal influences on, xiv, 15, 42, 230; stages of, 170; stress-related, 15, 34; treatment of, 32-33; understanding of, 14; uniqueness of patient, 84; and well-being, 15. *See also* disease

illness iceberg, 31-32

imaging, 107

incontinence, 187

independence, 144-53

industrialization, 47, 118

information: about illness, 33; accurate, 163; and adherence, 39-40; concealment of, 179, 213; emotion-laden, 177; gathering of, 166; giving of, 20, 23, 36, 38, 40, 49, 182; lack of, 180-82; in medical records, 5, 24-25; quality of, 163, 172; receiving of, 20, 33, 126; requiring of, 39; seeking of, 33; sharing of, 7, 174, 180-82; volunteering, 24; withholding of, 179, 201, 213

information transfer, 123